Pediatrics, Child and Adolescent Health

Pediatrics, Child and Adolescent Health is a book series with publications from a multidisciplinary group of researchers, practitioners and clinicians for an international professional forum interested in the broad spectrum of pediatric medicine, child health, adolescent health and human development.

Joav Merrick, MD, MMedSci, DMSc, born and educated in Denmark is Professor of Pediatrics affiliated with the Division of Pediatrics, Hadassah Hebrew University Medical Center, Mt Scopus Campus, Jerusalem, Israel, Kentucky Children's Hospital, University of Kentucky, Lexington, United States and Professor of Public Health at the Center for Healthy Development, School of Public Health, Georgia State University, Atlanta, United States, the former medical director of the Disability Administration, Ministry of Social Affairs and Social Services, Jerusalem and the founder and director of the National Institute of Child Health and Human Development in Israel. Email: jmerrick@zahav.net.il

nova
Medicine & Health
New York

Pediatrics, Child and Adolescent Health

Adventure Education and Positive Youth Development in Aotearoa, New Zealand
Damian Scarf (Editor)
2022. ISBN: 978-1-68507-753-2 (Softcover)
2022. ISBN: 978-1-68507-848-5 (eBook)

Chronic Disease and Disability: The Pediatric Kidney, Second Edition
Donald E. Greydanus, MD, Dr HC (Athens), FAAP, FIAP (HON) (Editor)
Vimal Master Sankar Raj, MD (Editor)
John D. Rowlett, MD (Editor)
Cheryl Dickson, MD (Editor)
Joav Merrick, MD, MMedSci, DMSc (Editor)
2022. ISBN: 978-1-68507-716-7 (Hardcover)
2022. ISBN: 978-1-68507-850-8 (eBook)

Why Do Children Die? Selective Perspectives on Thanatology in Pediatrics
Donald E. Greydanus, MD, Dr HC (Athens), FAAP, FIAP (HON) (Editor)
Dustin C. Rowland, MS (Editor)
Joav Merrick, MD, MMedSci, DMSc (Editor)
2022. ISBN: 978-1-68507-461-6 (Hardcover)
2021. ISBN: 978-1-68507-597-2 (eBook)

Preventing Child Abuse: Critical Roles and Multiple Perspectives
Vincent J Palusci, MD, MS (Editor)
Frank E. Vandervort, JD (Editor)
Donald E Greydanus, MD, Dr HC (Athens), FAAP, FIAP (HON) (Editor)
Joav Merrick, MD, MMedSci, DMSc (Editor)
2021. ISBN: 978-1-53619-268-1 (Hardcover)
2022. ISBN: 978-1-53619-696-2 (eBook)

Adolescence: International Aspects of Psychological Stress
Supa Pengpid, MPH, DrPH, MBA (Editor)
Karl Peltzer, MA Clin Psych, PhD (Editor)
Joav Merrick, MD, MMedSci, DMSc (Editor)
2021. ISBN: 978-1-53619-341-1 (Hardcover)
2021. ISBN: 978-1-53619-652-8 (eBook)

More information about this series can be found at
https://novapublishers.com/product-category/series/pediatrics-child-and-adolescent-health/

Donald E. Greydanus, Dilip R. Patel, Ahsan Nazeer, Roger W. Apple and Joav Merrick
Editors

Behavioral Pediatrics

Mental Health and Management. Fifth Edition

nova
Medicine & Health
New York

https://doi.org/10.52305/GBFG5410

Library of Congress Cataloging-in-Publication Data

ISBN: 979-8-88697-060-9

Published by Nova Science Publishers, Inc. † New York

Dedication for this 5th Edition

Helen D Pratt, PhD (1948-2020)

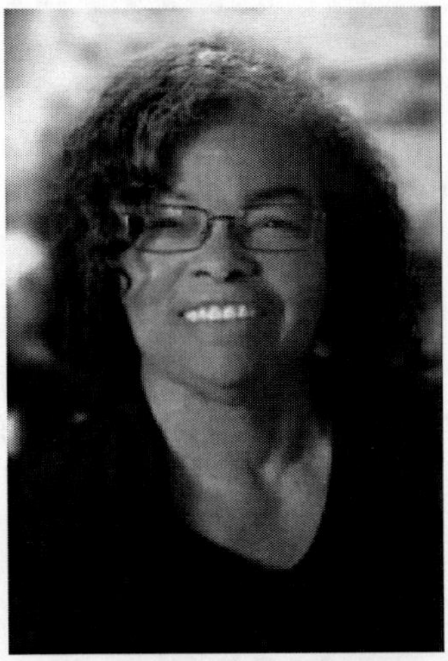

Photography courtesy of Bo Pratt photography

In 1991, Helen D Pratt, PhD became the founding faculty member and Director of Behavioral Pediatrics at Western Michigan University, Homer Stryker MD School of Medicine, formerly known as Michigan State University/Kalamazoo Center for Medical Studies. She remained in that role for nearly 25 years. In addition to her work as a clinician, Dr Pratt was a prolific writer, scholar, presenter and mentor. During her career, she published over 200 journal articles and book chapters. She presented her work at prestigious national and international professional conferences including the American Psychological Association. She was an inspiration to the countless psychology students, medical students and medical residents whom she mentored. She retired from Western Michigan University as Professor Emerita of Pediatric and Adolescent Medicine in 2015.

Starting college at age 30 years, Dr Pratt knew she had less time to pursue her career than traditional students. She was a dedicated, outstanding student who earned her undergraduate degree from the Lee-Honors College at Western Michigan University. She earned her master's and doctoral degrees in clinical psychology from Western Michigan University. Dr Pratt was proud of her accomplishments, valued professionalism, and pursued excellence, while encouraging others to do the same.

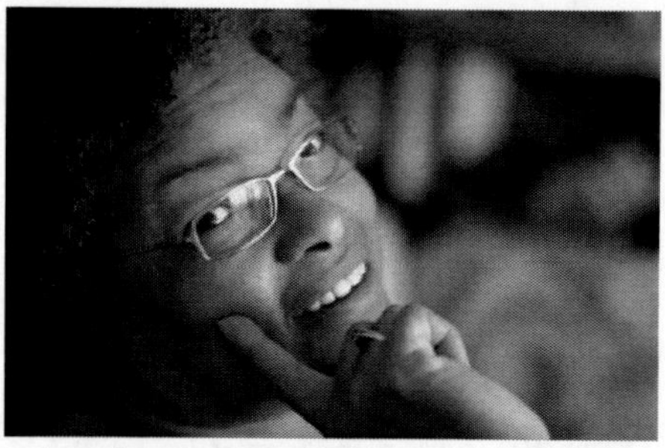

Photography courtesy of Bo Pratt photography

During the development of this book, I had the honor of speaking with her husband, Robert Pratt Jr, MA, and her daughter, Dr Brandy Brown. They told me that making the world a better place was a goal throughout Helen's life. Both her professional and personal life reflected her commitment to improving the world, one person at a time. In addition to supporting and guiding student mentees, Dr Pratt and her husband Bob fostered over fifty foster children; hosted seven international students; and guided, mentored, loved, and supported their own five children. Dr Pratt was especially proud of one of their exchange students from Ghana, Kwabena Oware Adu-Gyamfi. He was encouraged by Dr Pratt to pursue a medical degree when he returned home. He followed her advice, completed medical school, and returned to Michigan to become an outstanding resident at Western Michigan University, Homer Stryker MD School of Medicine.

In addition to her many accomplishments, her husband, Bob, spoke of several of her personal qualities: her wonderful smile, her laugh and her amazing ability to make all people feel comfortable and at ease. Daughter Brandy added that everyone could connect with her.

As I reflect on the legacy of Dr Pratt, it is these personal qualities that I remember most. Her ability to care for people was amazing. It allowed learners, like myself, to hear and accept critical feedback, and integrate that feedback into practice to become better psychologists.

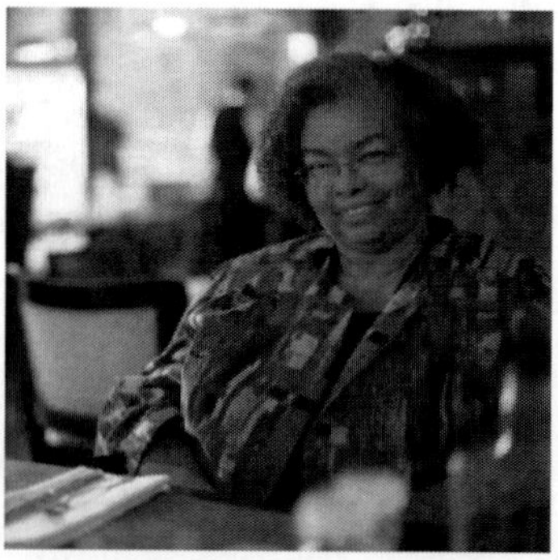

Photography courtesy of Bo Pratt photography

Thank you, Dr Pratt, from all of us whose lives you have touched. Your spirit lives on in how we teach and mentor young physicians, psychologists, family and friends.

Sincerely,

Roger W Apple, PhD

Contents

Forewords

First edition

Greydanus DE, Wolraich M, eds. Behavioral pediatrics, 1st edition. New York: Springer, 1992.

The origins of the term "behavioral pediatrics" are not clear, but we used it in the early 1970s at the University of Rochester to distinguish a program based in pediatrics from those based in child psychiatry. Most behavioral pediatrics programs involved child psychologists working with pediatricians. In the late 1970s the William T Grant Foundation funded 11 Behavioral Pediatrics Programs in the United States aimed at educating pediatric residents about behavioral problems in children. These programs were modeled on a program begun earlier by Dr. Stanford Friedman at the University of Maryland. A key element of all was that they were based in pediatric departments rather than in child psychiatry. This created some confusion and concern, especially among child psychiatrists. I see little reason for conflict, since, although there is some overlap, the two fields deal with different aspects of child behavior, and the very large need cannot be met by child psychiatry alone.

At the end of the Foundation's six years of support of these 11 programs, more than 35 pediatric training programs in the United States had divisions of behavioral pediatrics, and the field seemed well on its way to maturity. This was followed by the organization of the Behavioral Pediatric Society, and in the late 1980s, by the adoption of the Journal of Developmental and Behavioral Pediatrics as the official journal of the Society. All that is left to create a new specialty is a textbook and subspecialty boards. With this textbook, the first of these steps is achieved and the second, subspecialty boards, is now being proposed.

Some will object to a separate subspecialty of behavioral pediatrics. I take pride in being an academic general pediatrician, and I believe that this field includes adolescent medicine and behavioral pediatrics, as well as the area represented by the grandfather of these breakaway societies—the Ambulatory Pediatric Association. While I have had concerns about the separation of behavioral pediatrics from general pediatrics, and from the other pediatric research societies, I do have some difficulty in consistency, since I was one of the original "breakaway pediatricians" who formed the Ambulatory Pediatric Association. Behavioral pediatrics has come of age, and it deserves to be recognized as a separate subspecialty. The task is to integrate its knowledge and skills into the fabric of all pediatric training programs.

This book gives comprehensive coverage of the current status of the field of behavioral pediatrics. It deals very well with the general principles, the skills needed for assessment, and the management of the majority of clinical syndromes. It is authored, appropriately, by a group of authors from many disciplines, including pediatrics and psychology, and it touches on the psychologic aspects of chronic physical disease as well as family problems, including divorce, which puts children at risk. This coverage is very much in the tradition of most medical texts—oriented to the individual and family, and causes and treatments of the problems. There is relatively little in this or any other textbook of pediatrics on the social, cultural, and environmental origins of problem behaviors, or on social policies that may be necessary to prevent or effectively manage many of these problem behaviors of children and youth: better jobs for their parents and a hopeful future for themselves, better education, reduction of discrimination, and social violence. And, at the level of therapy, group approaches, peer counseling, community support groups, and community empowerment are interventions, I believe, the behavioral pediatrician will use more in the future, as well as the individual and family approach so well outlined in this book.

Since this text contains excellent chapters on schizophrenia and depression, which are usually considered the domain of child psychiatry, the question remains, how does behavioral pediatrics differ from child psychiatry? I offer my own idiosyncratic definition: "behavioral pediatrics is what the pediatrician does to diagnose, to treat, and most important, to prevent mental illness and problems behaviors in children." The field obviously overlaps with child psychiatry, but is still distinct. Some problems, such as teen pregnancy, failure to thrive, behavioral aspects of sports medicine, and sexually transmitted diseases, are rarely dealt with by child psychiatrists, and are clearly in the province of the behavioral pediatrician. On the other hand, schizophrenia, autism, and severe depression, while they may—and should—be picked up by the pediatrician, must usually be treated by the child psychiatrist. Given that behavioral pediatrics is a multidisciplinary field and has some overlap with child psychiatry and other disciplines, productive relations between these disciplines still need to be worked out in many institutions.

The challenge to the field of behavioral pediatrics is to learn to work effectively as a team, to develop advocacy skills to promote social policies that deal with the sociocultural causes of problem behaviors, and at the same time, develop the skills to relate to individual patients and their families and to diagnose and manage effectively those problems for which the pediatrician can become competent. This is a big order, but one that this book goes a long way toward helping to achieve. Unless pediatricians learn to deal effectively with these major problems, they will be unable to deal with most pressing and common problem faced by the children and their families today. With a textbook of its own, behavioral pediatrics has come of age.

Robert J Haggerty, MD
President, William T Grant Foundation, Clinical Professor of Pediatrics, New York Hospital/Cornell Medical Center, New York, United States of America

Second edition

Greydanus DE, Pratt HD, Patel DR, eds. Behavioral pediatrics, 2nd edition. New York: iUniverse Publishing, 2006.

When all's said and done, when the doors of the clinic or office close, the pediatrician, family doctor or nurse practitioner will drive home to a late dinner all the time thinking about the social and behavioral challenges presented by his or her young patients that day. The "medical" decision-making, diagnosis and treatment of the principal problems will, on the whole, have been made easy in comparison to the social and behavioral problems presented by the patients. For most practitioners, behavioral training (the psychosocial in the biopsychosocial) occurred years ago. The practitioner may not be conversant with contemporary diagnosis, treatment and psychological perspectives. So fortunately, within the pages of this volume, you will find expert articulation of the behavioral and social dimensions of your challenging cases as well as an excellent presentation of child and adolescent psychological and psychiatric diagnosis and treatment.

There are a number of features of this carefully edited volume that I recommend to you, the reader. The disciplinary "silos" of specialty and subspecialty are breached in a healthy way; the reader is presented with comprehensive coverage of behavior both normal and pathological in children and adolescents in clear prose writing by experts in many disciplines. The writing avoids specialty jargon while clarifying key concepts. This book is an asset not only for those seeking a deeper understanding but those interested in becoming more engaged in diagnosis and treatment of their behavioral disordered young patients. Increasing involvement by primary care clinicians in such treatment is essential in my view if we expect that access to treatment for these relatively common conditions will be available.

More important than the treatment is prevention. Primary prevention remains a "holy grail" awaiting more scientific discovery at least for the serious mental disorders but much is known about secondary prevention (reducing episodes of illness and morbidity) and tertiary prevention (reducing social disability). Prevention in many area of behavioral health can be linked to healthy family behaviors; for example, it is clear that drug use and dependence (including smoking) in adolescents is less common in families that closely monitor their children's activities. The same can be said for other risky behaviors with damaging consequences to health and well-being.

Family doctors, pediatricians, nurses and other primary care providers function as sentinels in the community for much that is happening in our culture and function, to use a current phrase, as "first responders." This volume can be a key resource for "first responders." The role of human behavior in illness and the human behavioral illnesses is so widely prevalent that, as a psychiatrist and a dean, it won't surprise the reader to know that I hope and even expect a high level of behavioral sophistication in those who care for children and adolescents.

Robert Haggerty in his Foreword to the first edition provided a brief history of behavioral pediatrics and attempts a definition of behavioral pediatrics that might distinguish child psychiatry from behavioral pediatrics. Since the first edition of this book, the American Board of Pediatrics (ABP) has recognized the subspecialty of Developmental and Behavioral Pediatrics. The American Board of Medical Specialties in the last several years supported the ABP's application for recognition and the provision of a subspecialty certificate. Behavioral pediatrics is here to stay. But the key question is not how child psychiatry and behavioral pediatrics are similar or different but "are patients better served" to have both. I have no doubt that they are! Dr Haggerty also emphasized the need for us to function in teams—certainly a challenge we have in medical schools—to create curricula that teach provision of care in cross-professional teams. This well-crafted volume covers behavioral pediatrics content and provides a context for effective team delivery of high quality behavioral care to children and adolescents.

Glenn C Davis, MD
Former Dean, College of Human Medicine, Michigan State University, East Lansing, Michigan, United States of America

Third edition

Greydanus DE, Pratt HD, Patel DR, eds. Behavioral pediatrics, Third edition. New York: Nova Biomedical, 2009.

Pediatrics (from two Greek words for child [*pais*] and healer [*iatros*]) is the field of medicine concerned with infants, children and adolescents, their growth and development along with their prospect to achieve full potentials as adults.

Abraham Jacobi (1830-1919), the father of American pediatrics and also the area of social pediatrics, is the name that comes up first to mind when you think about pediatrics. This German Jewish physician graduated from the University of Bonn in 1851, but when he traveled to Berlin to take his state medical exams, he was arrested and held in prison for nearly two years on a charge of promoting political and social reform in the German revolution of 1848. He left Germany and arrived in New York in 1853, where he practiced general medicine, surgery and obstetrics, but his early contributions to the New York Medical Journal helped establish the field of pediatrics. In 1857, Jacobi lectured on childhood diseases of the larynx at the College of Physicians and Surgeons, his first formal pediatric lecture, and in 1860, he accepted a position as professor of infantile pathology and therapeutics at New York Medical College. This appointment signaled a turning point as it was the first pediatric medical position and launched pediatrics as an academic discipline in the United States and during his lifetime all major medical centers in the United States established pediatric departments. He also established the bedside clinical teaching method, a landmark in medical education. In 1865 he accepted the position of clinical professor of diseases of children at New York Medical College and in 1870 the College of Physicians and Surgeons (Columbia University) appointed him professor of clinical pediatrics. He worked at almost every hospital in New York, but he concentrated on the Jews Hospital (later Mount Sinai Hospital), where he set up the first outpatient pediatric clinic in 1874. By 1878, the Jews Hospital had the first department of pediatrics in a United States general hospital.

But the fact is that already much earlier in time pediatrics had been the focus of several Persian physicians. In the 10th century, the famous Persian physician Rhazes (Muhammad ibn Zakariya Razi, 865-925) wrote the first book that we know about (diseases of children, one of his 184 publications) to deal with pediatrics as an independent field of medicine. His teacher Ali ibn Sahl Rabban al-Tabari (838-870), a modern convert of Jewish decent, who produced the first encyclopedia of medicine, was also a pioneer in the field of child development which was discussed in depth in his book, “Firdous al-Hikmah” (Paradise of wisdom). The first work on pediatrics in the Western world was the Book of Children, published in 1545 by Thomas Phaer (1510-1560). The first Hospital for Sick Children in Great Ormond Street in London that we know was founded in 1852 and still today considered one the best pediatric centers in the world.

So where and when does the field of behavioral pediatrics come into the picture? Some will go back to Charles Darwin (1809-1882), who in 1877 published his observations on his first child (A biographical sketch of an infant; Mind 1877; 2:285-94) as a study of human behavioral development. This and his other work inspired and influenced other scholars, which again resulted in major progress in cognition, personality, intelligence testing, learning, psychoanalysis and animal research on human development. In Europe and in Scandinavia, where I grew up and was trained, we would call this special field or area of interest for social pediatrics or even some would say that is it not a discipline, but rather a state of mind. In the

1980s this area in Europe (influenced a lot by the British discipline of community pediatrics) has developed into a field now called child public health involved with the organized efforts of society to develop public health policies to promote child and young people's health, to prevent disease in children and young people, and to foster equity for children and young people within a framework of sustainable development.

In the United States, the Society for Developmental and Behavioral Pediatrics was founded in 1982 in order to improve the health care of infants, children, and adolescents by promoting research and teaching in developmental and behavioral pediatrics. This society of pediatricians and other professionals have worked to encourage research in developmental and behavioral pediatrics with an emphasis on psychosocial issues arising in the context of questions and respond to issues that affect research, teaching, or program development in developmental and behavioral pediatrics and to promote an understanding of and particular interest in the social, educational and cultural influences on children. The work of this society and others resulted in the American Board of Pediatrics in 2002 to accept a subspecialty training in developmental and behavioral pediatrics.

The Journal of Developmental and Behavioral Pediatrics devoted to the developmental and psychosocial aspects of pediatric health care in now in 2009 in its 30th year of publication and this present textbook is now in its third edition.

The present book is a welcome addition to the field of behavioral pediatrics and it will be the textbook that will follow pediatricians interested in this field, in a career and subspecialty in behavioral pediatrics.

Professor Joav Merrick, MD, MMedSci, DMSc
Director, National Institute of Child Health and Human Development, Jerusalem Israel, Medical Director, Office of the Medical Director, Division for Mental Retardation, Ministry of Social Affairs, Jerusalem, Israel and Professor of Pediatrics, Kentucky Children's Hospital, University of Kentucky, Lexington, Kentucky, United States of America

Fourth edition

Greydanus DE, Patel DR, Pratt HD, Calles Jr JL, Nazeer A, Merrick J, eds. Behavioral pediatrics, 4th edition. New York: Nova Science, 2015.

Childhood and adolescence are periods critical for developing life-long good physical and mental health. According to Aristotle in the distant past and to the World Health Organization (WHO) nowadays, there is "no health without mental health," as both are inexorably intertwined. Indeed, poor physical and mental health in childhood and adolescence influence adversely both general health and social and economic outcomes across the lifespan.

The overall prevalence of mental disorders is quite high in the world population at all ages; it is estimated that 10-20% of young people worldwide experience mental health symptoms and express associated behavioral problems in childhood and adolescence. On the other hand, there is increasing recognition of the importance of mental health for the success of global development strategies, and, in particular, the achievement of the United Nations Millennium Development Goals, which include eradication of poverty, education for all, improvement of child and maternal health and combating sexually transmitted infections and other diseases.

Despite the above considerations, mental health promotion for children and adolescents remains a neglected public health issue worldwide.

Recently, the existing mental health "gap" has stimulated synergy in action plans and strategies endorsed by global organizations. The United Nations Educational, Scientific and Cultural Organization (UNESCO) Operational Strategy on Youth 2014-2021 aims to ensure youth access to skills and competencies development for their transition to adulthood. The WHO's Comprehensive Mental Health Action Plan 2013-2020 recognizes the essential role of mental health in achieving universal health and stresses the importance of prevention. In this action plan, the term "mental disorders" is used to denote a range of mental and behavioral disorders that include depression, bipolar disorder, anxiety disorders, schizophrenia, substance use disorders, intellectual disabilities, and developmental and behavioral disorders with onset usually occurring in childhood and adolescence, including attention deficit and hyperactivity disorder and autism. In this action plan, emphasis is placed on the provision of comprehensive, integrated mental health care services in community-based settings.

Many "mental health specialists," including psychiatrists, psychologists, family therapists, social workers, specially trained counselors, nurses, neuroscientists, developmental-behavioral pediatricians and adolescent medicine specialists, engage in the assessment and care of children and adolescents with mental health concerns. However, many primary care clinicians, including general pediatricians, are hesitant to engage in mental health screening, assessment, diagnosis, and treatment. The American Academy of Pediatrics in a Policy Statement in 2009 proposed the requisite competencies of pediatric primary care clinicians that enable them to provide mental health services in primary care settings.

We have only recently recognized that the boundaries between medical specialties are much more porous than originally perceived. Many clinicians are unfamiliar with contemporary evaluation, diagnosis, counselling and treatment of the wide range of developmental and behavioral difficulties faced by children, adolescents, and their families. "Behavioral pediatrics, 4th Edition," provides strong foundations for Developmental-Behavioral Pediatrics, moving away from the purely medical specialty-subspecialty model. The book has evolved through three major editions that have described the essential features of the full range of behavioral child and adolescent disorders. The current 4th edition builds on the goal of its predecessors to provide a deeper understanding of child and adolescent development and behavior and to shed light on deviations from the normal pattern. This carefully edited volume has been developed by a group of experts in Developmental-Behavioral Pediatrics, representing special expertise in their respective subareas. It begins with introducing concepts of normal vs. abnormal behavior and describing behavioral and psychological assessment, follows with description of disorders that more commonly manifest in early life and adolescence, and ends with chapters relevant to neglect and abuse, sexual offenders and concepts of family therapy and pharmacotherapy. The hot topics of assessment in primary care, child and adolescent behavior in chronic illness, and sexuality, are also addressed. A similar structure approach has been taken, where possible, within each chapter, to facilitate the comprehensive understanding of information and to improve its clinical utility to both specialists and non-specialists.

Mental health matters enormously and there is a long way ahead of us to achieve it universally. Childhood and adolescence are critical windows of plasticity from the developmental and behavioral perspectives, and prevention and intervention at these early times are critical. "Behavioral Pediatrics, 4th Edition", represents a timely, up-to-date, state-of-the-art academic effort ultimately aiming to improve the health outcomes of our children and adolescents.

George P Chrousos, MD, FAAP, MACE, MACP
Professor and Chairman, First Department of Pediatrics, Chairholder, UNESCO Chair in Adolescent Health Care, Athens University Medical School, Athens, Greece

Current fifth edition

This fifth edition of "Behavioral pediatrics" covers a wide range of pediatric behavioral conditions that may disrupt the optimal development of infants, children, adolescents and young adults. Approximately 20% of children and adolescents have behavioral/emotional problems. Donald E Greydanus, MD, the senior editor of this and earlier volumes, is a highly skilled academic pediatrician who has many years of experience caring for children and adolescents who have behavioral challenges as well as of training the next generation of child health providers to care for these children. Sadly, children's behavioral conditions are becoming more frequent among children and families over time as our society experiences unprecedented challenges resulting from general cultural unrest and the COVID pandemic that leave the developing child and family struggling during critical periods of children's development. These struggles may affect children's and families' health for years to come.

Behavioral pediatrics is a term coined in the mid-to-late 1960s and early 1970s by Drs Robert J Haggerty and Stanford B Friedman then of the Department of Pediatrics at the University of Rochester (New York). Dr. Friedman provided a broad definition of behavioral pediatrics as "an area within pediatrics which focuses on the psychological, social, and learning problems of children and adolescents" (1). The importance of behavioral problems was also recognized by pediatricians and child psychiatrists at Yale, Johns Hopkins, Boston Children's Hospital, the University of Indiana, and the University of California (UCSF).

Rush Rhees, former President of the University of Rochester, wrote in an introduction to a text on tonsillectomies in 1932: "No age has benefited more from scientific discoveries in medicine than that of childhood" (2). The impact of good nutrition, safe water, pasteurized milk, immunizations, and antibiotics all dramatically improved children's health and set the stage for the focus on the new morbidity of behavioral problems. That is, children's improving biologic health allowed greater attention to incorporating the definition of and treatment of behavioral and psychological problems into the practice of pediatrics. The "new pediatrics" was based partially on the biopsychosocial model of medicine created by George Engel in Rochester (3) with whose work Drs Haggerty and Friedman were aware resulting from their training in Rochester when Dr Engel was defining this model.

Today across the world, children's and adolescents' behavioral conditions are accelerating largely as a result of the unexpected COVID-19 pandemic leaving persons of all ages struggling to maintain and in some instances, retain any sense of equilibrium. Family life at its core is being disrupted, as the economy is uncertain and drew to a halt during the first peak of the pandemic. The economic consequences of complete shutdown of small and major businesses/industries left many wondering from where their very sustenance was coming. Working parents assumed the role of at-home untrained educators of their children with minimal direction from educators as disruption of all aspects of life occurred. The lack of predictability within families, schools, and communities has resulted in alarming anxiety, confusion, and depression among all age groups. The morbidity and mortality resulting from recurrences of COVID sweeping over the world resulted in greater uncertainty and anxiety. The critical importance of behavioral pediatrics now cannot be overemphasized.

This new volume is an important contribution to defining behavioral pediatrics further and providing child health care providers and educators of professionals new insights into the evolving conditions from which our children and their families suffer.

This book is a compendium of topics critical to health care providers' knowledge of optimal physical and emotional health of children, adolescents, and families as well as behavioral conditions resulting from disruptions in the pattern of normal growth and development. The initial section "sets the stage" with a review of normal child and adolescent development, behavioral assessment and follow-up care in the primary care providers' offices, and emerging strategies such as mindfulness to help resolve the children's symptoms. The next section clarifies the developmental disorders, disruptive disorders, and mood disorders and is an introduction to the sections that follow discussing conditions reflected in children's anxiety, depression, and mood disorders. Stress, anxiety, depression and mood disorders often are antecedents to destructive behaviors such as substance use/abuse, attention deficit disorder, suicidal behavior, eating disorders, and other conditions. Recognition of these antecedents is important with the hope of preventing further morbidity. The challenges of chronic illness are well-covered by discussing conditions such as cystic fibrosis and renal disease as models of chronic illness.

In the future, the negative effects psychologically of the COVID pandemic on developing children and adolescents, and their parents should make clearer the biologic and psychosocial manifestations of the conditions covered so clearly in this book. Additionally, we will begin to understand the short- and long-term effects of the immense stress on every age group and the toll resulting on the emotional health of all nations' children and families from a worldwide pandemic. Hopefully rather than destroying a generation of the world's children, we will learn how to strengthen children's and families' resilience.

This book illustrates the great of the field of behavioral pediatrics over six decades. With the addition to the literature of this updated volume, we expect that more primary care pediatric providers will provide improved screening and short-term intervention or referral to children burdened with behavioral conditions to assure that each child is a strong child. I congratulate Dr. Greydanus and his colleagues for this highly important and relevant addition to the literature on behavioral pediatrics.

Elizabeth R. McAnarney, MD
Distinguished University Professor, Chair Emerita, Department of Pediatrics, University of Rochester, Rochester, New York, United States of America

References

[1] Friedman SB, ed. Introduction: Symposium of behavioral pediatrics. Pediatr Clin North Am 1975; 22:55.

[2] Rhees, R. Foreword. In: Kaiser AD, ed. In or out: A critical study of the end results of tonsillectomy. Philadelphia, PA: JB Lippincott, 1932:v.

[3] Engel GL. The need for a new medical model: A challenge for biomedicine. Science 1975;196:129.

Preface

Pediatricians can provide a wide variety of care to children and adolescents with complex disorders, depending on their training as well as interests, but they need to work closely with professionals in psychiatry and psychology when dealing with complex issues in mental health disorders. Behavioral health screening is therefore an important task of pediatricians and behavioral pediatricians as they evaluate their pediatric patients.

Section one looks at what is called special issues in mental health that include suicide/self-harm in pediatrics, childhood-onset schizophrenia, child abuse/maltreatment, mental health issues of chronic disorders (i.e., diseases of the cardiovascular system, the kidneys and the liver), and behavioral/emotional effects of COVID-19 on children/adolescents (1).

In section two, we cover various aspects of substance use disorders (SUD) that include SUD neurobiology, substance use/abuse in adolescents, an overview on cannabis, psychosocial treatments of SUDs, pharmacologic management of SUDs, and pharmacology of tobacco abuse (2,3). Section three provides a critical look at mental health management that includes psychotherapeutic interventions (i.e., children, adolescents and families), behavioral/cognitive behavioral therapies and principles of psychopharmacologic management in pediatric persons (4).

Donald E Greydanus, MD, Doctor Honoris Causa (Athens, Greece)
Professor and Founding Chair, Department of Pediatric and Adolescent Medicine
Western Michigan University, Homer Stryker M.D. School of Medicine, Kalamazoo, Michigan, United States of America
Email: donald.greydanus@med.wmich.edu

Dilip R Patel, MD, MBA, MPH
Professor and Chair, Department of Pediatric and Adolescent Medicine, Western Michigan University, Homer Stryker MD School of Medicine, Kalamazoo, Michigan, United States of America
Email: Dilip.patel@med.wmich.edu

Ahsan Nazeer, MD
Associate Professor and Division Chief, Child and Adolescent Mental Health Services (CAMHS), Sidra Medicine, Doha, Qatar
Email: anazeer@sidra.org

Roger W Apple, PhD
Associate Professor, Chief, Division of Pediatric Psychology, Director, Autism Center, Department of Pediatric and Adolescent Medicine, Western Michigan University, Homer Stryker MD School of Medicine, Kalamazoo, Michigan, United States of America
Email: Roger.apple@med.wmich.edu

Joav Merrick, MD, MMedSci, DMSc
National Institute of Child Health and Human Development, Jerusalem, Israel, Department of Pediatrics, Mt Scopus Campus, Hadassah Hebrew University Medical Center. Jerusalem, Israel, Kentucky Children's Hospital, University of Kentucky, Lexington, Kentucky, United States, Center for Healthy Development, School of Public Health, Georgia State University, Atlanta, United States of America
Email: jmerrick@zahav.net.il

References

[1] Palusci VJ, Vandervoort FE, Greydanus DE, Merrick J, eds. Preventing child abuse: Critical roles and multiple perspectives. New York: Nova Science, 2022.
[2] Greydanus DE, Patel DR. The adolescent and substance abuse: Current concepts. Dis Mon 2005;51(7):387-432.
[3] Greydanus DE, Kaplan G, Patel DR, Merrick J, eds. Substance abuse in adolescents and young adults: A manual for pediatric and primary care clinicians, Second edition: New York: Nova Science Publishers, 2019: 389 pages.
[4] Schor EL; American Academy of Pediatrics Task Force on the Family. Family pediatrics: report of the Task Force on the Family. Pediatrics 2003;111(6 Pt 2):1541-71.

Section one: Special issues (editor: Donald E. Greydanus)

Chapter 1

Suicide and self-harm in children and adolescents

Finza Latif, MD, Karen Lim, MD and Ahsan Nazeer*, MD
Child and Adolescent Mental Health Services (CAMHS), Sidra Medicine, Doha, Qatar

Abstract

This discussion considers issues related to suicide and self-harm in pediatric persons. Suicide continues to be a leading cause of death in youth worldwide, and self-harm behaviors can lead to serious injury and increase the risks of eventual suicide. The concepts of this topic include epidemiology, risk, protective factors, prevention tools, and management strategies.

Introduction

Suicide is a leading cause of death among youth across the globe. Suicidality includes suicidal ideation, intent or plan to die, and suicidal attempts or behaviors. Non-suicidal self-harm may involve similar behaviors as a suicide attempt, but there is no intent to die. Suicide attempts and non-suicidal self-harm occur much more frequently than death by suicide in children and adolescents. Although self-harm behavior is not driven by the desire to die, it can still lead to serious injury and the risk of future death by suicide. Suicide in youth is multifaceted, with many drivers, including genetics, environmental issues, and personal factors (1).

Suicide prevention is a significant public health concern. The 2013 World Health Organization (WHO) Mental health Action Plan was devised to reduce suicide by 10% by 2020. Effective July 1, 2019, the US Joint Commission for hospital accreditation has mandated that all hospitals use standardized methods for screening and assessment of suicide and take measures to prevent self-injury in hospital settings (2). This review discusses the epidemiology, risk and protective factors, and prevention and treatment of suicide and self-harm in youth.

---

* ***Correspondence:*** Ahsan Nazeer, MD, Division Chief, Child and Adolescent Mental Health Services (CAMHS), Sidra Medicine, Doha, Qatar. Email: anazeer@sidra.org.

In: Behavioral Pediatrics
Editors: Donald E. Greydanus, Dilip R. Patel, Ahsan Nazeer et al.
ISBN: 979-8-88697-060-9

Epidemiology

Recent studies report rising rates of suicide in youth and young adults in the United States (3). The US Centers for Disease Control and Prevention (CDC) data showed a 30% increase in suicide rates of all ages from 2000 to 2017, while further trend analysis showed suicide rates in those 15-24-year-old increased to the highest point in 2017 (3). In 2017, 6,241 completed suicides occurred in individuals aged 15 to 24 years, of which 80% were male and 20% were female. For those ages 15 to 19 years, the rate of suicide was 11.8 per 100 000 youth (4). In 10-17-year-old youth, suffocation by hanging/strangulation (49%) was the most common means of suicide, followed by firearms (40%) (5).

The trend for self-harm in youth also revealed a rising trend from 2008 to 2015 in 10-24-year-old females while remaining stable in males, according to the National Electronic Injury Surveillance System—All Injury Program (6). Though higher rates of suicidal thinking were reported in white than non-white youth, recent literature has shown rising suicide rates in African American youth and closing this gap (7). Numerous studies have reported higher rates of suicidal thinking in females (7-9); male youth, however, are much more likely to die by suicide (4, 10, 11). This could be due to the higher use of irreversible means by males than females (12).

Global suicide rates

Analyzing global data on child and adolescent suicide is challenging due to the heterogeneity of data reporting among different nations. Therefore, global rates for youth suicide vary. In many cultures, suicide in adolescents is usually under-reported due to the desire to protect families from the stigma of suicide and to avoid social repercussions (13). According to the 1990 World Health Organization (WHO, Geneva, Switzerland) mortality database from 90 countries, suicide is the 4th leading cause of death among adolescent males and 3rd leading cause of death among adolescent females in the 15-19-year age range (14). This review estimated a suicide rate of 7.4/100,000 globally in youth ages 15-19 years (14).

A more recent review of the WHO database from 2010 onwards included 45 majority western countries and revealed a global suicide rate of 3.7/1000,000 in 10-19-year-old youth while the rate for 15-19-year-old subgroup was 6/100,000; this was similar to the estimate from 1990 (14, 15). Males were much more likely than females to die by suicide, while hanging and strangulation were the most commonly used methods (15). Disproportionately higher rates have been found in New Zealand, Estonia, and Uzbekistan (formerly part of the Russian Federation) (14, 15).

Suicide in young children

Death by suicide in children younger than ten years is a rare phenomenon. In 2019, the National Violent Death Reporting statistics showed a suicide rate of 5/1,000,000 for 5-9 years old children (5). Suicide has been ranked the 10th most common cause of death in children under 12 years of age (11). Demographically in the US, it has been reported as more likely to occur in black children in the elementary school age group (10). Researchers have suggested that a lower prevalence of suicidal intent and substance abuse problems in children, two major risk factors for suicide in adolescents, may account for lower suicide rates in children (12). Higher rates of suicidal behaviors have been reported in children with oppositional defiant disorder and attention deficit disorder, even in the absence of depression (16). Other associations with childhood suicide risk include relationship problems with family, parental opioid use, and childhood sexual abuse (1, 10, 17, 18).

Risk factors

Youth with psychiatric disorders carry a 5-fold increase in suicide risk compared to their peers (1). Research reveals that 89% of youth with suicidality have at least one diagnosed psychiatric disorder (12). The most common disorders associated with youth suicide are behavioral disorders, depressive disorders, and anxiety disorders (16, 19). Comorbidity of mood disorders with substance abuse substantially increases the risk for suicide attempts in youth (19). Conduct disorders are more common in male victims, while mood disorders are more common in female victims of suicide (12). Higher impulsivity and hopelessness are strongly associated with suicide attempts than suicidal ideation in youth (19).

Previous suicide attempts or self-harm behaviors

A history of a previous suicide attempt is the most critical predictor of subsequent suicidal behavior (20). Regarding the course of suicidal ideation, a longitudinal study in adults showed that 8.6% of individuals admitted for suicidal ideation eventually died by suicide, while 15% re-attempted suicide (21, 22). Compared to the general population, suicide risk remained elevated for one year after an initial attempt and then gradually declined (20). Ongoing suicidal intent and the potential lethality of the method used in the previous suicide attempt are other variables that impact the future course of suicidal risk. Youth who make highly lethal attempts and have serious suicidal intent are at extremely high risk for repeated attempts and completed suicide (4, 12). Although non-suicidal self-harm does not involve the intent to die, it is, however, a risk factor for subsequent completed suicide attempts (23).

Gender

Males and females do not differ in suicide intent. However, males are more likely to use lethal means for suicide resulting in higher rates of completed suicide attempts than females (12).

Sexual orientation

Studies have found a 2-6-fold increase in non-lethal suicidal behaviors among homosexual youth (24, 25). This risk is aggravated by comorbid depressive symptoms and substance use (24).

Familial factors

A family history of suicide behaviors is also a strong predictor of suicide in youth (12). First-degree relatives of suicide attempters have a two-fold increased risk of suicidal behavior than the general population (26). In addition, youth exposed to suicidal behavior from a friend or family member are more likely to attempt suicide (19). Children of parents with opioid abuse are at higher risk of suicide attempts, and therefore, care for adults using opioids should include mental health screening for their children (17).

Stressors

A higher number of lifetime stressful events increases the likelihood of suicide attempts compared to suicidal ideation in youth (19). Parent child-conflict is a vital risk factor for suicide in youth (1, 27). For example, other interpersonal difficulties, boyfriend/girlfriend conflict, are more commonly associated with adolescent suicide (1, 12). Early and lifetime physical and sexual abuse are significant risk factors for suicide, especially in young children and older adolescents (12, 18). Pediatric emergency department visits for self-harm are much higher while school is in session than during summer vacation, indicating that school may serve as a stressor for some youth leading to self-harm behaviors (28).

Access to lethal means

The presence of firearms at home is a risk factor for completed suicides. Access to firearms is a moderator for suicide globally, and 72% of those who die on their first suicide attempt have used a gun (15, 20).

Media and screen time

Recent literature reports an association between higher screen time and suicidality and a slightly higher risk of depression and anxiety in youth (1, 29). This may be due to the impact of cyberbullying or exposure to violence through social media. Additionally, the representation of suicidal acts dramatically and sensationally in the news and the movies has been known to increase suicidal behavior in vulnerable youth (30).

Protective factors

Protective factors decrease the likelihood of a suicide attempt, despite the presence of psychopathology.

Parental supervision

In children, higher parental supervision is associated with a lower risk of suicide. Therefore, improving parenting skills and increasing positive parent-child interaction could be a protective measure (1).

Social support

Social support, including the perception of family cohesion, is a protective factor for suicidal behavior. Adolescents who describe family life as emotionally supportive are less likely to engage in suicidal behavior than peers with the same mood psychopathology and life stress levels. In addition, school engagement serves as a protective factor (1). A positive school environment may increase the youth's sense of personal achievement and provide protective social support.

Religion

Religious beliefs against suicide can serve as a protective factor. Studies have shown similar rates of suicidal ideation in religious or secular groups; however, rates of suicide attempts are lower in religious groups than secular groups, independent of psychopathology or other social risk factors (31, 32).

Prevention

Suicide prevention is a public health priority, and national suicide prevention programs exist in many countries. Youth suicide prevention strategies aim to identify young people at risk of self-harm using universal, selective, or indicated approaches. Universal prevention efforts target all youth, while selective and indicated approaches focus on those identified as at-risk or presenting with suicide attempts. Traditionally, these measures are implemented in schools, communities, and healthcare systems.

Lethal means restriction

Evidence supports that restricting access to lethal means (e.g., guns) can effectively reduce the rate of suicide attempts (33-36). The World Health Organization (WHO) cites lethal means restriction as the most effective method to prevent suicide. Means reduction can include packaging changes for analgesics, withdrawal of toxic pesticides or restricting access, detoxifying gas, limiting access to jumping in cities, and reducing access to firearms (37). The evidence for firearm control legislation is mixed, as laws in certain countries, including Australian firearm control laws, were not associated with a decrease in suicide attempts in men (35). In the US, such restriction does not seem feasible (33).

While evidence for the older population is mixed, reducing access to firearms is still effective in preventing youth suicide by firearms (35, 37). Lethal means reduction counseling is designed for mental health professionals to counsel families on restricting access to lethal means for youth at risk of suicide. Lethal means reduction counseling for parents and guardians is also an effective preventive measure for at-risk youth (36).

School-based programs

School-based prevention programs follow the universal prevention approach. Components of school-based prevention programs include 1) Teacher or school personnel training, also referred to as 'gatekeeper training'; 2) Student education and skill-building; 3) Suicide risk screening programs to identify students at risk and provide a further assessment as well as treatment to students identified as at risk.

A large, randomized control trial showed that school-based prevention programs reduced both new suicide attempts and severe suicidal ideation in the intervention group compared to the control group (38). Another study from 9 schools in North America showed the efficacy of a classroom prevention strategy in reducing suicide attempts at a three-month follow-up (39).

School personnel training (gatekeeper training)

This training aims to increase knowledge and improve skills among school personnel about identifying students at risk and making referrals when needed. These programs have shown improvement in intervention and referral skills among school personnel and are well accepted by school principals (40). However, when studied on its own, gatekeeper training is less effective in prevention than when used in combination with student education and risk screening (37).

The Question, Persuade, and Refer (QPR) is a manualized gatekeeper training program for school personnel developed in the United States. The program includes training to recognize the risk of suicidal behavior in students and enhance teacher communication skills to motivate and help students at risk of suicide to seek mental health care (40).

Student education and skills training

Student education raises awareness of mental health problems, including depression and anxiety, and risk and protective factors associated with suicide. The focus is on teaching students that suicidal thoughts indicate underlying mental illnesses such as depression and are treatable. Students are asked to recognize signs and symptoms in others and learn the action steps to seek help. Skills training programs for students aim to strengthen cognitive and behavioral skills; also, there is an emphasis on problem-solving and coping skills to reduce the impact of suicide risk factors and enhance the effects of protective factors. Youth Aware of Mental Health (YAM) is an educational program for students. It teaches students about depression and anxiety and aims to improve the student's skills to cope with adverse life events and stress (41).

Suicide risk screening

Suicide risk screening in both schools and health care settings can improve the identification of children and adolescents at risk for suicide and enhance the use of mental health services. Arguments against screening include the poor positive predictive value of screening for subsequent suicide attempts. However, studies have found screening in health care settings feasible and acceptable with no adverse effect on youth (42, 43).

Commonly used screening tools include the Patient Health Questionnaire-9 (PHQ-9), the Patient Safety Screener (44), the Ask Suicide-Screening Questions (ASQ) (45), or the Columbia-Suicide Severity Rating Scale (CSSRS) (46). Signs of Suicide (SOS) is a US school-based prevention program that includes a curriculum that raises awareness of mental health and suicide and a brief screening for suicide risk and depression (39).

Community-based programs

Suicide hotlines via telephone or internet chat can be a low-cost, immediate method of indicated prevention. These hotlines aim to provide psychosocial support to youth in crisis (47, 48). However, there is limited information about the efficacy of hotlines in preventing youth suicide

(37). Other community interventions include contact after an initial attempt via email, postcards, or follow-up phone calls (43). This strategy can help support and reduce suicides in communities with low mental health resources.

Healthcare-based programs

Integration of mental health services within primary health care is feasible, acceptable, and effective compared with care as usual (49). Collaborative mental health care in primary care settings in the US is a relatively new strategy to improve access to mental health care. Mental health access programs in the United States are collaborative programs where community pediatricians can access mental health consultations, education, and help with community mental health referrals (50).

In addition, the education of community pediatricians to recognize depression and suicide risk can also be an effective method of identifying at-risk youth (43). Studies done in Europe to assess the impact of primary care provider education found a significant increase in the prescription of antidepressants and a reduction in suicide rates (43). Structured follow-up in outpatient mental health clinics after an initial suicide attempt also has evidence to reduce future attempts (37).

Media related prevention strategies

As noted above, the level of exposure to social media is associated with the risk of suicidal self-injury. News reporting that sensationalizes suicidal acts (especially involving celebrities) can provoke similar suicidal behaviors in youth, called the "copycat" phenomenon or "suicide contagion" (30). Evidence supports that responsible reporting that highlights the negative aspects of suicidal behaviors can have a protective effect (51). Therefore, improving the quality of reporting that highlights the detrimental impact of suicide on the individual, family, friends, and community can be a helpful preventive strategy against suicide contagion.

Assessment

Children and adolescents may not want to reveal suicidal thoughts due to fear of stigmatization, communication difficulties, or poor social and family support. It is essential to assess suicidality in private without the parent/caregiver present. It is also imperative to ask the parent/guardian about their observations regarding the adolescent, for example, any recent changes in mood or behavior. Studies report a higher lack of concordance between patient and parent reports regarding suicidality for younger children than adolescents (1).

Assessment of suicidal youth must include the following components: a) assessment of suicidal ideation (including duration, frequency, intensity, controllability, reasons for, and deterrents); b) assessment of suicidal behavior, including self-harm, the lethality of current or past attempts, whether attempts were interrupted by self or others; c) assessment of risk and protective factors discussed above.

Standardized assessment scales can be used as guides and include CSSRS Assessment Version, the ASQ Brief Suicide Severity Assessment, the Beck Scale for Suicide Ideation, and the Scale for Suicide Ideation-Worst (46, 52-54).

Treatment

The assessment of the severity of suicide risk is used to determine the location of treatment, including outpatient clinics, intensive outpatient programs (e.g., day hospitals), or inpatient psychiatry units. Outpatient treatment can further vary in intensity, such as frequency of contact with a therapist (e.g., weekly vs. biweekly). The two primary components for treatment are psychotherapy and pharmacological interventions.

Psychotherapy

Various psychotherapies have been shown to reduce suicide attempts in youth. The three most commonly studied are cognitive behavior therapy (CBT), dialectical behavior therapy (CBT), and mentalization-based treatment (MBT) (55-57). Both CBT and DBT can be used in individual, group-based, and family-oriented settings. Most studies recommend including a family component in individual therapy for adolescent suicidality (58, 59).

CBT builds skills for identifying thoughts, feelings, and behaviors that are problematic and teaches youth how to change negative thoughts and behaviors. Homework assignments for skill building are an essential focus in CBT.

DBT was first developed to treat adults with borderline personality disorders who self-harm. This was modified for adolescents with the addition of family components. DBT focuses on mindfulness, distress tolerance, and building emotion regulation and interpersonal skills (60).

MBT was also first developed for adults with borderline personality disorder and was later modified for adolescents with self-harming behaviors. Mentalization is the capacity to understand the feelings of others. MBT theorizes that emotional distress and self-harm in adolescents may stem from their inability to mentalize, confusing their negative feelings with the feelings of others. MBT seeks to improve adolescents' mentalization capacity and builds their capacity to understand their role in what another person may be feeling (61).

Pharmacological treatments

Youth suicidality is a multifaceted problem, and psychopharmacological treatment must be individualized according to the psychosocial context and underlying psychopathology. Psychopharmacology primarily plays a role in treating underlying psychiatric illnesses. Antidepressants are effective for treating adolescent depression and thus, may indirectly reduce suicidality. However, in 2004 the US Food and Drug Administration (FDA) issued a black box warning stating that antidepressants were associated with increased suicidal thoughts and behaviors in adolescents and young adults. This was followed by a trend of decrease in diagnosis of depression and prescription of antidepressants. Though it has been stated that there was also a trend of increase in suicide attempts, the rate of completed suicides did not change dramatically following the warning (62). In 2007, the FDA added that depression increases the risk of suicide; therefore, providers must weigh the benefit of antidepressant use for adolescent depression versus the risk of increased suicidal thinking.

Similarly, mood stabilizers for treating bipolar disorders can reduce associated suicide risk. Limited evidence exists for lithium in reducing suicidality in adults; however, insufficient evidence exists for this effect in youth (63). Preliminary evidence in adults also suggests that intravenous ketamine significantly reduces suicidal thoughts within one day, with effects lasting for up to 1 week (64). The evidence, however, in adolescents for efficacy and safety is still lacking.

Conclusion

Suicide remains a leading cause of death in adolescents worldwide, while suicide attempts and non-suicidal self-harm lead to an increased risk of serious injury and an increased risk of later suicide. Suicide has been ranked the 10th most common cause of death in children under 12 years of age.

A variety of factors influence suicidality in youth, including genetics, environmental factors, and personal issues. Research notes that 89% of youth with suicidality have at least one diagnosed psychiatric disorder (12). A history of a previous suicide attempt is the most critical predictor of subsequent suicidal behavior (20). Other factors increasing suicidality include a positive family history of suicide, exposure to lifetime stressors, and access to lethal means such as firearms.

Protective factors include strong parental supervision, good social support, and religious beliefs. Various preventive efforts have been identified in the school, community, and healthcare systems. Evidence supports that restricting access to lethal means (e.g., guns) can effectively reduce the rate of suicide attempts (33-36). Suicide risk screening in both schools and health care settings can improve the identification of children and adolescents at risk for suicide and enhance the use of mental health services.

Preventive suicide measures include a careful assessment by persons, including healthcare personnel, and management utilizes various psychotherapies that typically involve cognitive behavior therapy (CBT), dialectical behavior therapy (CBT), and mentalization-based treatment (MBT) (55-57). Psychopharmacology primarily plays a role in treating underlying psychiatric illnesses.

References

[1] Janiri D, Doucet GE, Pompili M, Sani G, Luna B, Brent DA, et al. Risk and protective factors for childhood suicidality: A US population-based study. Lancet Psychiatry 2020;7(4):317-26.

[2] Detecting and treating suicide ideation in all settings. Sentinel Event Alert 2016 Feb 24;(56):1-7.

[3] Hedegaard H, Curtin SC, Warner M. Suicide rates in the United States continue to increase. NCHS Data Brief 2018;309:1-8.

[4] Miron O, Yu KH, Wilf-Miron R, Kohane IS. Suicide rates among adolescents and young adults in the United States, 2000-2017. JAMA 2019;321(23):2362-4.

[5] Ertl A, Sheats KJ, Petrosky E, Betz CJ, Yuan K, Fowler KA. Surveillance for violent deaths - National Violent Death Reporting System, 32 States, 2016. MMWR Surveill Summ 2019;68(9):1-36.

[6] Mercado MC, Holland K, Leemis RW, Stone DM, Wang J. Trends in emergency department visits for nonfatal self-inflicted injuries among youth aged 10 to 24 years in the United States, 2001-2015. JAMA 2017;318(19):1931-3.

[7] Bridge JA, Goldstein TR, Brent DA. Adolescent suicide and suicidal behavior. J Child Psychol Psychiatry 2006;47(3-4):372-94.

[8] Goldman-Mellor S, Olfson M, Lidon-Moyano C, Schoenbaum M. Association of suicide and other mortality with emergency department presentation. JAMA Netw Open 2019;2(12):e1917571.

[9] Boeninger DK, Masyn KE, Feldman BJ, Conger RD. Sex differences in developmental trends of suicide ideation, plans, and attempts among European American adolescents. Suicide Life Threat Behav 2010;40(5):451-64.

[10] Sheftall AH, Asti L, Horowitz LM, Felts A, Fontanella CA, Campo JV, et al. Suicide in elementary school-aged children and early adolescents. Pediatrics 2016;138(4):e20160436.

[11] Centers for Disease Control and Prevention, National Center for Injury Prevention and Control Web-based Injury Statistics Query and Reporting System (WISQARS). Fatal injury reports, 2017, for national and regional. URL: https://www.cdc.gov/injury/wisqars/index.html.

[12] Brent DA, Baugher M, Bridge J, Chen T, Chiappetta L. Age- and sex-related risk factors for adolescent suicide. J Am Acad Child Adolesc Psychiatry 1999;38(12): 1497-505.

[13] Phillips MR, Li X, Zhang Y. Suicide rates in China, 1995-99. Lancet 2002; 359(9309):835-40.

[14] Wasserman D, Cheng Q, Jiang GX. Global suicide rates among young people aged 15-19. World Psychiatry 2005;4(2):114-20.

[15] Glenn CR, Kleiman EM, Kellerman J, Pollak O, Cha CB, Esposito EC, et al. Annual research review: A meta-analytic review of worldwide suicide rates in adolescents. J Child Psychol Psychiatry 2020;61(3):294-308.

[16] Dickerson Mayes S, Calhoun SL, Baweja R, Mahr F. Suicide ideation and attempts in children with psychiatric disorders and typical development. Crisis 2015;36(1):55-60.

[17] Brent DA, Hur K, Gibbons RD. Association between parental medical claims for opioid prescriptions and risk of suicide attempt by their children. JAMA Psychiatry 2019;76(9):941-7.

[18] Lopez-Castroman J, Melhem N, Birmaher B, Greenhill L, Kolko D, Stanley B, et al. Early childhood sexual abuse increases suicidal intent. World Psychiatry 2013; 12(2):149-54.

[19] Mars B, Heron J, Klonsky ED, Moran P, O'Connor RC, Tilling K, et al. What distinguishes adolescents with suicidal thoughts from those who have attempted suicide? A population-based birth cohort study. J Child Psychol Psychiatry 2019; 60(1):91-9.

[20] Bostwick JM, Pabbati C, Geske JR, McKean AJ. Suicide attempt as a risk factor for completed suicide: Even more lethal than we knew. Am J Psychiatry 2016; 173(11):1094-1100.

[21] Bostwick JM, Pankratz VS. Affective disorders and suicide risk: a reexamination. Am J Psychiatry 2000;157(12):1925-32.

[22] Owens D, Horrocks J, House A. Fatal and non-fatal repetition of self-harm. Systematic review. Br J Psychiatry 2002;181:193-9.

[23] Wilkinson P, Goodyer I, Non-suicidal self-injury. Eur Child Adolesc Psychiatry 2011;20(2):103-8.

[24] Silenzio VM, Pena JB, Duberstein PR, Cerel J, Knox KL. Sexual orientation and risk factors for suicidal ideation and suicide attempts among adolescents and young adults. Am J Public Health 2007;97(11):2017-9.

[25] Rutter PA, Soucar E, Youth suicide risk and sexual orientation. Adolescence 2002;37(146):289-99.

[26] Qin P, Agerbo E, Mortensen PB. Suicide risk in relation to family history of completed suicide and psychiatric disorders: a nested case-control study based on longitudinal registers. Lancet 2002;360(9340):1126-30.

[27] Saffer BY, Glenn CR, Klonsky ED. Clarifying the relationship of parental bonding to suicide ideation and attempts. Suicide Life Threat Behav 2015;45(4): 518-28.

[28] Plemmons G, Hall M, Doupnik S, Gay J, Brown C, Browning W, et al. Hospitalization for suicide ideation or attempt: 2008-2015. Pediatrics 2018; 141(6):e20172426.

[29] Khouja JN, Munafò MR, Tilling K, Wiles NJ, Joinson C, Etchells PJ, et al. Is screen time associated with anxiety or depression in young people? Results from a UK birth cohort. BMC Public Health 2019;19(1):82.

[30] Hong V, Ewell Foster CJ, Magness CS, McGuire TC, Smith PK, et al. 13 reasons why: Viewing patterns and perceived impact among youths at risk of suicide. Psychiatr Serv 2019;70(2):107-14.

[31] Burshtein S, Dohrenwend BP, Levav I, Werbeloff N, Davidson M, Weiser M. Religiosity as a protective factor against suicidal behaviour. Acta Psychiatr Scand 2016;133(6):481-8.

[32] Lawrence RE, Oquendo MA, Stanley B. Religion and suicide risk: A systematic review. Arch Suicide Res 2016;20(1):1-21.

[33] Mann JJ, Michel CA. Prevention of firearm suicide in the United States: What works and what Is possible. Am J Psychiatry 2016;173(10):969-79.

[34] Beautrais A, Fergusson D, Coggan C, Collings C, Doughty C, Ellis P, et al. Effective strategies for suicide prevention in New Zealand: a review of the evidence. NZ Med J 2007;120(1251):U2459.

[35] Klieve H, Barnes M, De Leo D. Controlling firearms use in Australia: has the 1996 gun law reform produced the decrease in rates of suicide with this method? Soc Psychiatry Psychiatr Epidemiol 2009;44(4):285-92.

[36] Miller M, Barber C, White RA, Azrael D. Firearms and suicide in the United States: is risk independent of underlying suicidal behavior? Am J Epidemiol 2013;178(6):946-55.

[37] Zalsman G, Hawton K, Wasserman D, van Heeringen K, Arensman E, Sarchiapone M, et al. Suicide prevention strategies revisited: 10-year systematic review. Lancet Psychiatry 2016;3(7):646-59.

[38] Wasserman D, Hoven CW, Wasserman C, Wall M, Eisenberg R, Hadlaczky G, et al. School-based suicide prevention programmes: the SEYLE cluster-randomised, controlled trial. Lancet 2015;385(9977):1536-44.

[39] Aseltine RH Jr, James A, Schilling EA, Glanovsky J. Evaluating the SOS suicide prevention program: a replication and extension. BMC Public Health 2007;7:161.

[40] Hangartner RB, Totura CMW, Labouliere CD, Gryglewicz K, Karver MS. Benchmarking the "Question, Persuade, Refer" program against evaluations of established suicide prevention gatekeeper trainings. Suicide Life Threat Behav 2019;49(2):353-70.

[41] Lindow JC, Hughes JL, South C, Minhajuddin A, Gutierrez L, Bannister E, et al. The Youth Aware of Mental Health Intervention: Impact on help seeking, mental health knowledge, and stigma in U.S. adolescents. J Adolesc Health 2020; 67(1): 101-7.

[42] Horowitz LM, Bridge JA, Pao M, Boudreaux ED. Screening youth for suicide risk in medical settings: time to ask questions. Am J Prev Med 2014;47(3 Suppl 2):S170-5.

[43] Mann JJ, Apter A, Bertolote J, Beautrais A, Currier D, Haas A, et al. Suicide prevention strategies: a systematic review. JAMA 2005;294(16):2064-74.

[44] Serrani Azcurra D. Psychometric validation of the Coumbia-Suicide Severity rating scale in Spanish-speaking adolescents. Colomb Med (Cali) 2017;48(4):174-82.

[45] Horowitz LM, Bridge JA, Teach SJ, Ballard E, Klima J, Rosenstein DL, et al. Ask Suicide-Screening Questions (ASQ): a brief instrument for the pediatric emergency department. Arch Pediatr Adolesc Med 2012;166(12):1170-6.

[46] Posner K, Brown GK, Stanley B, Brent DA, Yershova KV, Oquendo MA, et al. The Columbia-Suicide Severity Rating Scale: initial validity and internal consistency findings from three multisite studies with adolescents and adults. Am J Psychiatry 2011;168(12):1266-77.

[47] Doki S, Kaneko H, Oi Y, Usami K, Sasahara S, Matsuzaki I. Risk factors for suicidal ideation among telephone crisis hotline callers in Japan. Crisis 2016; 37(6):438-44.

[48] Mokkenstorm JK, Eikelenboom M, Huisman A, Wiebenga J, Gilissen R, Kerkhof AJFM, et al. Evaluation of the 113Online Suicide Prevention Crisis Chat Service: Outcomes, helper behaviors and comparison to telephone hotlines. Suicide Life Threat Behav 2017;47(3):282-96.

[49] Baum RA., King MA, Wissow LS. Outcomes of a statewide learning collaborative to implement mental health services in pediatric primary care. Psychiatr Serv 2019;70(2):123-9.

[50] Straus JH, Sarvet B. Behavioral health care for children: the Massachusetts child psychiatry access project. Health Affairs 2014;33(12):2153-61.

[51] Bohanna I, Wang X. Media guidelines for the responsible reporting of suicide. Crisis 2012;33(4):190-8.

[52] Toolkit, NA. ASQ brief suicide risk assessment, 2017; URL: https://www.nimh.nih.gov/research/research-conducted-at-nimh/asq-toolkit-materials/emergencydepartment/pdfs/bssa_155388.pdf.

[53] Steer RA, Kumar G, Beck AT. Self-reported suicidal ideation in adolescent psychiatric inpatients. J Consult Clin Psychol 1993;61(6):1096-9.

[54] Beck AT, Brown GK, Steer RA. Psychometric characteristics of the Scale for Suicide Ideation with psychiatric outpatients. Behav Res Ther 1997;35(11):1039-46.

[55] Hawton K, Witt KG, Taylor Salisbury TL, Arensman E, Gunnell D, Townsend E, et al. Interventions for self-harm in children and adolescents. Cochrane Database Syst Rev 2015(12:CD012013.

[56] Cox G, Hetrick S. Psychosocial interventions for self-harm, suicidal ideation and suicide attempt in children and young people: What? How? Who? and Where? Evid Based Ment Health 2017;20(2):35-40.

[57] McCauley E, Berk MS, Asarnow JR, Adrian M, Cohen J, Korslund K, et al. Efficacy of dialectical behavior therapy for adolescents at high risk for suicide: A randomized clinical trial. JAMA Psychiatry 2018;75(8):777-85.

[58] Asarnow JR, Mehlum L. Practitioner review: Treatment for suicidal and self-harming adolescents - advances in suicide prevention care. J Child Psychol Psychiatry 2019; 60(10):1046-54.

[59] Weinstein SM, Cruz RA, Isaia AR, Peters AT, West AE. Child- and family-focused cognitive behavioral therapy for pediatric bipolar disorder: Applications for suicide prevention. Suicide Life Threat Behav 2018;48(6):797-811.

[60] Miller AL. Dialectical behavior therapy: a new treatment approach for suicidal adolescents. Am J Psychother 1999;53(3):413-7.

[61] Rossouw TI. Mentalization-based treatment: can it be translated into practice in clinical settings and teams? J Am Acad Child Adolesc Psychiatry 2013;52(3):220-2.

[62] Friedman RA. Antidepressants' black-box warning--10 years later. N Engl J Med 2014;371(18):1666-8.

[63] Cipriani A, Hawton K, Stockton S, Geddes JR. Lithium in the prevention of suicide in mood disorders: updated systematic review and meta-analysis. BMJ 2013;346:f3646.

[64] Wilkinson ST, Ballard ED, Bloch MH, Mathew SJ, Murrough JW, Feder A, et al. The effect of a single dose of intravenous ketamine on suicidal ideation: A systematic review and individual participant data meta-analysis. Am J Psychiatry 2018;175(2):150-8.

Chapter 2

Psychotic disorders in children and adolescents

Burhan Ahmed Khan[1], MD, Zeeshan Mansuri[2], MD, MPH and Zheala Qayyum[3,*], MD MMSc

[1]Institute for Technology in Psychiatry, McLean Hospital, Harvard Medical School, Boston, Massachusetts, United States of America

[2]Child and Adolescent Psychiatry Fellow, Boston Children's Hospital, Harvard Medical School, Boston, Massachusetts, United States of America

[3]Child and Adolescent Psychiatry, Boston Children's Hospital, Harvard Medical School, Boston, Massachusetts, United States of America

Abstract

Psychotic disorders in children and adolescents include early-onset schizophrenia and childhood onset schizophrenia (COS). This discussion begins with a historical reflection and then proceeds to such concepts as definitions, epidemiology, etiology, pathogenesis, differential diagnosis, and principles of management. The differential diagnosis includes such disorders as substance use disorders (SUD) and drug intoxications, post-traumatic stress disorder (PTSD), autism spectrum disorders (ADS), schizoaffective disorder, mood disorder, and various medical conditions. It is important for clinicians to understand that delusional thinking and hallucinations can be seen in healthy nonpsychotic children and usually diminishes after age 6. Concepts for the evaluation of psychosis in children and adolescents are reviewed including history, physical examination, laboratory studies and others. Management concepts are presented that include principles of pharmacology for psychotic disorders.

Introduction

The first textbook on child psychiatry was written by Hermann Emminghaus (1845-1904) in 1887. This described child psychosis as cerebral neurasthenia and defined the disorder to be a "neurosis of the brain that is characterized by a reduction of cognitive abilities, mood changes,

* ***Correspondence:*** Zheala Qayyum, MD, MMSc, Training Director, Child and Adolescent Psychiatry Fellowship Boston Children's Hospital, Assistant Professor of Psychiatry, Harvard Medical School, Assistant Professor Adjunct, Yale School of Medicine, 100 Sudbury Street, Apt 3406, Boston MA 02114, United States. Email: Zheala.qayyum@childrens.harvard.edu.

In: Behavioral Pediatrics
Editors: Donald E. Greydanus, Dilip R. Patel, Ahsan Nazeer et al.
ISBN: 979-8-88697-060-9

sleep disturbances and manifold anomalies of innervation with a subacute or chronic course and different states of outcome" (1).

In 1926, August Homburger (1873–1930) described that childhood schizophrenia included withdrawal, negativism, and strange as well as unexpected behavior. These are now categorized as "negative" symptoms. It is also interesting to note that for much of the 20th century, autism has been a part of schizophrenia. It was Leo Kanner (1894-1981) in 1943 and Hans Asperger (1906-1980) in 1944 who separated two very well-known autistic syndromes - early infantile autism and autistic personality disorder, out of the group of schizophrenic psychosis. This then sparked a debate, which spanned decades and ultimately led to the delineation of autism and schizophrenia as well as their treatment as two separate disorders (2).

The term schizophrenia was introduced in 1911 by Eugen Bleuler (1857-1939), who spoke of different forms of schizophrenia that could be divided into groups and differentiated from each other. Childhood schizophrenia was described as a separate entity from adult schizophrenia in 1937 by Jacob Lutz (1903-1998) (3).

The term childhood-onset schizophrenia (COS) is reserved for children in whom the onset of symptoms begins before 13 years of age, whereas the term early onset schizophrenia is typically reserved for symptoms of schizophrenia that start prior to age 18 years (4). Also, adult-onset schizophrenia typically starts after the age of 18 years (included). There is ample evidence that pediatric schizophrenia is on a continuum with adult schizophrenia with premorbid cognitive abnormalities, chronic course and long-term morbidity as well as mortality.

Since the publication of the American Psychiatric Association's "Diagnostic and statistical manual, Third Edition (DSM-III-1980)," childhood-onset schizophrenia has been diagnosed using the adult criteria established by the DSM system that carries over to the current DSM-5 (2013). The DSM requires the presence of at least two of the following symptoms: delusions, hallucinations, disorganized speech, disorganized or catatonic behavior and negative symptoms (e.g., flat affect, poverty of speech and avolition) for a major part of one month during any six-month interval. DSM-5 also cautions that although the main symptoms of schizophrenia are the same in childhood, there are also important differences. In childhood schizophrenia, delusions are less elaborate and visual hallucinations are more common. These hallucinations should be distinguished from developmentally normal fantasies. DSM-5 has also removed the schizophrenia subtypes that were noted in DSM-IV-TR published in 2000. The following is a brief description of these symptoms.

Prodromal phase/Clinical high-risk phase

It is pertinent to mention clinically high-risk populations within this group, as not all children with symptoms resembling or preceding schizophrenia will develop psychosis; however, the probability of such a scenario is high. A meta-analysis showed that 22% of clinical high risk (CHR) patients convert to psychosis within one year, 29% within two years and 36% within three years (5). There are certain tools that help to establish the probability of conversion of CHR to psychosis which include scales such as CAARMS (Comprehensive Assessment of At-Risk Mental States) or SIPS (Structured Interview for Prodromal Syndromes). There is ongoing research that aims to establish and further the validity of these instruments in prediction of conversion, as early intervention in CHR has been shown to greatly improve therapeutics in these patient populations (6).

Delusions

Delusions refer to strongly held beliefs, which are not shared by other members of a family or community. They originate from a false interpretation of external reality and are not fitted to one's social or religious background. These can be complex to approach when dealing with a younger pediatric or adolescent population and must be evaluated in the appropriate developmental context.

Hallucinations

Hallucinations are false perceptions without identifiable external stimuli. In psychotic disorders, these misperceptions can occur in any of the five senses; therefore, psychotic individuals can present with auditory, visual, gustatory (taste-related), olfactory (smell-related), or somatic hallucinations. Auditory hallucinations ("hearing voices") are more commonly seen than visual hallucinations in children and teenagers with psychosis. Hallucinations are more likely to be seen in those with anxiety, depression, family dysfunction and inattention or hyperactivity. Just as delusions, as we shall discuss later as well, it is necessary that hallucinations be evaluated in the relevant developmental context or as part of a medical disorder in the child.

Disorganized speech

Individuals with psychotic disorders can present with abnormalities in the form or context of speech. Their speech may become completely incomprehensible, with inventions of new words (neologisms) or word salad (a jumble of meaningless or illogical words and phrases).

Disorganized behavior

Examples of disorganized behaviors include impaired ability to maintain adequate hygiene, intrusive behaviors, plan and achieve reasonable goals, or failure to respond in a socially appropriate manner.

Negative symptoms

Negative symptoms usually indicate an absence of normal behaviors. Examples of these symptoms include flat affect (lack of emotional expression); inability to experience pleasure (anhedonia); lack of or limited speech (alogia); and, lack of initiation (avolition).

Epidemiology

When considering these conditions in youth, misdiagnosis tends to become a serious issue. Early-onset schizophrenia and childhood onset schizophrenia have different criteria, which sometimes are hard to categorize, and misdiagnosis and its deleterious effects become particularly important. Considering the high prevalence rate (up to 5%) of psychotic symptoms in otherwise healthy children, early-onset schizophrenia and childhood-onset schizophrenia become relatively rare. The prevalence of early-onset schizophrenia has been estimated in epidemiologic studies at 0.5% of the population (7). However, it is hard to get a very accurate estimate as most of these studies are limited by differences in their definitions and criteria across studies, variations in usage of standardized diagnostic instruments as well as variations in diagnostic accuracies (8).

In childhood-onset schizophrenia specifically, the prevalence appears to be less common, with estimations around 0.04% in the United States (US). In the largest ever sample studied, the NIMH childhood-onset schizophrenia team identified over 350 patients nationwide in the US, with the age range of 6 to 18 years, who met the DSM-III-R criteria with onset of their symptoms before 12 years of age (9). Of these 350 patients, 98% were assessed in-person using structured interviews, and 28 of them were diagnosed with childhood-onset schizophrenia (9).

In comparing the prevalence of schizophrenia on a global level to the United States, onset later in life seems to have an equal prevalence with a possible increase in prevalence in urban populations. Studies also demonstrate an average male-to-female incidence of schizophrenia of 1.5-2.1; this ratio is continually re-examined and challenged (10).

To the best of our knowledge, no studies reporting on the overall prevalence of childhood onset schizophrenia in underdeveloped countries are available. A study in Nigeria of 49 pediatric patients with psychotic symptoms reported 40.8% of its patients to have schizophrenia with 8.1% being under the age of 12 (11).

Etiology

When considering the risk for developing a primary psychotic disorder, several factors must be taken into account as all of these can contribute towards development of psychotic disorders in adolescents and children. These factors include genetic vulnerability, environmental factors, obstetric complications, trauma, social adversities, and substance use, see Table 1.

Table 1. Etiologies and associated factors

Etiology	Associated Factors
Genetic Risk	1q21.1, 15q13.3, 22q11.2 deletion syndromes; DAOA, NRG1, DTNBP1 and GAD1, SOX10 genes
Neurodevelopmental and neuroanatomical abnormalities	Acquired neurodevelopmental damage during pregnancy and delivery suggests an increased vulnerability to schizophrenia later in life, particularly in combination with genetic risk; decrease in frontal and temporal gray matter volumes than healthy controls; loss of cortical thickness in prefrontal and temporal region; decreased whole brain and hippocampal volumes
Substance Abuse	Cannabis use at a young age (coupled with genetic vulnerability) may be a risk factor for schizophrenia onset

Etiology	Associated Factors
Infections	Viral CNS infections (mumps, cytomegalovirus) have shown correlations (further research is needed)
Immunology	Elevated platelet associated auto-antibodies are elevated in patients with COS; elevated IL-4 and IL-10 have also been implicated for involvement in early-onset schizophrenia

Childhood adversity

A meta-analysis with strong evidence reported that childhood adversity was linked with an increased risk of psychosis in adults, although these symptoms of psychosis may also be seen in cases of posttraumatic stress disorder (PTSD). Thus, in cases of children presenting with psychotic symptoms, a comorbid or a primary diagnosis of PTSD should be considered.

Genetic vulnerability

It is clear from several twin studies that childhood-onset schizophrenia may have a substantial genetic component. A study that examined twins with childhood-onset schizophrenia reported an 88.2 percent concordance in 17 monozygotic twins when compared to 22.9 percent concordance in 35 dizygotic twins using earlier diagnostic criteria for schizophrenia.

Pathogenesis

Over 45 genes have been highlighted demonstrating a positive association between schizophrenia and autism. Of these highlighted genes, 20 showed a positive association between the two disorders, and only 11 showed a correlation with schizophrenia. The pathological processes for childhood onset schizophrenia (COS) and early onset schizophrenia are thought to be quite like that of adult-onset schizophrenia. There are various neuroanatomic correlations in the structural brain alterations of patients diagnosed with childhood onset or early onset schizophrenia. A systematic review reporting on the neuroanatomical changes in COS reported a smaller overall brain volume for COS patients during initial imaging with a progressive decline in volume during adolescence. The review also reported on several studies finding COS to have larger ventricular volumes as well as greater increase in ventricular size compared to healthy controls. These findings describe some of the fundamental neurodevelopmental shifts in COS (12).

Differential diagnosis

Substance use disorders (SUD) and drug intoxications

Substance use disorders (SUD) can be comorbid with primary psychotic disorders and result in psychotic symptoms experienced by patients. SUD are acute, brief and will be related to usage of the drug. Symptoms and their timeline will also depend upon the drug in question.

Presentation of the patients will depend upon the nature of acute or chronicity of drug use. When contrasting primary psychotic disturbances with those due to substance use, physical symptoms associated with drug usage are helpful to differentiate between the two. Toxicology is not the ideal means to identify certain substance use disorders as many of the hallucinogenic drugs and newer synthetic agents do not appear on standard drug tests. Since SUD can elicit psychosis, drug use and withdrawal would need to be ruled out before a diagnosis of schizophrenia can be considered.

Post-traumatic stress disorder (PTSD)

In PTSD, signs and symptoms commonly include flashbacks, which tend to be misinterpreted by patients as auditory hallucinations. Symptoms of hypervigilance can be mistaken for signs of paranoia, which can make distinguishing between these two disorders a challenging task. When trying to differentiate PTSD from a primary psychotic disorder, in PTSD the symptoms are related to the trauma and there is a lower incidence of thought disturbances and disorganized thinking (13). A meta-analysis was able to demonstrate compelling evidence that childhood diversity is strongly linked to an increased risk for psychosis, hence PTSD should certainly be considered when the history of the youth being examined is indicative childhood diversity (13).

Autism spectrum disorders

Autism spectrum disorders (ASDs) must also be differentiated from psychotic disorders. Symptoms of psychosis in ASD can occur due to common features such as general impairment in social communication (which may be mistaken for negative symptoms of psychosis), or stereotyped language (which can be misinterpreted as disorganized speech). Investigation into developmental history and baseline thought process can be helpful in differentiating between the two conditions. Factors that are more in favor of a diagnosis of schizophrenia or a comorbid diagnosis of ASD and schizophrenia are the occurrence of new-onset delusions or hallucinations that last longer than one month, the presence of disordered or delusional thinking that is distinctly different from baseline, or deterioration in social and general functioning (14).

Schizoaffective disorders

It can be challenging to distinguish between schizoaffective disorder and early-onset schizophrenia as the psychotic symptoms continue to evolve as the youth grows and develops. Changes in symptoms can potentially lead to a change in diagnosis overtime. Studies looking at the clinical features and the functional outcomes, as well as neurocognitive testing in these populations tend to suggest the presence of overlapping characteristics of youth with these disorders (15).

Mood disorders

Mood disorders also need consideration as in severe cases they can present with psychotic features. Major depressive disorder with psychotic features, and bipolar disorder with psychosis are important considerations. A carefully elicited history looking at the mood episodes and their relation to the psychotic episodes/symptoms can help elicit a correct diagnosis. There is some evidence that extensive gray matter loss may be seen in those with childhood onset schizophrenia, although it might be unclear whether it is due to medication side effects or disease severity. There needs to be further investigation examining the neurobiological differences that exist between these disorders.

In the case of bipolar disorder, psychotic features are a prominent part of early onset bipolar disorder. Youth during the acute manic phase can be misdiagnosed with schizophrenia. Assessing the nature and quality of hallucinations and probing in detail for mood symptoms and their relation to the psychotic features can provide diagnostic clarity. Psychotic symptoms in bipolar disorder will be more mood congruent (elevated, grandiose mood). In schizophrenia, youth will have greater thought disturbances, deterioration in social and occupational functioning, delusions and/or hallucinations of age-appropriate themes. Furthermore, it is important to differentiate between negative symptoms of schizophrenia and symptoms of major depressive disorder.

Medical diseases

Certain medical diseases may also present with psychotic symptoms. Common medical conditions that present with psychotic symptomatology include seizure disorder, encephalitis, central nervous system (CNS) tumors, chromosomal abnormalities (22q11.2 deletion syndromes), autoimmune disorders (i.e., systemic lupus erythematosus), and metabolic disorders (i.e., Wilson disease, porphyria variegate).

Nonpsychotic Children

It is worth mentioning that delusional thinking, hallucinations and looseness of associations can be seen in healthy nonpsychotic children and usually diminishes after age 6 (16). We also see anxiety and related visual hallucinations commonly in preschool children (16). When examining the patient, a careful history focusing on decline in cognitive functioning, attention, and the presence of negative symptoms is helpful in diagnosing psychosis.

Evaluation

When approaching a case of pediatric psychosis, clinical assessments should begin with a thorough individual, medication, psychosocial and family history, see Table 2. The previously listed differential diagnosis should serve as guiding principles when navigating through the history and clinical interview sections. Physical examination should include a neurological exam. Once a diagnosis of childhood onset schizophrenia is suspected, there are several workup options that need to be considered to rule out other diagnostic considerations.

Laboratory studies are part of the assessment for psychotic disorders. A thorough workup should include complete blood count, serum electrolytes and glucose, hepatic and renal function, thyroid stimulating hormone, syphilis test, prolactin levels, hepatitis C, vitamin b12, folate and, serum ceruloplasmin, erythrocyte sedimentation rate, and antinuclear antibodies. Liver function studies, copper and ceruloplasmin are part of the workup of Wilson disease. Porphobilinogen levels would be helpful in excluding/including porphyria. In addition to these, HIV titers, Venereal Disease Research Laboratory (VDRL) testing, or heavy metal screening might also be needed.

If the patient's history and clinical assessment is suggestive for signs of intellectual disability or dysmorphic features, include a karyotype in the genetic assessment. One example is 22q11 deletion syndrome, or velocardiofacial syndrome (17). Some reports also suggest 5q involvement.

Table 2. Medical work-up and diagnostic approach considerations

History	Thorough history and clinical assessments with inquiring about medication use, psychosocial history and family history of mental illness. Differential diagnosis previously listed should serve as a guiding principle
Diagnostic clinical scales	Diagnostic Clinical Scales such as the CAARMS (Comprehensive Assessment of At-Risk Mental States), SIPS (Structured Interview for Prodromal Syndromes) and Kiddie Schedule for Affective Disorders and Schizophrenia (K-SADS)
Physical examination	Neurological exam, General Physical Examination for signs of General Medical Condition (GMC)
Laboratory studies	CBC, Serum Electrolytes and glucose, hepatic and renal function tests, thyroid stimulating hormone, syphilis test, prolactin level, hepatitis C, Vitamin B12, Folate, Serum Ceruloplasmin, Erythrocyte Sedimentation Rate, Antinuclear Antibodies, copper and ceruloplasmin levels, HIV testing
Developmental workup	If intellectual disability or developmental disorder are implicated, consider karyotype and genetic studies additionally
Imaging and neurological workup	MRI, EEG, LP

It is important to consider neuroimaging with MRI (CT if MRI not available) as part of the work-up when evaluating new-onset psychosis. MRI allows for exclusion of certain organic causes of psychosis. Demyelination would be observed in children with leukodystrophy, atrophy in children with neuronal ceroid lipofuscinosis. Although they are not considered diagnostic, ventricular enlargement and gray matter loss are consistent with childhood-onset schizophrenia.

It is important to obtain electroencephalography (EEG) if episodic symptoms or neurological signs are present when evaluating a child with psychosis. When considering prescribing clozapine in children, obtaining an EEG is useful due to the increased risk of seizures associated with clozapine. Further neurological workup may include lumbar puncture (LP) and cerebrospinal fluid (CSF) testing if indicated.

Approach considerations

The initial approach depends on the acuity of the presentation. Studies have estimated a lifetime risk of suicide between 4.9-10% (18). Suicide risk is higher during the initial years of the illness and immediately after discharge from the hospital. Furthermore, despite these high-risk phases, suicidal ideation tends to persist throughout the course of the disease. Thus, while interacting with these individuals, it is important to be vigilant about some of the warning signs such as verbal or physical aggression, restlessness, pacing, muted response to auditory or visual hallucinations, and sudden changes in mental status. Acute inpatient hospitalization is necessary for children with behaviors that are deemed dangerous to themselves or others for stabilization. A thorough suicide risk assessment and mental status examination are prudent to obtain in every case.

Consultations

For ideal outcomes, an essential component is to ensure that patients get all round support in the form of a team consultation. The team members can include:

- Case manager – To help the patient and family in facilitating outreach.
- Psychologist – For all kinds of therapy that are required.
- Dietician – To help the child and family in making healthier choices
- Child Neurologist – To rule out organic etiologies, if suspected.
- Ophthalmologist – For patients who are on thioridazine and chlorpromazine to check for retinal pathologies and for patients who take anticholinergics to rule out glaucoma, (although these agents are rarely used in the pediatric population).
- Other specialties like occupational therapy, speech therapy, language therapy and intellectual quotient/educational testing as required.

Pharmacotherapy

Pharmacotherapy is critical in the treatment of individuals with childhood-onset psychosis in addition to psychosocial interventions. Pharmacological treatment can be divided into two parts: Prodromal stage and first episode psychosis.

Prodromal stage

Children who have prodromal symptoms include disorganized behavior, paranoia or suspicion, or any unusual thoughts that are below the threshold of full-blown schizophrenia.

Medications for Prodromal stage

Three classes of medications have been tested in the children and adolescent population (cap) and young adults at a high risk of psychosis: antipsychotics, omega-3 fatty acids and antidepressants.

Antipsychotics

The use of antipsychotics to prevent psychosis in cap with psychosis is not supported by clinical trials.

Evidence

There was a clinical trial where 60 patients were randomly assigned to receive olanzapine 5 mg to 15 mg vs. placebo and followed over two years. In the first year, fewer patients on olanzapine converted to psychosis (17 vs. 40%) but the conversion rate did not differ in the subsequent year (19). Of note, the olanzapine group reported an average of a 9 Kg weight gain (19).

Omega-3 fatty acids

The clinical evidence of using omega-3 fatty acids is equivocal.

Evidence

A trial randomly assigned 81 youth aged 15 to 25 years with subthreshold psychosis to receive omega-3 polyunsaturated fatty acids (PUFA) (1 gram twice daily) vs. placebo for 12 weeks in addition to a nine-session psychosocial intervention. After 12 months, subjects assigned to receive omega-3 PUFAs were less likely to transition to a psychotic disorder compared with the placebo group (4.9 versus 27.5 percent) with no difference in adverse effects (20). A trial randomly assigned 304 youth/young adults (mean age 19 years) with high risk for psychosis to receive omega-3 PUFAs (1.4 grams daily) plus psychosocial intervention vs. placebo plus the psychosocial intervention. After six months, there was no difference in the rate of transition to psychosis (6.7 versus 5.1 percent) (21).

Antidepressants

Two studies found that treatment with antidepressants was associated with reduced rates of progression to a psychotic disorder in adolescents with prodromal symptoms.

Evidence

A prospective observational study of adolescents with prodromal symptoms found that 25 percent developed a psychotic disorder, with all converters having been prescribed second-generation antipsychotics. There were no conversions among antidepressant-treated adolescents; 11 of the 12 converters were non-adherent (22).

The Outreach and Support in South London (OASIS) 6-year naturalistic study found that the cognitive behavioral therapy (CBT) + antidepressant intervention was associated with a reduced risk of transition to psychosis, as compared with the CBT + antipsychotic intervention (hazards ratio = 0.129, 95% confidence interval 0.030-0.565, p = 0.007) (23).

Summary

Antipsychotics have no evidence in preventing the transformation of prodromal stage to full-blown schizophrenia or even delaying it. Omega 3 fatty acids have mixed results. However, given the low risk of side effects, omega 3 fatty acids are considered a safe option to try. Selective serotonin reuptake inhibitors (SSRIs) have shown some evidence in 2 naturalistic studies but do not have randomized control trials.

First episode psychosis

Antipsychotics are the first-line treatment for confirmed schizophrenia, in addition to psychosocial interventions, for first episode, maintenance treatment and subsequent episodes. Research has looked at the effect of antipsychotics on positive and negative symptoms:

Positive symptoms

Several randomized trials have shown that antipsychotics reduce positive symptoms of schizophrenia, such as hallucinations and delusions. Antipsychotics eliminate or reduce the symptoms to a tolerable level in about 70% of the patients with schizophrenia.

Negative symptoms

Negative symptoms of schizophrenia, such as diminished emotional expression or lack of motivation are more difficult to treat. Prior to starting any antipsychotic, the following baseline tests should be completed:

- Complete blood count
- Fasting glucose
- Cholesterol
- Triglycerides
- Transaminases
- HbA1c
- Electrocardiogram.

Most antipsychotics have been shown to cause QTc prolongation in limited studies, except for aripiprazole, which has been shown to improve the QTc (24-26). In children and adolescents, antipsychotics should generally be started at a low dose and titrated slowly using divided doses whenever possible. Table 3 lists antipsychotics with their commonly used doses. Once at that dose, it is prudent to wait three to five days for evidence of a clinical response in a patient with severe symptoms and up to two weeks in a patient with less severe symptoms. Table 4 provides factors to monitor for metabolic side effects of antipsychotic drugs. Table 5 provides potential adverse effects of antipsychotics with comments regarding their treatment.

Table 3. Antipsychotic dosing in children and adolescents with schizophrenia

Medication	Initial dose	Therapeutic range	Max dose
Second-generation antipsychotics			
Aripiprazole			
<13 years	2 mg	5 to 20 mg	20 mg
>=13 years	2 mg	10 to 30 mg	30 mg
Paliperidone			
<13 years	1.5 mg	6 mg	6 mg
>=13 years	3 mg	12 mg	12 mg
Risperidone			
<13 years	0.25 mg	2 to 3 mg/day	3 mg/day
>=13 years	0.25 mg twice daily	2 to 3 mg/day	6 mg/day
Clozapine			
<13 years	12.5 mg	150 to 900 mg	900 mg
>=13 years	25 mg	150 to 900 mg	900 mg
Olanzapine			
<13 years	2.5 mg	5 to 20 mg	20 mg
>=13 years	5 mg	10 to 30 mg	30 mg
Quetiapine			
<13 years	25 mg	100 to 400 mg	400 mg
>=13 years	25 mg twice daily	400 to 800 mg	800 mg
Lurasidone			
<13 years	20 mg	20 to 40 mg	40 mg
>=13 years	40 mg	40 to 80 mg	80 mg
First-generation antipsychotics			
Haloperidol			
<13 years	1 mg	0.5 to 6 mg	10 mg
>=13 years	1 mg	3 to 24 mg	24 mg
Chlorpromazine			
<13 years	50 mg	50 to 400 mg	400 mg/day
>=13 years	100 mg	100 to 400 mg	600 mg/day
Perphenazine			
<13 years	2 to 4 mg twice daily	16 to 36 mg/day	36 mg/day
>=13 years	4 to 8 mg three times daily	24 to 64 mg/day	64 mg/day

Table 4. Monitoring for metabolic side effects of antipsychotic drugs (all variables to be measured at baseline)

	1 month	2-months	3-months	Yearly
Waist circumference			+	+
Fasting lipid profile			+	
Weight (body mass index)	+	+	+	
Fasting plasma glucose	+			+
Blood pressure			+	+

Clinical trials have not consistently found any one antipsychotic more effective than the others except clozapine; however, due to a significant adverse effect profile it is reserved for use in treatment-resistant schizophrenia. The current recommendation is to start with a second-generation antipsychotic, except ziprasidone or clozapine. Ziprasidone has a negative trial and should only be used judiciously. Clozapine is reserved for treatment resistant cases due to multiple life-threatening side effects. Clinicians can select one amongst the above medications, based on patient age, family history, previous history of response, current medical comorbidities, comorbid psychiatric conditions, comorbid substance use disorders, intensity of psychosis and medication adverse effect profile.

Table 5. Adverse effects and treatment

Adverse effects	Comments
Dystonia	Anticholinergic medication is 1st line. Consider antihistamine next followed by Benzodiazepines
Parkinsonism (tremor, rigidity, bradykinesia)	Consider lowering the dose, changing the antipsychotic or adding an anticholinergic medication
Tardive dyskinesia	Lower dose. Consider Valbenazine or Deutetrabenazine (Generally used in adults). Clonazepam and Gingko Biloba can be considered. Consider Clozapine if patient has already failed 2 antipsychotics.
Akathisia	Consider lowering the dose, changing the antipsychotic or add Propranolol
Sedation	Consider dosing at night, reducing the dose or changing the antipsychotic. Using stimulant concomitantly has also been tried.
Sialorrhea	Behavioral modification-Sugarless candy and using pillow at night. Consider Ipratropium or atropine eye drops topically/sublingually, or scopolamine patch
Prolactin elevation	Evaluate the cause. Dose reduction or switching to a prolactin sparing antipsychotic. Adding low dose Aripiprazole has been found to be effective.
QT prolongation	Change antipsychotic and stop other QT prolonging drugs.
Orthostatic hypotension	Adjust dose, ensure adequate hydration or change antipsychotic
Myocarditis	Discontinue the antipsychotic and consult cardiology.
Anticholinergic effects (dry mouth, blurry vision, tachycardia, constipation)	Lower dose, treat symptomatically, stop the antipsychotic and avoid other medications that have anticholinergic properties
Weight gain, dyslipidemia	Diet and exercise. Consider Metformin very early.

Choosing the initial antipsychotic

Some tips for choosing the initial antipsychotic medication include:

- Typically, treatment is started with aripiprazole or risperidone. Risperidone is avoided in patients with gynecomastia or elevated prolactin and in late adolescent boys.
- Lurasidone is preferred in patients with increased weight as it is weight neutral. Aripiprazole was initially thought of as weight neutral but there have been several subsequent reports of significant weight gain.
- Aripiprazole is preferred in patients with comorbid mood disorder.
- Quetiapine or Olanzapine (in severe cases) is preferred in patients with insomnia.
- Olanzapine is preferred in patients with significant agitation.

Long-acting injectable (LAI) formulations

Initially, the use of long acting injectables in the child and adolescent population (cap) with psychosis was considered controversial. However, it is used, albeit less commonly in patients who have a difficulty in taking their daily oral dosing. The evidence base is still nascent.

Evidence

In a randomized clinical trial of 113 adolescents aged 12 to 17 years old with schizophrenia, participants were randomly assigned to paliperidone extended release vs. oral aripiprazole for eight weeks and no difference was seen in response rates between the two drugs (67.9 versus 76.3 percent). The risk of extrapyramidal symptoms was slightly higher in paliperidone extended release over aripiprazole (27). Case reports and open trials have described the use of LAI antipsychotics in 36 children (mean age of 12 years) with bipolar disorder or schizophrenia with 24 subjects receiving LAI risperidone and eight receiving paliperidone palmitate. Most cases reported clinical improvement with good tolerability (28). The dosing of LAI antipsychotics for pediatric schizophrenia has not been decided owing to the limited research.

Treatment resistant schizophrenia

The *Treatment of early-onset schizophrenia spectrum disorders (TEOSS)* study found that more than half of the participants did not respond to antipsychotic medication adequately after eight weeks of treatment, regardless of which antipsychotic was used (29). For patients with a confirmed diagnosis of schizophrenia who fail an adequate trial with 2 or more antipsychotics, a clozapine trial is recommended. An adequate trial is defined as a trial of six to eight weeks at the maximum tolerated dose.

Clozapine has demonstrated superior efficacy for treatment-resistant schizophrenia in three randomized clinical trials in youth in comparison with haloperidol and olanzapine (29-31). Due to its more severe side effect profile, its use is generally restricted to patients that have not responded to other antipsychotics. The side effect profile also brings a level of stigma against the medication and that leads to an underutilization of this medication. There is some preliminary evidence that clinical improvement in symptoms was directly correlated to the plasma level and hence obtaining a baseline and regular clozapine levels is useful. It also helps in understanding if deterioration is due to metabolism issues or due to not taking the medication (32). Children may be at greater risk for seizures when taking clozapine compared to the adult population. Some experts recommend a baseline electroencephalogram in patients with some evidence of neurological abnormalities or neurodevelopmental delay.

Side effects

Second-generation antipsychotics

Adverse effects associated with second-generation antipsychotics include QT interval prolongation, metabolic side effects (weight gain, diabetes, hyperlipidemia), akathisia, and tardive dyskinesia. They can also cause extrapyramidal side effects but generally at rates much lower than first-generation agents.

First-generation antipsychotics

Common adverse effects of first-generation antipsychotics include extrapyramidal side effects (i.e., tremor, bradykinesia, shuffling gait, akathisia), acute dystonic reactions, tardive dyskinesia, and hyperprolactinemia. Pimozide, thioridazine and intravenous haloperidol can prolong the QT interval, particularly at higher doses. These medications should be avoided in patients with cardiac disease, a family history of sudden death, and in conjunction with other medications that prolong the QT interval.

Side effect differences when compared to adults

Children and adolescents, compared to adults, are at a lower risk of tardive dyskinesias (0.4 versus 6.8 percent) (26, 33-37). The risk of tardive dyskinesia in children appears to be greatest with first-generation antipsychotics versus minimal risk with second-generation antipsychotics; some of these data, however, are extrapolated from adult studies. In contrast, children and adolescents carry a higher risk of side effects, including extrapyramidal side effects, withdrawal dyskinesias, elevated prolactin, weight gain, and metabolic abnormalities (26, 33-36). Serious side effects necessitating termination of the offending agent include neuroleptic malignant syndrome, agranulocytosis, myocarditis, and cardiomyopathy.

Treatment of side effects

Side effects in youth are treated in a similar way as in adults although the dosing is more conservative, especially if the child is younger than 13 years of age. The motto is, "Start low and go slow." Metformin has strong evidence in the form of randomized control trials in adolescents 10-17 years old, in preventing antipsychotic induced weight gain in patients on second generation antipsychotics.

Electroconvulsive Therapy (ECT)

Limited evidence supports the use of electroconvulsive therapy (ECT) in children and adolescents patients who do not adequately respond to, or cannot tolerate antipsychotic medications, or those with catatonia. The clinician must balance the relative risks and benefits of ECT against the morbidity of the disorder, the attitudes of the patient as well as the family, and the availability of other treatment options. Obtaining informed consent from the parents after a detailed discussion and obtaining an independent evaluation from a second psychiatrist is required before an ECT can be performed.

Psychosocial interventions

In 2008, the National Institute of Mental Health (NIMH) launched the *Recovery After an Initial Schizophrenia Episode (RAISE)* Project (38). RAISE was a large-scale research initiative that began with two studies examining different aspects of coordinated specialty care (CSC) treatments for first episode psychosis patients in adolescents and young adults. The RAISE Early Treatment Program (RAISE-ETP) was one of two research projects of the RAISE initiative. RAISE-ETP was a clinical trial that enrolled more than 400 people at 34 clinics across the U.S. It compared Navigate, a CSC treatment program for first episode psychosis vs. care typically found in community clinics (38).

Coordinated specialty care (CSC) is a recovery-oriented treatment program that promotes shared decision-making and uses a team of specialists who work with the patient to create a personalized treatment plan. The treatment modalities include psychotherapy, medication management, family education and support, case management, and work or education support, depending on the individual's needs and preferences. The CSC team works with the patient to make treatment decisions, involving family members as much as possible. The goal is to connect the patient with a CSC team swiftly after psychotic symptoms begin.

RAISE-ETP found that, over two years, clients at the Navigate clinics stayed in treatment longer; experienced greater improvement in their psychotic symptoms, their quality of life and interpersonal relationships; and were more involved in work or school compared to the control group (38).

Conclusion

The term early onset schizophrenia is typically reserved for symptoms of schizophrenia that start prior to age 18 while the term childhood-onset schizophrenia (COS) is reserved for children in whom the onset of symptoms begins before 13 years of age. There is ample evidence that pediatric schizophrenia is on a continuum with adult schizophrenia with premorbid cognitive abnormalities, chronic course and long-term morbidity as well as mortality. Factors of etiology include genetic vulnerability, environmental factors, obstetric complications, trauma, social adversities, and substance use. Studies have estimated a lifetime risk of suicide between 4.9-10% (18).

Diagnosis is made after a careful evaluation including laboratory and radiologic studies. Management includes a team approach with multiple specialists. Pharmacologic medications that are used include second-generation antipsychotics. Suggestions for their use are given along with consideration of their various adverse effects as well as treatment of these effects. Management of treatment-resistant schizophrenia include clozapine despite its known adverse profile, and electroconvulsive therapy (ECT). Psychosocial interventions are important in management of psychosis that includes the *Recovery After an Initial Schizophrenia Episode (RAISE)* Project that was introduced by the National Institute of Mental Health (NIMH) in 2008 (38).

References

[1] Emminghaus H. [Die Psychischen Störungen Des Kindesalters, Vol 2]. Tübingen: H Laupp, 1887.

[2] Remschmidt HE, Schulz E, Martin M, Warnke A, Trott GE. Childhood-onset schizophrenia: history of the concept and recent studies. Schizophr Bull 1994;20(4):727-45.

[3] Nicolson R, Giedd JN, Lenane M, Hamburger S, Singaracharlu S, Bedwell J, et al. Clinical and neurobiological correlates of cytogenetic abnormalities in childhood-onset schizophrenia. Am J Psychiatry 1999;156(10):1575-9.

[4] Tamnes CK, Agartz I. White matter microstructure in early-onset schizophrenia: A systematic review of diffusion tensor imaging studies. J Am Acad Child Adolesc Psychiatry 2016;55(4):269-79.

[5] Fusar-Poli P, Bonoldi I, Yung AR, Borgwardt S, Kempton MJ, Valmaggia L, et al. Predicting psychosis: meta-analysis of transition outcomes in individuals at high clinical risk. Arch Gen Psychiatry 2012;69(3):220-9.

[6] Yoviene Sykes LA, Ferrara M, Addington J, Bearden CE, Cadenhead KS, Cannon TD, et al. Predictive validity of conversion from the clinical high risk syndrome to frank psychosis. Schizophr Res 2020;216:184-91.

[7] Ritsner MS. Handbook of schizophrenia spectrum disorders. Vol Ii: Phenotypic and Endophenotypic presentations, Vol 2. Berlin: Springer Science Business Media, 2011.

[8] Maloney AE, Yakutis LJ, Frazier JA. Empirical evidence for psychopharmacologic treatment in early-onset psychosis and schizophrenia. Child Adolesc Psychiatr Clin North Am 2012;21(4):885-909.

[9] Rapoport JL, Gogtay N. Childhood onset schizophrenia: support for a progressive neurodevelopmental disorder. Int J Dev Neurosci 2011;29(3):251-8.

[10] Okkels N, Vernal DL, Jensen SO, McGrath JJ, Nielsen RE. Changes in the diagnosed incidence of early onset schizophrenia over four decades. Acta Psychiatr Scand 2013; 127(1):62-8.

[11] Okewole AO, Ogunwale A, Mosanya TJ, Ojo BM. A 12 year chart review of childhood and adolescent onset psychosis at a Nigerian tertiary mental health facility. J Child Adolesc Ment Health 2016;28(3):189-97.

[12] Ordóñez AE, Luscher ZI, Gogtay N. Neuroimaging findings from childhood onset schizophrenia patients and their non-psychotic siblings. Schizophr Res 2016;173(3):124-31.

[13] Braakman MH, Kortmann FA, van den Brink W. Validity of 'post-traumatic stress disorder with secondary psychotic features': a review of the evidence. Acta Psychiatr Scand 2009; 119(1):15-24.

[14] Cochran DM, Dvir Y, Frazier JA. “Autism-plus” spectrum disorders: intersection with psychosis and the schizophrenia spectrum. Child Adolesc Psychiatr Clin North Am 2013; 22(4):609-27.

[15] Hooper SR, Giuliano AJ, Youngstrom EA, Breiger D, Sikich L, Frazier JA, et al.. Neurocognition in early-onset schizophrenia and schizoaffective disorders. J Am Acad Child Adolesc Psychiatry 2010;49(1):52-60.

[16] Dominguez MDG, Garralda ME. Assessing and managing hallucinations in children and adolescents. BJPsych Adv 2016;22(6):380-90.

[17] Bassett AS, Chow EW, AbdelMalik P, Gheorghiu M, Husted J, Weksberg R. The schizophrenia phenotype in 22q11 deletion syndrome. Am J Psychiatry 2003;160(9):1580-6.

[18] Palmer BA, Pankratz VS, Bostwick JM. The lifetime risk of suicide in schizophrenia: a reexamination. Arch Gen Psychiatry 2005;62(3):247-53.

[19] McGlashan TH, Zipursky RB, Perkins D, Addington J, Miller T, Woods SW, et al. Randomized, double-blind trial of olanzapine versus placebo in patients prodromally symptomatic for psychosis. Am J Psychiatry 2006;163(5):790-9.

[20] Amminger GP, Schäfer MR, Papageorgiou K, Klier CM, Cotton SM, Harrigan SM, et al. Long-chain omega-3 fatty acids for indicated prevention of psychotic disorders: a randomized, placebo-controlled trial. Arch Gen Psychiatry 2010;67(2):146-54.

[21] McGorry PD, Nelson B, Markulev C, Yuen HP, Schäfer MR, Mossaheb N, et al. Effect of ω-3 polyunsaturated fatty acids in young people at ultrahigh risk for psychotic disorders: The NEURAPRO Randomized Clinical Trial. JAMA Psychiatry 2017;74(1):19-27.

[22] Cornblatt BA, Lencz T, Smith CW, Olsen R, Auther AM, Nakayama E, et al. Can antidepressants be used to treat the schizophrenia prodrome? Results of a prospective, naturalistic treatment study of adolescents. J Clin Psychiatry 2007;68(4):546-57.

[23] Fusar-Poli P, Frascarelli M, Valmaggia L, Byrne M, Stahl D, Rocchetti M, et al. Antidepressant, antipsychotic and psychological interventions in subjects at high clinical risk for psychosis: OASIS 6-year naturalistic study. Psychol Med 2015;45(6):1327-39.

[24] McNally P, McNicholas F, Oslizlok P. The QT interval and psychotropic medications in children: recommendations for clinicians. Eur Child Adolesc Psychiatry 2007;16(1):33-47.

[25] American Academy of Child and Adolescent Psychiatry. AACAP official action. Summary of the practice parameters for the assessment and treatment of children and adolescents with schizophrenia. American Academy of Child and Adolescent Psychiatry. J Am Acad Child Adolesc Psychiatry 2000;39(12):1580-2.

[26] Correll CU. Antipsychotic use in children and adolescents: minimizing adverse effects to maximize outcomes. J Am Acad Child Adolesc Psychiatry 2008;47(1):9-20.

[27] Savitz AJ, Lane R, Nuamah I, Gopal S, Hough D. Efficacy and safety of paliperidone extended release in adolescents with schizophrenia: a randomized, double-blind study. J Am Acad Child Adolesc Psychiatry 2015;54(2):126-137.

[28] Lytle S, McVoy M, Sajatovic M. Long-acting injectable antipsychotics in children and adolescents. J Child Adolesc Psychopharmacol 2017;27(1):2-9.

[29] Sikich L, Frazier JA, McClellan J, Findling RL, Vitiello B, Ritz L, et al. Double-blind comparison of first- and second-generation antipsychotics in early-onset schizophrenia and schizo-affective disorder: findings from the treatment of early-onset schizophrenia spectrum disorders (TEOSS) study. Am J Psychiatry 2008;165(11):1420-31.

[30] Shaw P, Sporn A, Gogtay N, Overman GP, Greenstein D, Gochman P, et al. Childhood-onset schizophrenia: A double-blind, randomized clozapine-olanzapine comparison. Arch Gen Psychiatry 2006;63(7):721-30.

[31] Kumra S, Kranzler H, Gerbino-Rosen G, Kester HM, DeThomas C, Cullen K, et al. Clozapine versus "high-dose" olanzapine in refractory early-onset schizophrenia: an open-label extension study. J Child Adolesc Psychopharmacol 2008;18(4):307-16.

[32] Piscitelli SC, Frazier JA, McKenna K, Albus KE, Grothe DR, Gordon CT, et al. Plasma clozapine and haloperidol concentrations in adolescents with childhood-onset schizophrenia: association with response. J Clin Psychiatry 1994;55(Suppl B):94-7.

[33] Correll CU, Penzner JB, Parikh UH, Mughal T, Javed T, Carbon M, et al. Recognizing and monitoring adverse events of second-generation antipsychotics in children and adolescents. Child Adolesc Psychiatr Clin North Am 2006;15(1):177-206.

[34] Correll CU, Carlson HE. Endocrine and metabolic adverse effects of psychotropic medications in children and adolescents. J Am Acad Child Adolesc Psychiatry 2006; 45(7):771-91.

[35] Correll CU. Weight gain and metabolic effects of mood stabilizers and antipsychotics in pediatric bipolar disorder: a systematic review and pooled analysis of short-term trials. J Am Acad Child Adolesc Psychiatry 2007;46(6):687-700.

[36] Correll CU, Manu P, Olshanskiy V, Napolitano B, Kane JM, Malhotra AK. Cardiometabolic risk of second-generation antipsychotic medications during first-time use in children and adolescents. JAMA 2009;302(16):1765-73.

[37] Correll CU, Leucht S, Kane JM. Lower risk for tardive dyskinesia associated with second-generation antipsychotics: a systematic review of 1-year studies. Am J Psychiatry 2004; 161(3):414-25.

[38] Recovery after an initial schizophrenia episodde (RAISE). URL: https://www.nimh.nih.gov/health/topics/schizophrenia/raise.

Chapter 3

Recognizing and treating the emotional and behavioral effects of child maltreatment

Olga Jablonka[*], PhD, Chanelle Coble, MD and Vincent J Palusci, MD, MS

Frances L Loeb Child Protection and Development Center, Bellevue Hospital Center, New York University Grossman School of Medicine, New York, United States of America

Abstract

The experience of the past sixty years has established a solid foundation in preparation for the work that clinicians need to address to improve the physical and emotional health outcomes after child abuse and maltreatment. This discussion serves as a primer for professionals who, regardless of their individual interests and fields of expertise, can improve the growth and development of children by understanding and responding to the behavioral as well as emotional issues related to abuse and neglect. It provides an overview of the extent of the behavioral and other mental health issues after all types of maltreatment, how to identify them, and the best ways to treat them. It focuses on extent of the problem, screening, evaluation, and treatment for these issues as they relate to child abuse and neglect to assist the clinician in recognizing as well as providing services to improve children's lives and that help them reach their full potential after their victimization.

Abbreviations

AAP:	American Academy of Pediatrics;
CM:	child maltreatment;
CBT:	cognitive behavioral therapy;
CPS:	child protective services;
DSM:	Diagnostic and Statistical Manual of Mental Disorders;
ICD	International Classification of Diseases
IPV:	intimate partner violence;
NCANDS:	National Child Abuse and Neglect Data System;

[*] Corresponding Author's Email: olga.jablonka@nyulangone.org.

In: Behavioral Pediatrics
Editors: Donald E. Greydanus, Dilip R. Patel, Ahsan Nazeer et al.
ISBN: 979-8-88697-060-9

NIS:	National Incidence Studies of Child Abuse and Neglect;
NOFTT:	non-organic failure to thrive;
PM:	psychologic maltreatment;
PTSD:	posttraumatic stress disorder;
SSRIs:	selective serotonin reuptake inhibitors;
TCAs:	tricyclic antidepressants;
TF-CBT:	trauma-focused cognitive behavioral therapy;
TIF:	trauma-informed care;
WHO:	World Health Organization

Introduction

In the sixty years since the publication of C Henry Kempe's (1922-1984) landmark article, "The battered child syndrome" (1), the subject of child maltreatment has become a universal topic, not restricted to one community or to one type of provider. Childhood abuse is thought to adversely affect adult health through the pathway of toxic stress, leading to increased risk for depression, trauma and stress-related disorders, participation in harmful activities, difficulty in forming and sustaining healthy relationships, and negative beliefs as well as attitudes towards others (2). We are only beginning to use methods derived from economics to understand the medical and nonmedical costs of victimization as well as the long-term emotional and mental health effects. As the field has grown, professionals have had to broaden their intellectual and personal perspectives to not only identify maltreatment when it occurs but to recognize and treat the behavioral as well as emotional issues and to prevent further harm. The goal of professionals dedicated to this field is to optimize a child's physical and mental health and to ensure that child abuse, like many other adverse childhood experiences and social determinants of health, will be improved or eradicated in the near future.

While each state in the United States (US) defines child maltreatment in its child welfare and criminal statutes, broad definitions have been developed for the US Child Abuse Prevention and Treatment Act (3) and by the World Health Organization (WHO) (4) (see Table 1). While child abuse overall pertains to the variety of acts committed or omitted by parents or caretakers for children, the quality of the parent-child relationship and nurturing is often left out of state laws. Sexual abuse, for example, has been defined as sexual contacts or exploitation of children by adults that cannot be consented to by the child and which violate social laws or taboos; however, the emotional effects far outweigh the physical findings (5). Similarly, all of the major types of child maltreatment carry their emotional and behavioral harms. In the broader sense, the WHO qualitative definitions add context to this relationship and the broader nature of caring for children (4).

Table 1. World Health Organization Definitions (4)

Child Abuse - Child abuse or maltreatment constitutes all forms of physical and/or emotional ill-treatment, sexual abuse, neglect or negligent treatment or commercial or other exploitation, resulting in actual or potential harm to the child's health, survival, development, or dignity in the context of a relationship of responsibility, trust or power.
Physical Abuse - Physical abuse of a child is that which results in actual or potential physical harm from an interaction or lack of an interaction, which is reasonably within the control of a parent or person in a position of responsibility, power or trust. There may be a single or repeated incidents.

Emotional Abuse - Emotional abuse includes the failure to provide a developmentally appropriate, supportive environment, including the availability of a primary attachment figure, so that the child can establish a stable and full range of emotional and social competencies commensurate with her or his personal potentials and in the context of the society in which the child dwells. There may also be acts towards the child that cause or have a high probability of causing harm to the child's health or physical, mental, spiritual, moral or social development. These acts must be reasonably within the control of a parent or person in a position of responsibility, power or trust. Acts include restriction of movement, patterns of belittling, denigrating, scapegoating, threatening, scaring, discriminating, ridiculing or other non-physical forms of hostile or rejecting treatment.
Neglect and negligent treatment - Neglect is the failure to provide for the development of the child in all spheres: health, education, emotional development, nutrition, shelter and safe living conditions, in the context of resources reasonably available to the family or caretakers and causes or has a high probability of causing harm to the child's health or physical, mental, spiritual, moral or social development. This includes the failure to properly supervise and protect children from harm as much as is feasible.
Sexual abuse - Child sexual abuse is the involvement of a child in sexual activity that he or she does not fully comprehend or is unable to give informed consent to, or that violates the laws or social taboos of society. Child sexual abuse is evidenced by this activity between a child and an adult or another child who by age or development is in a relationship of responsibility, trust or power, the activity being intended to gratify or satisfy the needs of the other person. This may include but is not limited to: • The inducement or coercion of a child to engage in any unlawful activity • The exploitative use of a child in prostitution or other unlawful sexual practices • The exploitative use of children in pornographic performances and materials
Exploitation - Commercial or other exploitation of a child refers to the use of the child in work or other activities for the benefit of others. This includes, but is not limited to, child labour and child prostitution. These activities are to the detriment of the child's physical or mental health, education, or spiritual, moral or social-emotional development.

In the effort to allow diagnostic coding for physicians in medical systems and for medical examiners as well as coroners for state public health statutes, the International Classification of Disease (ICD) Codes have been developed applicable to child abuse and neglect. ICD-9 lists individual types as well as external modifiers related to perpetrator relationship ("E codes"). A revised set of codes (ICD-10) is increasingly being used (6, 7), and comparisons of the two systems are listed in Table 2.

Table 2. International National Classification of Disease Codes Applicable to Child Abuse (6, 7)

ICD-9	ICD-10
995.50 Child abuse, unspecified	T74.92 Unspecified child maltreatment
995.51 Child emotional/psychological abuse	T74.32 Child psychological abuse
995.52 Child neglect (nutritional)	T74.02 Child neglect or abandonment
995.53 Child sexual abuse	T74.22 Child sexual abuse
995.54 Child physical abuse	T74.12 Child physical abuse
995.55 Shaken infant syndrome	T74.4 Shaken infant syndrome

Extent of the problem

The victimization of children through maltreatment remains an all-too-common occurrence. In the United States, 1-2% of children are confirmed victims of abuse or neglect each year, while young children and infants have the highest rates. More than one-third (37.4%) of all US children will experience a CPS investigation by age 18 years (8). Maltreated children suffer from a variety of behavior problems and mental disorders in addition to physical injuries (9, 10). The Adverse Childhood Experiences study has noted the powerful relationship between adverse childhood experiences and several conditions of adulthood, including risk of suicide, alcoholism, depression, illicit drug use, and other lifestyle changes (11, 12).

While the exact pathways are still being explored, childhood abuse is thought to affect adult physical and mental health by putting people at risk for depression, trauma and stress-related disorders, difficulties in relationships, destructive behaviors, and negative beliefs as well as attitudes towards others. Most children will experience some type of trauma during childhood, and many children suffer from significant adversities. Research in genetics, neuroscience, and epidemiology all provide evidence that these experiences have effects at the molecular, cellular, and organ level, with consequences on physical, emotional, developmental, and behavioral health across the life span. Trauma-informed care translates that science can inform and improve pediatric care and outcomes. In order to practically address trauma and promote resilience, pediatric clinicians need tools to assess childhood trauma and adversity experiences as well as practical guidance, resources, and interventions. The American Academy of Pediatrics (AAP) has recently offered advice for rendering trauma-informed care across varied medical settings (13).

Two large administrative sources provide information about the US annual incidence of child maltreatment; these are the National Child Abuse and Neglect Data System (NCANDS) and the National Incidence Studies of Child Abuse and Neglect (NIS). NCANDS contains aggregate and case-level data on child abuse reports received by state Child Protective Service (CPS) agencies, and almost all US states and territories provide information annually about the outcomes of child abuse reports, types of maltreatment, child and family factors and services being provided (14). National estimates of the overall numbers of victims (substantiated or indicated CPS reports) as well as victims identified with physical and sexual abuse show decline over the 20+ years of nationally collected data in NCANDS (see Figure 1) following similar trends in other national crime statistics (15).

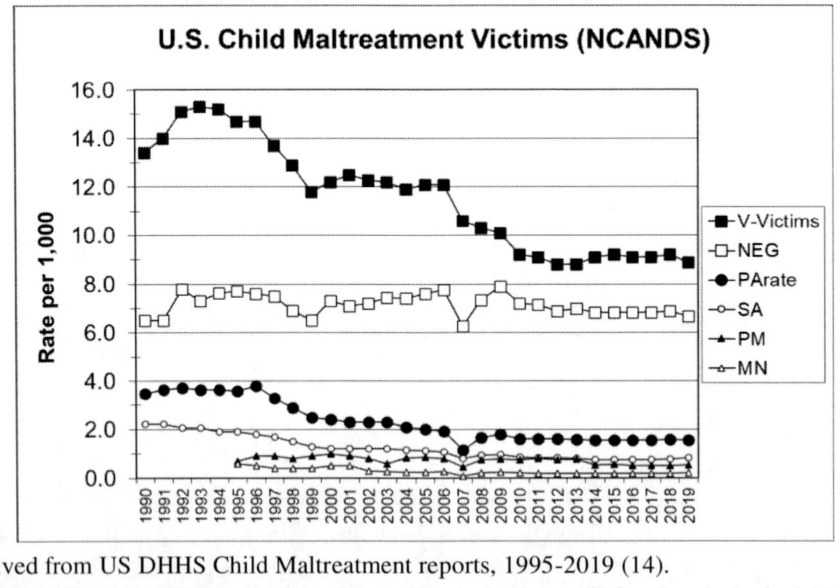

Note. Derived from US DHHS Child Maltreatment reports, 1995-2019 (14).

MN = Medical Neglect; NEG = Neglect; PA = Physical Abuse; PM = Psychological Maltreatment; SA = Sexual Abuse.

Figure 1. U.S. child maltreatment victims, rates per 1,000, 1990-2019.

The most recent year available for NCANDS includes 709,748 confirmed reports of child abuse and neglect (14). When broken down by age and major type of child maltreatment, it is apparent that most CM occurs in very young children, and most CM is neglect (see Figure 2). Neglect was the most frequent type of CM confirmed in all age groups. This pattern continues with older children, but the number falls dramatically. For sexual abuse, more older children are affected, peaking in the 10–14-year age group. Medical neglect, in contrast, affects mostly children younger than five years. Young children are the highest proportion for all CM types, except sexual abuse. Although the focus of concern about maltreatment is usually the younger child, statistics show that 30 to 50% of all reported cases involve adolescents.

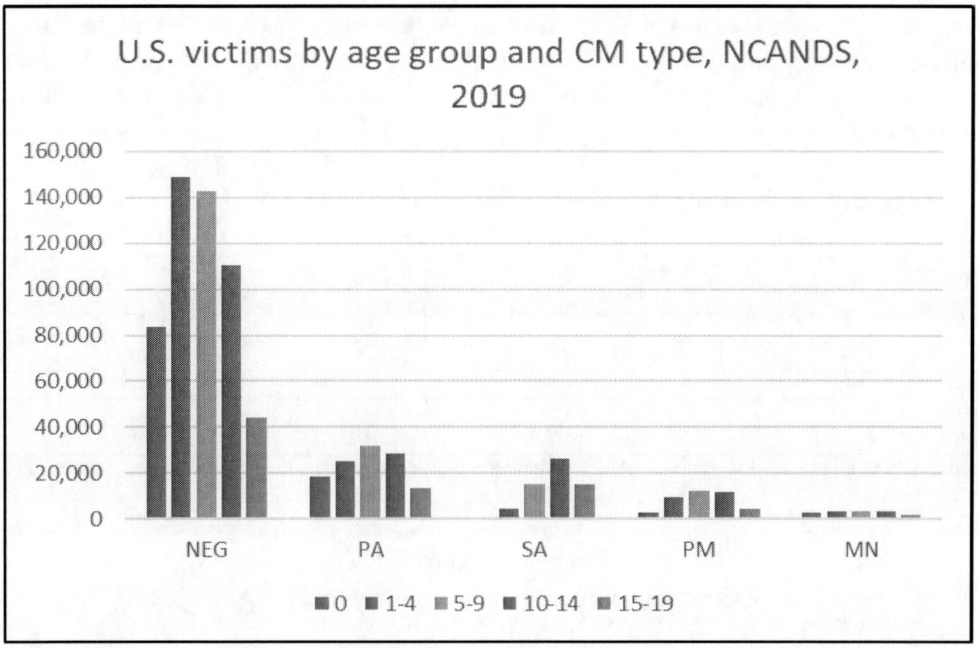

MN = Medical Neglect; NEG = Neglect; PA = Physical Abuse; PM = Psychological Maltreatment; SA = Sexual Abuse. Derived from (111).

Figure 2. U.S. victims by age group and maltreatment type, NCANDS, 2019.

In contrast, NIS samples sentinel counties to identify under two standards: the harm standard (relatively stringent in that it generally requires that an act or omission result in demonstrable harm in order to be classified as abuse or neglect) and the endangerment standard (which allows children who were not yet harmed by maltreatment to be counted if the CM was confirmed by CPS or identified as endangerment by professionals outside CPS, either by their parents or other adults) (16). The Fourth National Incidence Study of Child Abuse and Neglect (NIS–4) also shows an overall decrease in the incidence of maltreatment since the NIS–3, as well as decreases in some specific maltreatment categories and increases in others. Using the stringent Harm Standard definition, more than 1.25 million children (an estimated 1,256,600 children) experienced maltreatment during the NIS–4 study year (2005–2006). A large percentage (44%) or an estimated total of 553,300 were abused, and most of these abused children experienced physical abuse (58%).

Screening for depression and anxiety, with tools such as the PHQ-9 adapted for adolescents, has found that over 25% of high school students reported experiencing unwanted sexual contact; in clinical populations, the rates are even higher (17). A prospective study demonstrated that child maltreatment is an independent predictor of later adolescent pregnancies, with birth rates highest for sexually abused and neglected females when compared to a matched cohort (18). Repeated sexual contact and pregnancy places teenagers at increased risk for several health harms. Repeated sexual contact has been associated with younger ages of sexual initiation, higher rates of depression, anxiety, substance abuse and delinquency. When the frequency of CM types for each age group is stratified by the number of CM types confirmed in a report, the most cases are found in children ages 5-9 years, followed by 1-4 years and 10-14 years (see Table 3). Those with 2 or more types exceed 10% of the total. Using confirmed reports as a guideline suggests that there are, at a minimum, more than 600,000 children in all age groups who should be screened for behavioral and emotional problems each year in the US (14).

Table 3. Frequency of CM types* by age group in United States, NCANDS, 2019

Age Group	Single	2 types	3 or more
0	93,184	7,221	419
1-4 y	158,085	14,880	1,202
5-9 y	164,509	18,376	1,537
10-14 y	138,197	18,535	1,813
15-19 y	59,290	8,834	819
TOTAL	613,265	67,846	5,790

*Confirmed CM types included: physical abuse, sexual abuse, psychological maltreatment, neglect and medical neglect; derived from (111).

Table 4. Children with behavior problems in NCANDS, 2019, by age group and confirmed maltreatment type, NCANDS, 2019

Age Group	PA	SA	PM	MN	N	2 types	3 +	Total***
Total*	4207	2097	1131	614	15885	2468	266	34981
%**	5.35	4.53	5.27	7.95	5.15	6.94	7.30	10.48
0-1 years	73	0	17	23	1345	51	5	1398
%	0.53	0.00	1.33	1.56	2.42	1.18	1.85	2.00
1-4 y	365	68	72	86	2088	228	26	2395
%	2.12	1.99	1.62	4.36	2.30	2.75	3.21	2.12
5-9 y	1226	412	277	152	4204	673	73	5452
%	6.0%	3.59	4.30	8.52	5.23	7.24	7.30	47.81
10-14 y	1579	894	506	215	5166	937	107	21139
%	8.6%	4.52	7.67	13.30	8.75%	10.17	9.83	21.74
15-19 y	964	723	259	138	3082	579	55	4597
%	10.81	6.41	9.68	15.70	13.58	12.97	11.58	10.86

Note. Not all states and territories include behavior problems (N = 333,637); derived from (111).
PA = physical abuse; SA = sexual abuse; PM = psychological maltreatment; MN = medical neglect; N = neglect.
*number of children in age group with behavior problems for each maltreatment type.
**percent of children in age group with behavior problems for each maltreatment type.
***total unduplicated cases.

NCANDS reports two variables recorded by child protective services agencies that can inform this review. "Behavior problem-child" is defined as behaviors in the school and/or the community that adversely affects socialization, learning, growth, and moral development. These may include adjudicated or non-adjudicated behavior problems, including a child's running away from home or other placement. Not all states reported this variable, and those that did contributed 47% of the confirmed reports in NCANDS 2019 (14). Cases with confirmed neglect associated with behavior problems almost equal all other CM types combined, with the sum of cases with 2 or more CM types approaches 8% of the total (see Table 4). Peaks are noted among 5-9y and 10-14y are groups. Behavior problems are noted in 5-10% of cases overall, but are much higher (>10%) among 10–15-year-olds and among children with medical neglect, physical abuse and psychological maltreatment.

Table 5. Children with emotional problems in NCANDS, 2019, by age group and confirmed maltreatment type

Age Group	PA	SA	PM	MN	N	2 types	3+	Total***
Total*	3147	2144	1515	451	9588	2032	298	14612
%**	6.68	5.65	8.88	8.07	4.01	7.48	13.26	4.34
0-1 y	42	0	0	5	85	13	0	128
%	0.39	0.00	0.00	0.43	0.20	0.40	0.00	0.24
1-4 y	190	44	69	31	878	138	11	1102
%	1.51	1.54	2.09	2.36	1.25	2.24	2.84	1.28
5-9 y	876	330	326	104	2626	520	69	3690
%	5.84	3.49	6.52	8.29	4.19	7.49	12.02	4.20
10-14	1302	974	740	200	3719	879	145	5868
%	90.29	5.98	13.27	16.45	8.06	12.13	18.90	7.65
15-19 y	737	796	380	111	2280	482	73	3824
%	10.19	8.80	16.13	17.10	12.69	13.43	19.26	11.28

Note: Not all states and territories include emotional problems (N = 337,779); derived from (111).
PA = physical abuse; SA = sexual abuse; PM = psychological maltreatment; MN = medical neglect; N = neglect.
*number of children in age group with emotional problems for each maltreatment type.
**percent of children in age group with emotional problems for each maltreatment type.
***total unduplicated cases.

"Emotional disturbance-child" is defined as a clinically diagnosed condition exhibiting one or more of the following characteristics over a long period of time and to a marked degree: an inability to build or maintain satisfactory interpersonal relationships; inappropriate types of behavior or feelings under normal circumstances; a general pervasive mood of unhappiness or depression; or a tendency to develop physical symptoms or fears associated with personal problems. The term includes schizophrenia and autism. The diagnosis is based on the 2013 "Diagnostic and statistical manual of mental disorders, 5th edition (DSM-5)" (19). Not all states reported this variable, and those that did contributed 48% of the confirmed reports in NCANDS 2019. Even with the under-ascertainment using confirmed cases, there are more than 35,000 children in the US with behavior problems and more than 14,000 children with emotional problems identified by CPS (see Tables 4-5). Most are in the 5-9- and 10-14-years age groups with confirmed neglect or physical abuse. Fewer are identified with two or more types of confirmed CM in their report, but these numbers are similar to the number of children with sexual abuse. The frequencies identified in NCANDS should serve as a baseline national estimate for the number of children needing diagnosis and treatment for behavioral and emotional problems related to CM.

Table 6. Multivariable logistic regression models* ($p < 0.01$) for behavior and emotional problems

	Behavior Problems		Emotional Problems	
Factor**	**OR**	**95%CI**	**OR**	**95%CI**
5-9y	5.725	4.900, 6.689	4.531	3.882, 5.289
10-14y	10.649	9.161, 12.379	9.154	7.888, 10.623
15-19y	10.013	15.388, 21.086	11.541	9.839, 13.537
Female child	1.739	1.604, 1.885	2.174	1.802, 2.622
Native American	2.889	2.391, 3.491	1.440	1.307, 1.587
White	1.468	1.332, 1.619	0.598	0.541, 0.660
Hispanic	0.815	0.743, 0.894	NS	--
Military	0.440	0.204, 0.950	NS	--
Physical Abuse	0.171	0.123, 0.238	0.372	0.323, 0.430
Sexual Abuse	0.130	0.093, 0.182	0.510	0.442, 0.588
Medical Neglect	0.093	0.061, 0.142	0.437	0.334, 0.572
Neglect	0.073	0.053, 0.102	0.282	0.249, 0.320
Psychologic Maltreatment	0.091	0.064, 0.129	NS	--
2 types	10.405	7.345, 14.742	2.802	2.432, 3.228
3+types	101.682	49.021, 210.915	9.295	6.762, 12.777
Family violence	0.834	0.747, 0.931	NS	--
Money problems	2.628	2.371, 2.913	1.211	1.085, 1.352
Public assistance	1.365	1.237, 1.506	2.135	1.952, 2.335
Child Alcohol	1.695	1.266, 2.269	NS	--
Child Drug	3.770	3.217, 4.419	2.065	1.751, 2.435
Child Behavior	NS	--	9.680	8.797, 10.653
Child Emotional	11.183	10.020, 12.482	NS	--
Child Learning	6.717	5.862, 7.697	2.728	2.362, 3.149
Child Medical	2.885	2.458, 3.387	2.341	2.030, 2.698
Child Visual	NS	--	2.684	2.042, 3.528
Family Drug	0.560	0.497, 0.632	0.667	0.596, 0.748
Family Emotional	1.369	1.168, 1.604	5.674	5.063, 6.359
Family Learning	1.625	1.261, 2.094	0.479	0.357, 0.643
Family Medical	1.344	1.111, 1.626	1.332	1.113, 1.595
Fam Retardation	0.303	0.175, 0.522	1.772	1.269, 2.476
Family Visual	1.928	1.230, 3.022	NS	--
Service referrals	2.764	2.514, 3.040	2.781	2.522, 3.067

Note: Behavior Problems: N = 163,105; Emotional Problems: N = 189,627; derived from (111).
OR = odds ratio; 95%CI = 95% confidence interval.
*Additional variables removed by stepwise backward regressions: Infant age, age 1-4y, Black race, Pacific Island race, public housing, child learning problem, child retardation, child physical problems, family alcohol problems, family physical problems.
**All factors in model $p<0.01$ except where noted (NS = not significant, [>0.01]).

When child and family factors are included in regression models, several are together significantly associated with CPS findings of behavior and emotional problems (see Table 6). Child age group is increasingly associated with these issues, with increasing odds ratios as children age. Teens were 10-12 times more likely to have these problems. Specific types of abuse had odd ratios less than 1, with multiple types ranging from 10.4 and 2.8 for 2 types (behavior and emotional problems respectively) to >100 and 9.3 for 3 or more. This highlights that fact that, while smaller in number, children with multiple forms of CM have much greater risk. Behavioral and emotional problems also interacted and had increased risk for each other. Other factors associated with elevated risk are child drug exposure, family emotional problems, and the need for service referrals.

Behavioral issues for young children

Maltreated children present with significantly more internalizing as well as externalizing problems than do non-maltreated children and have greater risk for developing co-morbid medical and/or psychiatric conditions that may further derail normal development (20-22). Clinical presentations may vary regardless of the identified trauma. Common emotional symptoms include fear, sadness, anger, and/or extreme difficulties in emotion regulation (23). Young children, who may have more difficulty verbalizing their feelings as compared to older children, may present with notable behavioral difficulties, such as oppositional and/or defiant behavior, aggression, separation anxiety, and/or sexualized behavior (24). In addition, children may exhibit behavioral avoidance, a hallmark symptom of PTSD (23).

For instance, a child who witnessed his mother being robbed at a train station may refuse to enter that train station or take that train altogether. Over time, these reminders can generalize and lead to secondary problems (i.e., the child may refuse to take any train, and as a result may miss out on previously enjoyed activities or opportunities for socialization with peers). In turn, this avoidance can lead to an increase in emotional symptoms (i.e., feelings of sadness, loneliness, and isolation) and negatively impact the child's functioning. In addition, the child's refusal to take the train or enter the train station, particularly when accompanied by tantrum behavior, may be conceptualized as oppositional or defiant behavior, when it would be better understood as a trauma reaction. Parents, who may be unaware of trauma triggers or common childhood responses to trauma, may respond negatively to their child's behavior, which may contribute to the child's ongoing difficulties.

Identifying mental health issues, and specifically posttraumatic stress disorder (PTSD), in maltreated children under the age of six years is particularly difficult given their limited abilities to report on their psychological symptoms (25-27). The diagnostic criteria for PTSD in the most recent DSM (19) identifies four categories of posttraumatic stress symptoms: 1) intrusion symptoms, 2) avoidance symptoms, 3) negative alterations in thoughts and feelings that developed or worsened following the trauma, and 4) arousal and reactivity trauma-related alterations; many of these require language or highly attuned parent report. In addition, some research indicates that very young children may experience additional trauma symptoms that are not captured by the current DSM criteria, such as constriction of play, regression to earlier functioning, aggression, separation anxiety, and development of new fears (27). A thorough assessment of the child and their behavior is warranted following trauma exposure.

More than two-thirds of children report experiencing a trauma before age 16 years (28). Short-term distress following trauma exposure is common, and it is important to note that the majority of children return to their prior levels of functioning. Current estimates suggest that 3% to 15% of girls and 1% to 6% of boys who are exposed to trauma will develop PTSD (10). Factors that may increase risk for PTSD include female gender, previous trauma exposure or multiple traumas, prior psychiatric history and especially past history of anxiety, family adversity or parent psychopathology, as well as low social support. When working with youth who have experienced a trauma, it is important to conduct a thorough evaluation of symptoms and history to better understand their clinical needs.

Behavioral issues for adolescents

Child maltreatment is given as a comorbid factor in a spectrum of adolescent problems, such as substance abuse, truancy, runaways and psychiatric disorders (29, 30). According to findings from a longitudinal project examining the effects of maltreatment in adolescents, adolescents that experience CM were more likely to meet the clinical criteria for at least one mental health problem (e.g., depression, anxiety, externalizing problems, PTSD, and psychological impairment) than were their non-maltreated peers (31, 32).

Adolescents who experience maltreatment are also more likely to engage in sexual risk behaviors. Maltreated adolescent males have reported significantly younger age at first consensual intercourse and higher number of lifetime sexual partners, and were more likely to report 'one-night stands' in comparison to other youth. Additionally, females with sexual abuse history were at high risk of having sex under the influence of alcohol or drugs, and experienced teen pregnancy more than non-maltreated females (31). Most adolescent rape and sexual assault is perpetrated by an acquaintance or relative of the adolescent, with younger adolescents having assailants more likely from the extended family. Increased rates of sexual assault are seen in adolescents with disabilities, alcohol use and other family dysfunction (33). Males are less likely to report sexual assault, less likely to receive treatment, and more likely to become perpetrators themselves after being victimized than were female adolescents (34).

There has been considerable growth in treatments available for victims of child abuse and neglect, but adolescents face the additional burdens of developing risk-taking behaviors or paraphilias, or becoming perpetrators as the result of their victimization, if not appropriately treated (17, 34). Sexual abuse in particular appears to be a strong risk factor for subsequent perpetration, influencing adolescents and young adults to develop an orientation that is abusive to other children (35). An adolescent's exposure to a pervasive atmosphere of violence in the home is a key risk factor of future perpetration and suggests the need to address the specific behaviors and risks in the child as well as the overall environment.

There is a proper focus on the need to confront offending behavior while taking into account the developing cognitive and social abilities of the adolescent. Sex offenders report more histories of maltreatment, both physical and sexual, compared to generally conduct-disordered young people. Thus, any treatments must consider the adolescent's victimization as well as their developing patterns of perpetration and their environment. When young people are identified as being responsible for committing abusive acts against others, it is essential to assess and intervene in their own victimization experiences to prevent post-traumatic stress and other emotional effects (35). Clinicians need to be sensitive to the psychological needs of the adolescent and provide initial psychological support after sexual assault while making referrals to appropriate mental health professionals as well as community resources for longer-term assessment and counseling (33).

Issues related to the COVID-19 pandemic

The SARS-CoV-2 coronavirus (COVID-19) pandemic has radically changed the lives of individuals around the globe. Aside from the health concerns related to infection, disease, and death, the pandemic has brought stay-at-home orders, school closures, and unemployment that abruptly and significantly upheaved the daily lives of youth and their families. These challenges have increased parental stress and burnout, and subsequently increased the risk of family violence, including domestic violence as well as child abuse and maltreatment (36, 37).

A study examining patterns of parent stress in the US in 2020 has shown that parents experienced a substantial increase in stress in the spring of 2020 and had not yet returned to pre-COVID-19 levels by fall of 2020 (38). The most common stressor was a change in children's daily structure and routines that placed an increased demand on parental time and resources. A mismatch between the demands of parenting and the resources available for parents to meet those demands defines parental burnout (36), which is a key factor that has been linked to child abuse as well as neglect.

Although rates of reported child abuse appear to be declining during the pandemic as of this writing, this is likely due to limited contact with mandated reporters. Research on prior disasters such as 2017's Hurricane Harvey demonstrated that families already experiencing family violence pre-disaster had higher rates of both domestic violence and child abuse during and after the natural disaster (39). In addition, preliminary data from a level I pediatric trauma center in Maryland indicated an increase in the proportion of traumatic injuries caused by physical child abuse during the COVID-19 pandemic (40). While more severe forms of child maltreatment may be caught, it is likely the case that the majority of cases are going undetected, and a surge of newly diagnosed victims will emerge once social distancing measures are relaxed (37).

Evaluation

Several health effects of child maltreatment have been identified. While there is considerable overlap, specific health effects and injuries are often related to a major subtype of child abuse, and the diagnostic evaluation varies with the type of child maltreatment as well as the physical injuries of concern.

Medical evaluation (Medical history, examination and diagnosis)

At a minimum, the clinician caring for children should be able to recognize and report potential child maltreatment, using standard methods for obtaining history, physical examination and selected laboratory and imaging tests. This clinician must also be cognizant that multiple forms of maltreatment may co-exist, understand the importance of certain risk factors, assist in choosing the appropriate location as well as timing of evaluation, and appropriately refer children and families to specialized medical and social services. In health care, a clinical assessment of child victimization begins with a medical encounter that usually follows information-gathering, physical assessment, testing, and clinical diagnosis followed by treatment and referral. It is important to realize that children being evaluated may have experienced significant trauma in their lives and would benefit from trauma informed care (TIC) that includes specific trauma assessments and clinical approaches to minimize any additional trauma from the evaluation (13).

TIC is defined by the National Child Traumatic Stress Network as medical care in which all parties involved assess, recognize, and respond to the effects of traumatic stress on children, caregivers, and health care providers (13). This includes attention to secondary traumatic stress, the emotional strain that results when an individual hears about the first-hand trauma experiences of another. In the clinical setting, TIC includes the prevention, identification, and assessment of trauma, response to trauma, and recovery from trauma as a focus of all services. Much of the information needed to integrate TIC into practice may be obtained as part of the routine health evaluation. Social, developmental, and medical history are all opportunities to identify risks, stressors, and strengths.

The health history provides an opportunity to assess child and family resilience factors, social connectedness, parenting attitudes, and skills. The review of systems allows the medical provider to collect symptoms of trauma that may not have been identified in the chief complaint but that can offer valuable insight into the current impact of trauma on the patient. Symptoms may be functional, neurodevelopmental, or related to immune function. It is important to obtain as much of this information as possible before proceeding with the evaluation. Collecting this data is often done best by members of the team with expertise in medicine, social work, psychology and forensic interviewing, as well as those preparing the child for physical examination.

Medical diagnosis of child abuse and neglect follows commonly accepted practices for other medical diagnoses. Pediatricians should consult current clinical procedural terminology for coding for encounters and "International classification of disease" codes for diagnosis as in **table 2**. Medical history, a cornerstone of medical diagnosis, plays the most important part in the diagnosis of child abuse and neglect. It is the history, taken with the physical examination and lab and imaging studies, that offers a sound basis for diagnosis and treatment recommendations for the child and family. Inquiring and recording the specific complaints and disclosures of maltreatment by the child and parent, if any, in their own words is vitally important to the ultimate protection of the child. Behavioral and emotional issues are equally important in this assessment. Certain non-specific behaviors, developmental delays, and history of trauma should be recorded as part of the medical history; this history aids in assessing harm and planning for appropriate treatment (5). The practitioner then arrives at an assessment or diagnosis, usually utilizing schema of diagnostic categories. Documentation must be objective, with appropriate use of psychological screening, testing and mental health referrals as part of the comprehensive evaluation.

Skin lesions in physical abuse

The most common visible injuries from physical abuse affect the skin by bruising or burning. Recognition and documentation require complete undressing of the child and comprehensive physical examination that may be emotionally traumatic. Skin lesions should be described by location, size, color, depth, and integrity of the epidermis and may be documented using notes, hand-drawn diagrams or photographs. If photographs are taken, the clinician should also contemporaneously document skin injuries that are identified (41). Additionally, specific statements by the family and child should also be copied verbatim in the medical record for potential use later in the legal system.

In the case of bruising, standard coagulation tests should be ordered to objectively assess platelet count and function as well as coagulation (41). Any skin lesion beyond temporary reddening should be considered as potential physical abuse when 1) the injury is inflicted and nonaccidental, 2) the pattern of injury fits biomechanical models of abusive trauma, 3) the pattern corresponds to infliction with an instrument that would not occur through play or in the environment, 4) the history provided is not in keeping with the child's development, or 5) the history does not explain the injury.

The aging of bruises in children has received considerable attention and current guidelines are severely limited in their ability to precisely time when an injury occurred. Pattern, depth (degree), and healing helps in determining their specificity for maltreatment. Developmental and other considerations need to be entertained as there are a host of potential confounders or 'mimics' which need to be reviewed when coming to a diagnosis. The distribution of lesions can be a critical factor in determining if a child has been abused. Certain sites are highly correlated with abuse, such as buttocks, the lower back, the posterior aspects of the extremities and the ears (42). Bruising at other sites, such as the bony prominences of the forehead, the elbows and lower legs, are consistent with the normal childhood trauma seen in mobile children. Sugar, Taylor & Feldman noted "those who don't cruise, rarely bruise," signaling we should be concerned when non-walking infants or motor delayed children have bruising (43). Inflicted bruising may have clear patterns or may be non-specific. Bruises of the torso, ears or neck in a child under 4 years are considered "sentinel" injuries and markers for children with increased risk for more serious injury or later death (44).

When an object is used, the pattern of the injury may clearly show the outline of the object. Another form of patterned bruising comes from biting. A careful inspection and measurement of the lesion can determine if a bite is human or animal, adult or child, or self-inflicted. Since the most common skin manifestation of physical abuse is multiple bruises in different stages of healing, it is imperative to use a diagram and appropriate imaging to document the color, distribution and pattern of these injuries.

A burn is the destruction of skin and underlying tissue caused by the application of a physical agent. These agents may be chemicals, heat, cold, or electrical in nature. Since the spectrum of burns can range from a simple isolated injury to the involvement of major portions of the child's body, the clinician should assess the type of agent, the distribution and extent of the burn, and the history given of how the burn occurred (45). Many burns in childhood are accidental but are also the result of poor judgment or the failure of the caretaker to provide adequate supervision. Here, as in other forms of maltreatment, the developmental age and the size of the child are very important. Inflicted burns often have very specific patterns such as those seen with immersion or dunking. Burns may result from splash, immersion, or contact with a heated instrument or utensil, a flame, a chemical/caustic agent or an electrical source.

Accidental burns/scalds commonly involve hot liquids in contact with a child's face, neck, and upper chest. If a child pulls down a cup of hot water, this will produce a different pattern than if he had pulled down a cup of thick liquid. The action may be modified by the height from which the hot liquid fell, the vehicle that contained the hot substance, and the child's size. Immersion burns present with distinctive patterns that result from placing the child in hot water. The patterns include stocking/glove burns that are symmetrical burns of the extremities.

Forced immersion of the child in a tub can produce a burn pattern with well-demarcated lesions and little or no evidence of splash. Contact burns can present with identifiable object patterns such as an iron or a cigarette lighter. A child can easily have contact with an iron left on the floor or by pulling the cord. Other sources of contact burns are room heaters, hair curling irons, electric cooking utensils, and radiators which can each produce distinctive lesions. Lit cigarettes can produce lesions that can be difficult to distinguish from chicken pox or impetigo given the similarity of the size and distribution.

Acute fractures may be clinically apparent as bruising or soft tissue swelling over a fracture site, a deformity of the involved limb, or as a decrease in movement with or without external bruising. Infants may present with irritability and/or not using an affected limb. Healing fractures may be identified as palpable lesions consistent with callus formation, especially over the ribs. The absence of swelling or bruises near a fracture site is not uncommon in fractures of the extremities and ribs. There is no fracture type that is pathognomonic for abuse, and all fracture types can potentially result from inflicted injury.

The diagnosis of inflicted fracture must be made through careful correlation of the history provided by the caregiver with the child's developmental level and physical as well as radiographic findings. Classic metaphyseal lesions, rib fractures (particularly posteriorly), scapular fractures, vertebral spinous process fractures, and sternal fractures all have a high specificity for abuse (46). Further assessment for fractures requires appropriate skeletal imaging as outlined by the American College of Radiology and the American Academy of Pediatrics Section on Radiology (47-51).

Sexual abuse

The prime injury of sexual abuse is emotional. While most young children with proven sexual abuse have few physical injuries, patterns of anogenital injury and sexually transmitted diseases have been identified (17). Assessing sexual abuse requires detailed knowledge of anogenital anatomy and sexually transmitted infections in children, both of which have important differences from adults; also, specialized skills and examination techniques have had to be developed (5). It has become apparent that most physicians have little knowledge about prepubertal genital anatomy and cannot identify key landmarks when abusive injury occurs.

When confronted with concerns of potential sexual abuse, the clinician should obtain key elements of the history (such as type, frequency and timing of contact) and physically assess the child for gross injuries or infection. Definitive assessment and treatment are increasingly handled by referral to clinicians with specialized experience in testing, interpretation, and documentation of anogenital findings. Procedures such as colposcopy and videocolposcopy offer a way to better document and record trauma, to allow the child to be more relaxed as well as cooperative during examination, and to begin the process of emotional healing. Early work suggested that these procedures are not emotionally traumatic and are well-tolerated (52).

It is beyond the scope of this review to detail all of the findings associated with sexual abuse, and research suggests that only limited findings have high specificity, such as lacerations and transections of the hymen and bruising or other injury to the anus as well as genitals (5, 17). Several findings which were once thought to indicate trauma are now considered non-specific, accidentally acquired, or congenital variations. This suggests that the appropriate physical evaluation should not be rushed and should be done at a place and time with the most expert clinicians available; this should be followed unless there are concerns about acute pain, significant physical injury, sexually transmitted infection transmission or collection of forensic trace evidence. These will need to be addressed, prevented if possible, and treated before long term emotional effects can be addressed. Follow-up examinations will be vital for evaluating certain lesions, determining the course of healing, assessing treatment efficacy, and making mental health referrals.

Psychological maltreatment

Psychological maltreatment (PM) is commonly associated with other forms of abuse but may also occur in isolation in a small number of cases. By definition, PM is a repeated pattern of interaction between a parent and child that harms the child's emotional well-being (53). Spurning, belittling, degrading, ridiculing, or shaming a child is considered harming a child's self-worth. Terrorizing and otherwise exploiting the child increases the harm further. The shear denial of emotional closeness leads to physical and developmental delays in young children as well as failure to thrive in infants. Rejection, isolation, and inconsistent parenting styles lead children to feel insecure in their home and relationships. PM occurs when a child witnesses violence in the home, including spousal violence, intimate partner violence (IPV), community violence, or even violence on television or movies. PM is seldom the focus of CPS investigation and has increasingly been coupled with other forms of CM in CPS reports (54, 55).

PM is, however, associated with a variety of negative and lasting effects. Shaffer et al. suggested that the effects of PM (also called emotional maltreatment) are disabling and enduring, with adjustment outcomes varying according to the type of psychological maltreatment (i.e., emotional abuse, emotional neglect), gender, and other factors (56). PM is strongly linked to depression and problems with relationships as well as attachment; also, it predicts more rapid onset of major and minor mental illness in a dose-dependent manner (57-60). PM and recurrent PM in childhood and adolescence represent important risk factors for increased victimization; in addition, children with high levels of co-occurring internalizing and externalizing symptoms are particularly likely to experience increased exposure to peer victimization, maltreatment, and sexual victimization, thereby escalating physical and mental harm (61, 62). Psychological neglect has been significantly associated with behavior problems and poor cognitive development, even while controlling for poverty and services put in place (63, 64).

The effects of psychological maltreatment may be very difficult to recognize in the medical office. Sometimes the poor parent-child relationship is seen and the verbal stigmata of PM exposed, but often there are little or no physical findings demonstrating the emotional harm, other than weight loss or excessive weight gain. The quiet, depressed child is not often identified as a victim of neglect as readily as is the hyperactive, aggressive child (65). The child's clinician needs to evaluate the harm or potential harm to the child's mental health, while realizing that it may take several years for such harm to become apparent, and the effects are often confounded with exposure to other violence.

Behavioral changes in the child are early but non-specific events, and assessment should include multiple domains, including function at home, school and at play. The psychological effects are further modified by the intensity, type, frequency, and severity of exposure as well as the developmental stage and resiliency of the child (53, 63). One study noted that fewer than 25% of families received counseling, mental health or other services after PM; also, the study noted that service referrals varied significantly based on family race, ethnicity, poverty and co-occurring child maltreatment (61). When offered, counseling was associated with a 54% reduction in PM recurrence, and other services were not associated with significant reductions (62).

Physical and medical care neglect

Child neglect is the most common form of child maltreatment, affecting 50% or more of children reported annually to child protective services (14). Ray Helfer (1930-1992) reminded pediatricians about the significant harms caused by the 'litany of smoldering neglect' and the de-emphasis of neglect that has caused mandated reporters to have second thoughts about reporting neglect because little, if anything, could supposedly be done by overwhelmed, understaffed child protective services agencies (66). Neglect is the omission or lack of a minimal level of care by the parents or caretakers that results in actual or potential harm to the child. Neglect is often associated with poverty, but poor families are not necessarily neglectful (67).

Many subtypes of neglect often occur concurrently, but our understanding of its outcome is often aided by identifying subtypes that can direct potential interventions (68). Physical neglect is the lack of food, clothing or shelter; emotional neglect is a form of psychological maltreatment, and educational neglect refers to the lack of proper educational resources. The morbidity and mortality associated with neglect are substantial (69). Physical conditions caused by neglect include injuries, ingestions, inadequately treated illnesses, dental problems, malnutrition, and neurological as well as developmental deficits. Manifestations in neglectful families include noncompliance or non-adherence to medical recommendations, delay or failure in seeking appropriate health care, hunger, failure to thrive and unmanaged morbid obesity, poor hygiene and physical as well as medical conditions contributing to poor cognitive and educational achievement (70).

Poor supervision is less defined but has been broken down into broad categories, consisting of not watching the child closely enough, inadequate substitute childcare, failure to protect from third parties, knowingly allowing the child to participate in harmful activities, and driving recklessly or while intoxicated. A comprehensive response requires that the pediatrician address the actual or potential harms that have occurred to the child and to make appropriate referrals to community services to address a variety of social as well as economic issues in the family (71).

Management of neglect first centers on properly identifying the sources contributing to neglect. For example, while malnutrition is medically addressed through proper provision of fluids, calories, and protein as dictated by commonly accepted parameters, the child's clinician must also assess the lack of appropriate food, the provision of that food to the child, and the explanation, if any, as to why it was not provided. Important screening questions that can elicit further avenues of intervention include inquiring about the family's access to food, their access to appropriate medical as well as dental services and medicines, substance abuse during and after pregnancy, homelessness, housing and environmental safety, depression, domestic violence, and degree of supervision (70). Multiple missed medical appointments, unreasonable delay in seeking medical treatment, abandonment, illnesses that could be prevented by routine medical care, and inadequate care have been identified as potential minimal criteria for a neglect report.

The AAP has offered a working definition with five required standards for diagnosing medical neglect: 1) a child is harmed or is at risk of harm because of lack of health care; 2) the recommended health care offers significant net benefit to the child; 3) the anticipated benefit of the treatment is significantly greater than morbidity, so that reasonable caregivers would choose treatment over non-treatment; 4) it can be demonstrated that access to health care is available and not used; and 5) the caregiver understands the medical advice given (71).

Failure to thrive associated with malnutrition due to neglect has historically been grouped into organic, non-organic (NOFTT), and mixed varieties (72). In addition to the short-term and long-term physical effects, the effects on emotional development and bonding are protean.

While a full discussion of the evaluation of NOFTT is beyond the scope of this discussion, it is important to emphasize that the findings on a comprehensive history and physical examination should guide management as well as initial laboratory testing. In the face of normal basic metabolic measurements, a careful observation of parental feeding practices and the child's intake and output is often illuminating. Height and weight need to be precisely measured over multiple visits and compared to currently accepted norms, some of which are modified by genetics, prematurity or other medical conditions. With acceptable weight gain under direct observation and lack of significant medical cause for malnutrition, a presumptive diagnosis of NOFTT can be made and community resources activated.

Mental health screening and evaluation

The need for a thorough and accurate assessment of mental health symptoms and behaviors is critical for the identification as well as implementation of appropriate therapeutic interventions. While diagnostic evaluations are typically completed by trained mental health professionals, the objective of this section is to provide clinicians with tools to obtain an initial snapshot of symptoms that can then inform treatment referrals.

The primary challenge in screening young children, particularly those under the age of 7y, is their limited capacity to adequately self-report on the severity, intensity, and duration of their symptoms and subsequent functional impairment (27, 73). As a result, parent/caregiver report is often the primary source of information. When possible, collateral contact is encouraged, since teachers and extended family members can provide a glimpse into how the child functions in different settings. In addition, behavioral observations during medical visits should be considered.

Given the high rates of suicide among youth, and the significant risk factor that child abuse as well as maltreatment poses in increasing a child's risk for suicide, it is imperative for clinicians to conduct suicide screenings even for young children as part of their evaluations (74). A brief screening tool, like the Patient Health Questionnaire (PHQ-9), which has been adapted for adolescents and most recently for younger children, can increase the chances of identifying youth at-risk and establishing safety.

PTSD assessment measures for pre-school aged children

Aside from gathering information via an informal interview, standardized assessment measures should be used to aid with diagnosis, provide a baseline measure of their symptomatology, and serve as a tool to track symptom progression. However, assessment measures evaluating PTSD symptoms in children under five years of age are limited (75). The Pediatric Emotional Distress Scale (PEDS) is used to detect elevated levels of symptoms and behaviors in children ages 2 to 10 following exposure to a stressful or traumatic experience (76). This 21-item parent/caregiver report scale provides an overall total scale score, as well as three subscale scores (Anxious or Withdrawn, Fearful, and Acting Out). While it is not intended to be a diagnostic instrument, it can provide valuable information regarding a child's symptom presentation following exposure to trauma. The PSTD in Preschool Aged Children (PTSD-PAC), which is another brief parent/caregiver report, can be used to screen and diagnose PTSD in children ages 2-5y; however, the items were based on an older version of the DSM (26). Given these limitations, many clinicians use more generalized measures of childhood behavior, which will be covered later, along with the most recent DSM criteria to screen and evaluate children under the age of 7y.

PTSD assessment measures for school-aged children

Assessment measures for school-aged children are more common and widely accessible. The Child Trauma Screen (CTS) is a brief and free screener for children ages 6 to 17 years that can be administered by pediatric providers (77). The first four items use developmentally appropriate language to assess for common traumatic events (i.e., physical abuse, sexual abuse, witnessing domestic violence) and the remaining six items evaluate common reactions that can be a preliminary marker of PTSD symptomatology. While it is not a comprehensive tool, it is empirically supported and user-friendly. The Child PTSD Symptom Scale for DSM-5 (CPSS-V SR) is a more comprehensive measure that evaluates PTSD diagnosis and measures symptom severity in the past month for children ages 8 to 18 years (78). It is a self-report measure that has strong empirical support, is available online for no cost, and versions are available in English, Hebrew, Portuguese, Slovenian, Spanish, and Swedish.

General assessment measures for youth

Many providers will administer general measures of childhood behavior, along with specific measures that evaluate internalizing or externalizing problems. The Child Behavior Checklist (CBCL) is a standardized measure that yields scores on both internalizing and externalizing problems in youth ages 6 to 18 years (79). The CBCL is comprehensive and well researched, with parent-report, youth-report, and teacher-report options. At this time, the measure is available for purchase and requires specialized training for scoring.

The Revised Children Anxiety and Depression Scale (RCADS) is a 47-item self-report and parent-report questionnaire that focuses specifically on internalizing symptoms and yields subscales on separation anxiety disorder, social phobia, generalized anxiety disorder, panic disorder, obsessive compulsive disorder, and low mood (80). The measure, which is intended for youth ages 8 to 18 years, takes between five to ten minutes to administer, has good psychometric properties, and is available for free online. For providers interested in evaluating major depressive symptoms specifically, the Beck Depression Inventory-II (BDI-II) is a brief and psychometrically sound measure that can be used with teens ages 13 years and older (81).

With respect to measures of externalizing behavior, the Eyberg Child Behavior Inventory (ECBI) is a brief and well validated measure of frequent child behavior problems (82). The instrument can be completed by parents or teachers of youth between the ages of 2 and 16 years, can be scored easily by hand, and is currently available in English and Spanish. Lastly, the Strengths and Difficulties Questionnaire (SDQ) is a 25-item tool that evaluates emotional symptoms, conduct problems, hyperactivity/ inattention, peer relationship problems, and prosocial behavior (83). There are parent-report and teacher-report forms for youth aged 2 to 17, as well as self-report forms for youth aged 11-17 and 18 years and older. The SDQ is one of the most widely and internationally used measures of child mental health and has been translated into more than 80 languages.

Mental health screening and PTSD evaluation for adolescents

The issues surrounding abuse are compounded during adolescence. Adolescents who have experienced maltreatment have been found to have higher rates of depression, anxiety, and posttraumatic stress disorder (PTSD) than their non-abused peers (32). Youth with PTSD often carry dual psychiatric diagnosis, making it difficult for clinicians to distinguish between overlapping symptoms (84). The challenges in the assessment of PTSD in children and adolescents are related to the diverse symptomology of PSTD-related behaviors across ages, and developmental and cognitive functioning of this diverse group (32). There are a number of validated tools have been used to assess PSTD in children and adolescents (see Table 7) (85-91).

Table 7. Testing alternatives for children and adolescents

Diagnostic Interview for Children and Adolescents (85)
Kiddie Schedule for Affective Disorder and Schizophrenia for School-age Children Present and Lifetime version (86)
Clinician Administered PTSD Scale for Children and Adolescents (85)
Child Posttraumatic Stress Disorder Reaction Index (86)
PTSD Symptom Scale (87)
Traumatic Symptom Checklist for Children Posttraumatic Stress scale (88)
Impact of Event Scale-Revised (89).

Reporting

Clinicians have legal responsibilities to report their concerns of child abuse and neglect to appropriate state or local agencies in all states and territories in the United States (14). Although the forms of the legislation vary, these "child protection laws" stipulate that certain professionals must report their concerns of child abuse and neglect to appropriate governmental agencies. The reporting requirements of these laws supersede the confidentiality of medical records and the patient-provider relationship. These "mandated reporters" generally include physicians, nurses, and other medical professionals, in addition to a variety of other licensed professionals who include teachers, counselors, law enforcement officers, and mental health professionals. Clinicians should be knowledgeable about legal definitions and reporting requirements while providing preventive screening for emotional and behavioral effects of CM.

Treatment

There are a variety of psychological and psychopharmacological interventions available for the treatment of PTSD in youth (see Table 8). A full review of these treatments is beyond the scope of this discussion, but interested clinicians are strongly encouraged to familiarize themselves with these interventions to better guide their referrals. Child health clinicians who are not formally trained to provide trauma therapy may express concern and apprehension about managing the mental health effects of their patients. Aside from gathering information related to patient symptomatology, without needing full access to the details of the trauma exposure, clinicians caring for children can play a critical role in providing psychoeducation on trauma, discussing basic coping strategies, and conducting safety planning. In addition, engaging and mobilizing the non-offending caregiver is vital as perceived parent support is a major protective factor for children (92, 93). This section provides a brief summary of shared treatment components, presents briefly on empirically supported treatments, and explores psychopharmacological options. In addition, guidance is provided for pediatricians who are supporting youth as they are waiting to be connected to mental health treatment.

Table 8. Treatment alternatives

Young Children
Attachment and Biobehavioral Catch-up
Child Parent Psychotherapy
Parent-Child Interaction Therapy, and Trauma-Focused Cognitive-Behavioral Therapy
School-age children
Alternatives for Families: A Cognitive Behavioral Therapy
Bounce Back
Cognitive Behavioral Interventions for Trauma in Schools
Eye Movement Desensitization and Reprocessing
Grief and Trauma Intervention
Narrative Exposure Therapy for Children, Parent-Child Interaction Therapy
Trauma-Focused Cognitive Behavioral Therapy
Adolescents
Cognitive Processing Therapy,
Eye Movement Desensitization and Reprocessing
Narrative Exposure Therapy for Children
Prolonged Exposure for Adolescents
Trauma-Focused Cognitive Behavioral Therapy.

Shared treatment components

Trauma-informed treatments may include one or more or a combination of the following components: psychoeducation, affective identification, emotion regulation, cognitive coping, parent training and behavior management, exposure via conducting a narrative or engaging in *in-vivo* exposure exercises, safety planning, and relapse prevention. In addition, therapists often conduct risk assessments, utilize motivational interviewing, engage patients as well as families in addressing barriers to services, monitor treatment progress, collaborate with collateral contacts, and advocate on behalf of patients. These treatment components aim to educate, empower, and avert revictimization, a common occurrence for children with a history of abuse (94).

Pharmacologic treatment

Research into the pharmacologic treatment of youth with PTSD is emerging but more data is needed in maltreated youth (32). Pharmacologic treatment often focuses on the maladaptive behaviors and emotional symptoms after stress that include depression and anxiety symptoms (32). These treatments often focus on the primary neurotransmitter symptoms involved in PTSD that include catecholamines, serotonin, and gamma amino butyric acid. Pharmacologic treatment of child-abuse related PTSD can include the use of selective serotonin reuptake inhibitors (SSRIs) and tricyclic antidepressants (TCAs) (29). Other medications have been shown to have some effectiveness in adults with PTSD; these include clonidine, guanfacine, mirtazapine, propranolol, risperidone, nefazadone, citalopram, and carbamazepine (95-98).

A 2019 meta-analysis of the pharmacological treatment of PSTD and acute stress disorder found several studies that used hydrocortisone with some potentially promising results as a treatment of PSTD in adults (98). Finally, a United Kingdom-based research group has found some promising results in the effective treatment of 'refractory to treatment' PTSD in adults with the use of a MDMA (3,4-methylenediometham-phetamine) for drug-assisted psychotherapy (99). Current research does not support use of SSRIs or other pharmacologic treatment as first-line treatment for PTSD. Pharmacologic treatment in practice is commonly used as an adjunctive therapy in the treatment of individuals with PTSD (100).

Unlike in the pharmacologic treatment of PTSD, selective serotonin reuptake inhibitors (SSRIs) are an important treatment tools for moderate-severe depression and other disorders (100). Two significant multisite, placebo-controlled trials concluded that the combination of SSRI and psychotherapy was superior to either alone in the treatment of anxiety and depression in children and adolescents (101, 102). These trials are the Treatment of Adolescents with Depression Study (101) and the Child/Adolescent Anxiety Multimodal Study (102). Specific SSRIs that have been FDA approved for use in children and adolescents include sertraline, fluoxetine, escitalopram, and fluvoxamine. Additionally, citalopram is another SSRI that is not FDA approved in children and adolescents that is also used to treat depression and anxiety (100).

Empirically supported non-pharmacologic treatment

Cognitive behavioral therapy (CBT) has the strongest research support for the treatment of PTSD in children. CBT is an active, goal-oriented, and collaborative treatment that explores the connections between our thoughts, feelings, and behaviors. CBT therapists work collaboratively with their clients to identify the various parts of their emotional experience (i.e., thoughts, body sensations, and action urges), find alternative ways of thinking about situations, and engage in more effective behavior. Treatment can be delivered in various modalities (i.e., individual, individual with parent involvement, and group) and is short-term (i.e., can range from 8-25 sessions).

Trauma-focused cognitive behavioral therapy (TF-CBT) is an evidence-based treatment specifically designed for children and adolescents who have been impacted by trauma (103). Backed by decades of research, it is a short-term, structured treatment model that significantly improves a range of trauma-related outcomes. Treatment components include psychoeducation, parenting skills, relaxation, affective identification as well as modulation, cognitive processing, trauma narration and processing, in-vivo mastery of trauma reminders, conjoint parent child sessions, and safety planning. TF-CBT has been shown to be effective for single and chronic episodes of trauma, with youth of different developmental levels, and across different cultures.

Youth who have experienced multiple traumas and/or prolonged traumatic stress may also benefit from comprehensive treatment frameworks, such as Attachment, Self-Regulation, and Competency (ARC) or Trauma Systems Therapy (TST) that provide a broader context in addressing the child's social environments and/or systems of care (104, 105). ARC is grounded in both attachment theory as well as early childhood development and focuses on 'building blocks' of attachment (such as attunement), regulation (such as identification of emotions), and competency (such as executive functions) via multiple modalities such as individual, group, as well as family treatment, parent workshops, milieu/systems intervention, and home-based prevention programs. TST is a 3-phase treatment (Safety Focused Treatment, Regulation Focused Treatment, and Beyond Trauma Treatment) that is specifically designed to address the complex needs of traumatized youth and families via understanding the child's symptoms in the context of their world, focusing on the family's strengths, and breaking down barriers between service systems. Both treatment approaches emphasize parent engagement, interdisciplinary team collaboration, and fostering resiliency in youth as well as their families.

Prevention of child abuse and maltreatment is often at the forefront for clinicians treating at-risk families. Positive parenting practices are often discussed and encouraged, yet implementation of newly acquiring skills based on empathy and less use of corporal punishment are limited (68). Parent-child interaction therapy (PCIT), is an evidenced-based treatment for children ages 2-7 years designed to reduce externalizing child behavior problems, increase child social skills, and improve the parent/caregiver-child relationship, It includes live coaching sessions with the parent/caregiver and child via a transmitter-receiver system and a one-way mirror. PCIT is a highly specific type of parent management training that has been researched extensively with various populations, including children with histories of maltreatment. Parents/caregivers who have completed PCIT report improvements in parent/caregiver-child communication, less stress, and decreased use of corporal punishment as well as coercive means to control their children (106-108).

Conclusion

Pediatricians and other child-care clinicians play a vital role in the assessment, care, and treatment of victims of child abuse and neglect. Physicians, nurses, and other health professionals have developed increasingly sophisticated techniques for diagnosing and documenting physical abuse, abusive head trauma, fractures, anogenital trauma, and sexually transmitted infections. However, it has become increasingly clear that the long-term behavioral and mental health effects of abuse and neglect far outshadow the physical effects of many forms of maltreatment. This discussion serves as an introduction to not only the physical manifestations but also the importance of screening and treating these emotional sequelae.

While C. Henry Kempe first taught us about the battered child in 1962, we still have a long way to go in solving the problems and treating the behavioral as well as emotional effects of child abuse and neglect (1). The effects of child maltreatment are now well-established, and we now know that chronic childhood maltreatment exposure is associated with psychopathology that can be detected in childhood and that extends into emerging adulthood (109). We also know which therapies are most beneficial, and TF-CBT remains the best- supported treatment for children and adolescents following child maltreatment with new evidence that symptom improvements are maintained at longer-term follow up (110).

Despite this, many segments of our population do not understand the compounding effects of higher rates of poverty, unique health concerns, and other special circumstances of children and their need for specialized physical as well as mental health services. Our response to the needs of abused and neglected children requires earnest dedication by all medical and mental health professionals in clinical care, training, research, as well as advocacy to identify, treat, and prevent the devastating emotional and behavioral consequences of child maltreatment.

References

[1] Kempe CH, Silverman FN, Steele BF, Droegemueller W, Silver HK. Landmark article July 7, 1962: The battered-child syndrome. By C. Henry Kempe, Frederic N. Silverman, Brandt F. Steele, William Droegemueller, and Henry K. Silver. Reprinted JAMA. 1984;251(24):3288-94.

[2] Shonkoff JP, Boyce WT, Levitt P, Martinez FD, McEwen B. Leveraging the biology of adversity and resilience to transform pediatric practice. Pediatrics 2021;147(2):e20193845.

[3] Child Welfare Information Gateway. About CAPTA: A legislative history. Washington, DC: US Department of Health and Human Services, Children's Bureau, 2019.

[4] Consultation on Child Abuse Prevention, World Health Organization. Violence and Injury Prevention Team & Global Forum for Health Research. Report of the consultation on child abuse prevention, 29-31 March 1999. Geneva: World Health Organization, 1999. URL: https://apps.who.int/iris/handle/10665/65900.

[5] Jenny C, Crawford-Jakubiak JE; Committee on Child Abuse and Neglect; American Academy of Pediatrics. The evaluation of children in the primary care setting when sexual abuse is suspected. Pediatrics 2013;132(2):e558-67.

[6] US Department of Health and Human Services, Centers for Disease Control and Prevention, National Center for Health Statistics. ICD-10: International statistical classification of diseases and related health problems, tenth revision. Washington, DC: US Government Printing Office, 1998.

[7] American Academy of Pediatrics. Coding Fact Sheet for Treating Trauma, Jan 2016. URL: https://www.aap.org/.../healthy-foster-care-america/Pages/Trauma-Guide.aspx.

[8] Kim H, Wildeman C, Jonson-Reid M, Drake B. Lifetime prevalence of investigating child maltreatment among US children. Am J Public Health 2017;107:274-80.

[9] Kaplan SJ, Sunday SR, Labruna V, Pelcovitz D, Salzinger S. Psychiatric disorders of parents of physically abused adolescents. J Fam Viol 2009;24(5):273-81.

[10] US Department of Veteran Affairs. PTSD in children and adolescents, 2019. URL: https://www.ptsd.va.gov/understand/common/common_children_teens.asp.

[11] Dube SR, Anda RF, Felitti VJ, Chapman DP, Williamson DF, Giles WH. Childhood abuse, household dysfunction and the risk of attempted suicide throughout the lifespan: Findings from the Adverse Childhood Experiences Study. JAMA 2001;286,3089-96.

[12] Dube SR, Felitti VJ, Dong M, Giles WH, Anda RF. The impact of adverse childhood experiences on health problems: Evidence from four birth cohorts dating back to 1900. Prev Med 2003;37(3):268-77.

[13] Forkey H, Szilagyi M, Kelly ET, Duffee J; Council on Foster Care, Adoption, and Kinship Care, Council on Community Pediatrics, Council on Child Abuse and Neglect, Committee on Psychosocial Aspects of Child and Family Health. Trauma-informed care. Pediatrics 2021; 148(2):e2021052580.

[14] U.S. Department of Health and Human Services, Administration on Children, Youth and Families, Children's Bureau. Child maltreatment 2019: Reports from the states to the national child abuse and neglect data system. Washington, DC: US Government Printing Office, 2020. URL: https://www.acf.hhs.gov/cb/resource/child-maltreatment-2019.

[15] Finkelhor D, Jones L, Shattuck A. Updated trends in child maltreatment, 2011. Durham, NH: University of New Hampshire Crimes Against Children Research Center, 2013. URL: www.unh.edu/ccrc/pdf/Updated trends 2016.pdf.

[16] Sedlak AJ, Mettenburg J, Basena M, Petta I, McPherson K, Greene A, et al. Fourth National Incidence Study of Child Abuse and Neglect (NIS–4): Report to Congress. Washington, DC: US Department of Health and Human Services, Administration for Children and Families, 2010. URL: https://www.acf.hhs.gov/sites/default/files/opre/nis4_report_congress_full_pdf_jan2010.pdf.

[17] Adams JA, Kellogg ND, Farst KJ, Harper NS, Palusci VJ, Frasier LD, et al. Updated guidelines for the medical assessment and care of children who may have been sexually abused. J Pediatr Adolesc Gynecol 2016;29(2):81-7.

[18] Noll JG, Shenk CE. Teen birth rates in sexually abused and neglected females. Pediatrics 2013131(4):e1181-7.

[19] American Psychiatric Association. Diagnostic and statistical manual of mental disorders, 5th ed. (DSM-5). Arlington, VA: American Psychiatric Publications, 2013.

[20] Cohen JA, Berliner L, Mannarino A. Trauma focused CBT for children with co-occurring trauma and behavior problems. Child Abuse Negl 2010;34:215-24.
[21] Humphreys KL, LeMoult J, Wear JG, Piersiak HA, Lee A, Gotlib IH. Child maltreatment and depression: A meta-analysis of studies using the Childhood Trauma Questionnaire. Child Abuse Negl 2020;102:104361.
[22] Milot T, Éthier LS, St-Laurent D, Provost MA. The role of trauma symptoms in the development of behavioral problems in maltreated preschoolers. Child Abuse Negl 2010;34: 225-34.
[23] Cohen JA, Mannarino AP, Deblinger E. Treating trauma and traumatic grief in children and adolescents. New York: Guilford, 2016.
[24] Chu AT, Lieberman AF. Clinical implications of traumatic stress from birth to age five. Ann Rev Clin Psychol 2010;6:469-94.
[25] Levendosky AA, Bogat GA, Martinez-Torteya C. PTSD symptoms in young children exposed to intimate partner violence. Violence Against Women 2013;19(2):187-201.
[26] Levendosky AA, Huth-Bocks AC, Semel MA, Shapiro DL. Trauma symptoms in preschool-age children exposed to domestic violence. J Interpers Viol 2002;17:150-64.
[27] Scheeringa MS, Zeanah CH, Myers L, Putnam FW. New findings on alternative criteria for PTSD in preschool children. J Am Acad Child Adolesc Psychiatry 2003;42(5):561-70.
[28] American Psychological Association. Children and trauma: Update for mental health professionals, 2008. URL: https://www.apa.org/pi/families/resources/children-trauma-update.
[29] Cohen JA, Mannarino AP, Zhitova AC, Capone ME. Treating child abuse-related posttraumatic stress and comorbid substance abuse in adolescents. Child Abuse Negl 2003; 27(12):1345-65.
[30] Fergusson DM, Horwood LJ, Lynskey MT. Childhood sexual abuse, adolescent sexual behaviors and sexual revictimization. Child Abuse Negl 1997;21(8):789–803.
[31] Negriff S, Gordis EB, Susman EJ, Kim K, Peckins MK, Schneiderman JU, et al. The Young Adolescent Project: A longitudinal study of the effects of maltreatment on adolescent development. Devel Psychopathol 2020;32(4):1440-59.
[32] Kearney CA, Wechsler A, Kaur H, Lemos-Miller A. Posttraumatic stress disorder in maltreated youth: A review of contemporary research and thought. Clin Child Fam Psychol Rev 2010;13(1):46-76.
[33] Kaufman M; American Academy of Pediatrics Committee on Adolescence. Care of the adolescent sexual assault victim. Pediatrics 2008;122(2):462-70.
[34] Pratt H, Patel D, Greydanus DE, Dannison L, Walcott D, Sloane M. Adolescent sexual offenders: Issues for pediatricians. Int Pediatr 2001;16(2):1-12.
[35] Bentovim A. Preventing sexually abused young people from becoming abusers, and treating the victimization experiences of young people who offend sexually. Child Abuse Negl 2002; 26(6-7):661-78.
[36] Griffith AK. Parental burnout and child maltreatment during the COVID-19 pandemic. J Fam Viol 2020;23:1-7.
[37] Rodriguez CM, Lee SJ, Ward KP, Pu DF. The perfect storm: Hidden risk of child maltreatment during the COVID-19 pandemic. Child Maltreat 2021;26(2):139-51.
[38] Adams EL, Smith D, Caccavale LJ, Bean MK. Parents are stressed! Patterns of parent stress across COVID-19. Front Psychiatry 2021;12:626456.
[39] Serrata JV, Alvarado MH. Understanding the impact of Hurricane Harvey on family violence survivors in Texas and those who serve them. Austin, TX: Texas Council on Family Violence, 2019.
[40] Kovler ML, Ziegfeld S, Ryan LM, Goldstein MA, Gardner R, Garcia AV, et al. Increased proportion of physical child abuse injuries at a level I pediatric trauma center during the Covid-19 pandemic. Child Abuse Negl 2020;104756.
[41] Christian CW, Committee on Child Abuse and Neglect, American Academy of Pediatrics. The evaluation of suspected child physical abuse. Pediatrics 2015;135(5):e1337-54.
[42] Maguire S, Mann MK, Sibert J, Kemp A. Are there patterns of bruising in childhood which are diagnostic or suggestive of abuse? A systematic review. Arch Dis Child 2005;90:182-6.
[43] Sugar NF, Taylor JA, Feldman KW. Bruises in infants and toddlers: Those who don't cruise rarely bruise. Puget Sound Pediatric Research Network. Arch Pediatr Adolesc Med 1999; 153(4):399-403.

[44] Sheets LK, Leach ME, Koszewski IJ, Lessmeier AM, Nugent M, Simpson P. Sentinel injuries in infants evaluated for child physical abuse. Pediatrics 2013;131(4):701-7.

[45] Maguire S, Okolie C, Kemp AM. Burns as a consequence of child maltreatment. Paediatrics Child Health 2014;24(12):557-61.

[46] Kleinman PK, Perez-Rossello JM, Newton AW, Feldman HA, Kleinman PL. Prevalence of the classic metaphyseal lesion in infants at low versus high risk for abuse. Am J Roentgenol 2011;197(4):1005-8.

[47] Flaherty EG, Perez-Rossello JM, Levine MA, Hennrikus WL; American Academy of Pediatrics Committee on Child Abuse and Neglect; Section on Radiology, American Academy of Pediatrics; Section on Endocrinology, American Academy of Pediatrics; Section on Orthopedics, American Academy of Pediatrics; Society for Pediatric Radiology. Evaluating children with fractures for child physical abuse. Pediatrics 2014;133(2):e477-89.

[48] Servaes S, Brown SD, Choudhary AK, Christian CW, Done SL, Hayes LL, et al. The etiology and significance of fractures in infants and young children: a critical multidisciplinary review. Pediatr Radiol 2016;46(5):591-600.

[49] Wood JN, Fakeye O, Feudtner C, Mondestin V, Localio R, Rubin DM. Development of guidelines for skeletal survey in young children with fractures. Pediatrics 2014;134(1):45-53.

[50] Wood JN, Henry MK, Berger RP, Lindberg DM, Anderst JD, Song L, et al. Use and utility of skeletal surveys to evaluate for occult fractures in young injured children. Acad Pediatr 2019; 19(4):428-37.

[51] Expert Panel on Pediatric Imaging, Wootton-Gorges SL, Soares BP, Alazraki AL, Anupindi SA, Blount JP, Booth TN, et al. ACR appropriateness criteria® suspected physical abuse-child. J Am Coll Radiol 2017;14(5S):S338-49.

[52] Palusci VJ, Cyrus TA. Reaction to videocolposcopy in the assessment of child sexual abuse. Child Abuse Negl 2001;25(11):1535-46.

[53] Kairys SW, Johnson CF; Committee on Child Abuse and Neglect. The psychological maltreatment of children--technical report. Pediatrics 2002;109(4):e68. doi: 10.1542/peds.109.4.e68.

[54] Trickett PK, Mennen FE, Kim K, Sang J. Emotional abuse in a sample of multiply maltreated, urban young adolescents: issues of definition and identification. Child Abuse Negl 2009;33(1):27-35.

[55] Turner HA, Finkelhor D, Ormrod R, Hamby SL. Infant victimization in a nationally representative sample. Pediatrics 2010;126(1):44-52.

[56] Shaffer A, Yates TM, Egeland BR. The relation of emotional maltreatment to early adolescent competence: Developmental processes in a prospective study. Child Abuse Negl 2009;33(1):36-44.

[57] Liu RT, Alloy LB, Abramson LY, Iacoviello BM, Whitehouse WG. Emotional maltreatment and depression: Prospective prediction of depressive episodes. Depress Anxiety 2009;26(2): 174-81.

[58] Reyome ND. Childhood emotional maltreatment and later intimate relationships: Themes from the empirical literature. J Aggress Maltreat Trauma 2010;19:224-42.

[59] Steinberg JA, Gibb BE, Alloy LB, Abramson LY. Childhood emotional maltreatment, cognitive vulnerability to depression, and self-referent information processing in adulthood: Reciprocal relations. J Cognit Psychother 2003;17(4):347-58.

[60] Uhrlass DJ, Gibb BE. Negative life events, self-perceived competence, and depressive symptoms in young adults. Cogn Ther Res 2007;31:773–83.

[61] Turner HA, Finkelhor D, Ormrod R. The effects of adolescent victimization on self-concept and depressive symptoms. Child Maltreat 2010;15(1):76-90.

[62] Palusci VJ, Ondersma SJ. Services and recurrence after psychological maltreatment confirmed by child protective services. Child Maltreat 2012;17(2):153-63.

[63] Dubowitz H, Papas MA, Black MM, Starr RH Jr. Child neglect: Outcomes in high-risk urban preschoolers. Pediatrics 2002;109(6):1100-7.

[64] Liu J, Raine A, Venables PH, Dalais C, Mednick SA. Malnutrition at age 3 years and lower cognitive ability at age 11 years: Independence from psychosocial adversity. Arch Pediatr Adolesc Med 2003;157(6):593-600.

[65] Wright MO, Crawford E, Del Castillo D. Childhood emotional maltreatment and later psychological distress among college students: The mediating role of maladaptive schemas. Child Abuse Negl 2009;33(1):59-68.

[66] Helfer RE. The neglect of our children. Pediatr Clin North Am 1990;37(4):923-42.

[67] Block RW, Krebs NF; American Academy of Pediatrics Committee on Child Abuse and Neglect; American Academy of Pediatrics Committee on Nutrition. Failure to thrive as a manifestation of child neglect. Pediatrics 2005;116(5):1234-7.
[68] Palusci VJ, Crum P, Bliss R, Bavolek SJ. Changes in parenting attitudes and knowledge among inmates and other at-risk populations after a family nurturing program. Child Youth Serv Rev 2008;30(1):79-89.
[69] Knight LD, Collins KA. A 25-year retrospective review of deaths due to pediatric neglect. Am J Forensic Med Pathol 2005;26(3):221-8.
[70] Dubowitz H, Giardino A, Gustavson E. Child neglect: guidance for pediatricians. Pediatr Rev 2000;21(4):111-6.
[71] Jenny C; Committee on Child Abuse and Neglect, American Academy of Pediatrics. Recognizing and responding to medical neglect. Pediatrics 2007;120(6):1385-9.
[72] Black MM, Dubowitz H, Casey PH, Cutts D, Drewett RF, Drotar D, et al. Failure to thrive as distinct from child neglect. Pediatrics 2006;117(4):1456-8.
[73] Stover CS, Berkowitz S. Assessing violence exposure and trauma symptoms in young children: A critical review of measures. J Traumatic Stress 2005;18:707-17.
[74] Ngai M, Delaney K, Limandri B, Dreves K, Tipton MV, Horowitz LM. Youth suicide risk screening in an outpatient child abuse clinic. J Child Adolesc Psychiatr Nurs 2021 Jun 10. doi: 10.1111/jcap.12335.
[75] Strand VC, Sarmiento TL, Pasquale LE. Assessment and screening tools for trauma in children and adolescents: A review. Trauma Viol Abuse 2005;6:55-78.
[76] Saylor CF, Swenson CC, Reynolds SS, Taylor M. The pediatric emotional distress scale: a brief screening measure for young children exposed to traumatic events. J Clin Child Psychol 1999;28(1):70-81.
[77] Lang JM, Connell CM. Development and validation of a brief trauma screening measure for children: The Child Trauma Screen. Psychol Trauma 2017;9(3):390-8.
[78] Foa EB, Asnaani A, Zang Y, Capaldi S, Yeh R. Psychometrics of the Child PTSD Symptom Scale for DSM-5 for trauma-exposed children and adolescents. J Clin Child Adol Psychol 2018;47:38-46.
[79] Achenbach TM, Rescorla L. Manual for the ASEBA school-age forms & profiles: An integrated system of multi-informant assessment. Burlington, VT: Aseba, 2001.
[80] Chorpita BF, Yim L, Moffitt C, Umemoto LA, Francis SE. Assessment of symptoms of DSM-IV anxiety and depression in children: A revised child anxiety and depression scale. Behav Res Ther 2000;38:835-55.
[81] Beck AT, Steer RA, Brown G. Beck depression inventory–II. Psychological Assessment. San Antonio, TX: Psychological Corporation, 1996.
[82] Eyberg S, Pincus D. Eyberg Child Behavior Inventory & Sutter-Eyberg Student Behavior Inventory-Revised: Professional Manual. Odessa, FL: Psychological Assessment Resources, 1999.
[83] Goodman R. Psychometric properties of the strengths and difficulties questionnaire. J Am Acad Child Adol Psychiatr 2001;40:1337-45.
[84] Hawkins SS, Radcliffe J. Current measures of PTSD for children and adolescents. J Pediatr Psychol 2006;31(4):420-30.
[85] Reich W, Leacock N, Shanfeld C. Diagnostic interview for children and adolescents-revised (DICA-R). St Louis, MO: Washington University, 1994.
[86] Kaufman J, Birmaher B, Brent D, Rao UM, Flynn C, Moreci P, et al. Schedule for affective disorders and schizophrenia for school-age children-present and lifetime version (K-SADS-PL): Initial reliability and validity data. J Am Acad Child Adol Psychiatr 1997;36(7):980-8.
[87] Newman E, Weathers FW, Nader K, Kaloupek DG, Pynoos RS, Blake DD, et al. Clinician-Administered PTSD Scale for Children and Adolescents (CAPS-CA). Los Angeles, CA: Western Psychological Services, 2004.
[88] Pynoos RS, Frederick C, Nader K, Arroyo W, Steinberg A, Eth S, et al. Life threat and posttraumatic stress in school-age children. Arch Gen Psychiatr 1987;44(12):1057-63.
[89] Foa EB, Riggs DS, Dancu CV, Rothbaum BO. Reliability and validity of a brief instrument for assessing post-traumatic stress disorder. J Traumat Stress 1993;6(4):459-73.

[90] Briere J. Trauma symptom checklist for children. Odessa, FL: Psychological Assessment Resources, 1996:00253-8.

[91] Weiss DS, Marmar CR. Assessing psychological trauma and PTSD. New York: Guildford, 1997;399–411.

[92] McLaughlin KA, Lambert HK. Child trauma exposure and psychopathology: mechanisms of risk and resilience. Curr Opin Psychol 2017;14:29-34.

[93] Scoglio AA, Kraus SW, Saczynski J, Jooma S, Molnar BE. Systematic review of risk and protective factors for revictimization after child sexual abuse. Trauma Viol Abuse 2021;22: 41-53.

[94] Classen CC, Palesh OG, Aggarwal R. Sexual revictimization: A review of the empirical literature. Trauma Viol Abuse 2005;6:103-29.

[95] Cohen JA, Mannarino AP, Rogal S. Treatment practices for childhood posttraumatic stress disorder. Child Abuse Negl 2001;25(1):123-35.

[96] Donnelly CL. Pharmacologic treatment approaches for children and adolescents with posttraumatic stress disorder. Child Adolesc Psychiatr Clin 2003;12(2):251-69.

[97] Stein DJ, Ipser J, McAnda N. Pharmacotherapy of posttraumatic stress disorder: a review of meta-analyses and treatment guidelines. CNS Spectr 2009;14(1 Suppl 1):25-31.

[98] Wright LA, Sijbrandij M, Sinnerton R, Lewis C, Roberts NP, Bisson JI. Pharmacological prevention and early treatment of post-traumatic stress disorder and acute stress disorder: A systematic review and meta-analysis. Translat Psychiatr 2019;9(1):334.

[99] Sessa B. MDMA and PTSD treatment: "PTSD: From novel pathophysiology to innovative therapeutics". Neurosci Lett 2017;649:176-80.

[100] Southammakosane C, Schmitz K. Pediatric psychopharmacology for treatment of ADHD, depression, and anxiety. Pediatrics 2015;136(2):351-9.

[101] March J, Silva S, Petrycki S, Curry J, Wells K, Fairbank J, et al. Fluoxetine, cognitive-behavioral therapy, and their combination for adolescents with depression: Treatment for Adolescents With Depression Study (TADS) randomized controlled trial. JAMA 2004; 292(7):807-20.

[102] Piacentini J, Bennett S, Compton SN, Kendall PC, Birmaher B, Albano AM, et al. 24-and 36-week outcomes for the Child/Adolescent Anxiety Multimodal Study (CAMS). J Am Acad Child Adol Psychiatr 2014;53(3):297-310.

[103] Cohen JA, Mannarino AP. Trauma-focused cognitive behavioral therapy for traumatized children and families. Child Adol Psychiatr Clin 2015;24(3):557-70.

[104] Blaustein ME, Kinniburgh KM. Treating traumatic stress in children and adolescents: How to foster resilience through attachment, self-regulation, and competency. New York: Guilford, 2018.

[105] Saxe GN, Ellis BH, Brown AD. Trauma systems therapy for children and teens. New York: Guilford, 2015.

[106] Chaffin M, Funderburk B, Bard D, Valle LA, Gurwitch R. A combined motivation and parent-child interaction therapy package reduces child welfare recidivism in a randomized dismantling field trial. J Consult Clin Psychol 2011;79(1):84-95.

[107] McNeil CB, Hembree-Kigin TL, Anhalt K, Hembree-Kigin TL. Parent-child interaction therapy. New York: Springer, 2010.

[108] Timmer SG, Urquiza AJ, Zebell NM, McGrath JM. Parent-child interaction therapy: Application to maltreating parent-child dyads. Child Abuse Negl 2005;29:825-42.

[109] Russotti J, Warmingham JM, Duprey EB, Handley ED, Manly JT, Rogosch FA, et al. Child maltreatment and the development of psychopathology: The role of developmental timing and chronicity. Child Abuse Negl 2021;120:105215.

[110] Bennett RS, Denne M, McGuire R, Hiller RM. A systematic review of controlled-trials for PTSD in maltreated children and adolescents. Child Maltreat 2021;26(3):325-43.

[111] Children's Bureau, Administration on Children, Youth and Families, Administration for Children and Families, US Department of Health and Human Services. National Child Abuse and Neglect Data System (NCANDS) Child File, FFY 2019. Washington, DC: National Data Archive on Child Abuse and Neglect, 2019. doi: 10.34681/7gy0-e516.

Chapter 4

Mental health and chronic disease: Issues in cardiovascular disease

Nelli El-Ghazal[1], PhD, Christina Helen Vlahos[2], PhD and Ahsan Nazeer[2,*], MD

[1]Child and Adolescent Psychiatry, Department of Psychiatry, Sidra Medicine, Doha
[2]Department of Psychiatry, Weil Cornell Medical School, Doha, Qatar

Abstract

This discussion reflects on mental health issues in pediatric persons with cardiovascular disorders. Research notes that chronic diseases, including cardiovascular illness, may lead to the development of mental health conditions, which have a negative social and academic impact on the lives of pediatric persons. Though more research is needed, clinicians need to be aware of these issues so that they can intervene in a timely manner to improve the quality of life of these patients and families.

Introduction

Cardiovascular disease (CVD) in children, whether occurring congenitally, as a result of viral infections, or acquired later in childhood, brings with it a slew of medical and non-medical concerns (1). Advancements in the medical field, particularly in diagnosing and treating heart conditions in children, have resulted in 90% of children surviving into adolescence and adulthood. During the last decade, concerns have been gaining attention regarding these children's development, exercise, quality of life (QoL), psychosocial functioning, and cognitive development (2, 3). Children with CVD have been identified as having more cognitive, developmental, psychological, and behavioral concerns than their same-age peers. However, in many cases, the presence of the disease in and of itself is not necessarily related to other non-medical complications; indeed, it is more so the interaction of the disease with treatment, environmental, and demographic variables related to these deficits (3).

* ***Correspondence:*** Ahsan Nazeer, MD, Division Chief-Child and Adolescent Psychiatry, Sidra Medical and Research Center, C2M 224, 2nd Mezzanine, OPC, POBox 26999, Al Luqta Street, Education City North Campus, Qatar Foundation, Doha, Qatar. Email: anazeer@sidra.org.

In: Behavioral Pediatrics
Editors: Donald E. Greydanus, Dilip R. Patel, Ahsan Nazeer et al.
ISBN: 979-8-88697-060-9

Of all the types of CVD in children, congenital heart defects (CHD) are the most common physical disability and occur in approximately 1% of live births. Of those born with CHD, about 25% will require medical intervention such as surgery to survive, adding another risk factor to their overall quality of life (4). The majority of the available research on the developmental and psychological impact of heart disease is mostly in the context of CHD, as opposed to general cardiovascular disease (5).

Quality of Life

As CHD patients live longer, it is imperative to recognize the quality of life in the context of overall life expectancy as a measure of the success of their treatment (6). Quality of life is a subjective experience that accounts for overall life satisfaction while integrating emotional, physical, and social wellbeing. Given that the manifestation and severity of CHD can vary, the restrictions and adjustments to everyday life that CHD patients will have to make, per their disease, will also vary. These restrictions may affect one or multiple aspects, including the patient's life's social, environmental, or physical domains (7).

In general, there is no consensus on whether CHD significantly impairs patients' quality of life compared to their healthy peers. This inconsistency is due to the complex nature of both CHD and the quality of life as observable and measurable factors. Fortunately, the mere presence of a CHD does not seem to be enough of a predictor of impairment in quality of life. Instead, the personal and medical experiences along the CHD treatment path are more likely to contribute to the patient's perceptions of their quality of life.

In studies of adult patients, researchers have found that the quality of life in CHD patients is proportionate, if not better, than in healthy controls (8). However, no similar pattern has arisen in children with CHD. One possible reason may be the variation in perspectives of families whose children have CHDs, with more positive attitudes being directly related to a positive quality of life outcomes. Along with the above, the quality and intensity of medical treatment and parents' satisfaction with care may also be tied to varying reports of quality of life.

A sense of the low quality of life in patients is linked to cardiac instability, increased disease severity, impaired motor functioning, and decreased autonomy (9, 10). Furthermore, increased medical and surgical interventions are also related to lower quality of life ratings. For example, operative procedures create a significant interruption to life, including day-to-day activities and experiences that would otherwise be identified as 'typical' for children. It is, therefore, not surprising that the above children have a more negative outlook on their overall functioning and quality of life (11).

Furthermore, postoperative complications, length of hospital stay, and need for ongoing medication use are also linked to lower quality of life reporting. There are conflicting reports on whether the duration and number of certain medical procedures (e.g., the duration of circulatory arrest or cardiopulmonary) impact the quality of life. Further research is needed to address the above question (12, 13).

Regardless of whether CHD patients undergo surgery, parents of children with CHD may lower their expectations and underestimate their child's physical ability. Such increased limitations on children's behavior and experiences, with or without surgery, are generally related to lower quality of life. This issue is particularly pertinent when children are withheld from desirable activities their peers engage in.

Another concern is the loss of known health and psychological benefits of exercise and the reduced access to social interactions. Despite the drawbacks of increased limitations, authors understand that, at times, caution about daily functioning may be warranted for complicated patients. This is why it is essential that the decisions about the extent of physical activity should only be taken on a case-by-case basis and only after extensive consultation with the patients' cardiologists.

In one study, physical functioning scores on the Pediatric Quality of Life Inventory (PedsQoL), as reported by parents and children, were lower for children with severe cardiovascular disease than in children with less severe disease (5). Patients and their parents rated physical symptoms much more consistently, particularly with increased CHD severity. However, non-physical symptoms were different. Parent ratings of physical appearance, treatment anxiety, and their children's communication were related to disease severity, whereas patients' self-report ratings were not associated with disease severity (5).

The degree of disease severity is also a risk factor for the poor quality of life ratings, not only due to the limitations imposed on the child but also because of the physical discomfort experienced and the amount of medical intervention necessary. Another notable disease characteristic is whether the amount of oxygen in the body is lowered due to the CHD (cyanotic), as it is generally related to a lower quality of life than when the oxygen amount is not impacted.

Another essential factor to consider is the impact of CHD on school attendance, which is particularly salient with increased CHD severity and medical interventions. Poor school attendance also raises concerns regarding patients' acquisition of knowledge and availability for learning, which is then linked to lower quality of life ratings. However, the academic experience is more than just the academic and learning components of the school; it also encompasses the children's social integration and functioning.

Time away from school because of medical necessity also means time away from opportunities to develop social skills and relationships. Because of the above, CHD students miss out on a fundamental shared experience with other children. Though the lack of social support is a risk factor in the QoL ratings, its presence is a protective factor and increases the reported quality of life. Therefore, social opportunities must be intentionally sought out and tailored to the patient's limitations.

Demographic risk factors have also been examined concerning the QoL. Some studies have reported a positive relationship between patient age and quality of life, which may be linked to the patients' ability to understand and manage the disease more independently. Although some self-report ratings indicated a positive relationship between age and quality of life, parent ratings have indicated the opposite, i.e., age and quality of life are negatively related. This is another area where a clear understanding has not yet developed, and further studies are needed.

Higher intelligence quotient (IQ) was also related to higher levels of quality of life, potentially for the same reason that underlies the relationship with older age. There are inconsistent findings concerning the relationship between gender and quality of life, but data indicate that males do better in this regard. Although the reason for this relationship is unclear, it may be beneficial to examine behavioral and physical activity limitations placed on CHD patients through a gender norm lens to determine whether lower limitations are present for male patients, which would inadvertently be related to a higher quality of life ratings.

Family factors have also been found to be related to patient quality of life. Parental unemployment and inter-familial conflicts because of family stress are related to lower quality of life ratings. Family socioeconomic status has been examined, but results are inconsistent with regard to its relation to the quality of life. It is important to note that the parents more often report quality of life impairments than noted by the child. In particular, parents who have children with developmental, language, or cognitive delays, tend to report more psychological problems (11, 14, 15). This trend may be because children do not have a point of comparison or may not have the cognitive skills to understand the extent of their deficits. However, these findings may also be overestimated if the parents are overprotective of their child.

Emotional and behavioral difficulties

Chronic illness has generally been established as a factor related to emotional or psychological distress; this finding is consistent for patients with CHD. These children are at a higher risk for emotional, behavioral, and psychological difficulties than the general population (16). Compared to the general population, where one in five adults has a psychiatric disorder, one in three CHD patients is noted to have a psychiatric disorder (5, 14-17).

Some data indicate that the prevalence of lifetime psychopathology in the CHD population is 18.7%, with double the rates in females than in males. These psychological difficulties are typically classified within the broader categories of behavior that are *internalizing* (i.e., withdrawal, anxiety, depression, dysphoria, etc.) and *externalizing* (i.e., defiance, impulsivity, hyperactivity, disruptiveness, aggression, and antisocial features) (7, 11). It is important to note that even if patients present with externalizing behaviors, they are generally more at risk for major depression, bipolar disorder, and substance abuse in the future (2). In another study, feeling angry was the most frequent emotional problem noted by both parents and children with CHD (5). One (12.5%) in 8 children among the study sample also reported worrying about the future, while parents' and patients' most common cognitive problems were related to memory and attention (5).

There have also been connections made between CHD and attention-deficit/hyperactivity disorder, internalizing problems, limitations in socialization, and low self-esteem (3). As the children grow into adolescence, peer acceptance and participation in activities with peers become increasingly important. Fear of the unexpected nature of CHD and the possibility of a sudden cardiac event may also contribute to stress in these patients. These differences between CHD patients and their healthy peers have been established in multiple countries, including the United States, Canada, China, Norway, and Germany; such results indicate that irrespective of cultural differences, these difficulties seem to be prevalent in the population of patients with CHD (3, 6, 7).

Surgery has also been identified as a potential risk factor with regard to patient psychological/behavioral functioning and development (3, 11). Except for patients with transposition of the great arteries (TGA), children who have undergone other surgical repairs have more psychological difficulties; this difference in the outcome may be because of the better postoperative prognosis or because of the low incidence of genetic disorders in TGA group (11, 16). Postoperatively, most of the psychological complications tend to be attentional, social, and somatic. One study indicated that 5 to 10-year-olds who had undergone surgery as newborns were rated as "clinically significant" on inattention and hyperactivity at a rate of 3-4 times the general population (16, 18).

Some findings indicate that older age at the time of surgery may also be a risk factor. The number of surgical procedures and the duration of the hospital stay were also a predictor of externalizing problems. The relationship between CHD and the development of internalizing, externalizing, attention, and social difficulties may be associated with the level of intensity of the treatment (i.e., the more intense the treatment, the greater the behavioral problems) (11). Despite the positive relationship between treatment severity and psychological and behavioral difficulties, there is an inconsistency in the available data on whether a relationship exists between disease severity and the level of psychological and cognitive functioning.

Some specific treatments or conditions may also be related to greater psychological or behavioral difficulties. For example, there are some indications that deep hypothermic circulatory arrest (DHCA) seems to be linked to long-term behavioral and emotional issues; however, this association should be taken with caution because of the limitations in the research methodology. Prolonged hypoxia is also a risk factor in developing psychological difficulties in TGA patients; however, like many other findings, this is also not consistent across studies.

Another factor that has been identified to impair psychological functioning is premature birth. In one study, parents of 3.5-year-olds who met this criterion reported more internalizing problems than parents of the control group (16). Low birth weight and less than 36-week gestation are added risk factors to a number of surgeries and deep hypothermic circulatory arrest in predicting future internalizing problems.

Demographic factors have also been found to be related to psychological and behavioral functioning. Some studies have found that older adolescents have had more difficulty adjusting, but this has not been consistent. Patients aged 12 to 17 years have been reported to be more withdrawn, while older patients (19-26 years) were reportedly more anxious, had more difficulty with attention, and had more externalizing problems. Conversely, younger children have reported fewer externalizing and internalizing behaviors than controls.

Based on parent reports in one study, children aged 5 to 7 showed no differences from their same-age peers, whereas those 13-18 years show psychological functioning significantly below their peers. Therefore, age may be more related to psychological problems than the presence or severity of CHD. This is consistent with other chronic illnesses and maybe because adolescents have greater exposure to risk factors throughout their lifetime than younger children. Additionally, the hormonal and brain changes that occur in adolescence may trigger the expression of genetic vulnerabilities in conjunction with stressful experiences related to CHD.

It is essential to note the numerous variables that affect the results of available studies. First, there are noted to be inconsistencies among parents, teachers, and self-report measures of psychological and behavioral difficulties. When rating CHD patients' functioning, parents report fewer symptoms than their children, and teachers report less deviant behaviors than parents. The difference between parent and self-report may be due to the potentially unobservable nature of internalizing behaviors also, as parents have more insight into their child's functioning than teachers; hence, the discrepancy in ratings.

The discrepancy can also occur with the use of the Child Behavior Checklist (CBCL); this is an instrument to access psychological functioning, is commonly used in studies accessing QoL, and consists of an internalizing scale that includes physical symptoms items. Since these children already have a physical condition, this scale may not accurately reflect their internalizing feelings, as they may endorse specific items based on actual physical symptoms. In contrast, the item may measure a somatic complaint in a healthy child.

Finally, some family factors may be linked to behavioral difficulties; these include early parental distress, maternal fear, poor parental behavior management skills, high maternal worry about their children, and maternal psychological symptoms. Because parental well-being is related to the psychological adjustment of CHD patients, an integrated family approach to care and wellness is imperative.

Cognitive and academic impact

Another area that has received an increased focus is the cognitive and academic functioning of CHD patients (6, 14, 15). Because this area is still emerging, the research remains inconsistent concerning identifying a clear or consistent relationship between CHD and cognitive functioning. One salient point to note is that the majority of cognitive testing in study samples is conducted in persons between the ages of four and eighteen. As the reliability and validity of cognitive testing are low in younger children, the research findings need to be interpreted in this context.

Unlike difficulties with emotional functioning or quality of life, the presence of CHD has been identified as a predictor of developmental delays; this is especially true when complications occur at birth (19). The presence of CHD is often accompanied by other symptoms such as trouble breathing, fatigue, dizziness, low weight, frequent respiratory infections, arrhythmias, and cyanosis. Depending on the degree of these symptoms, children with CHD can experience physical and motor constraints that directly impact their cognitive and emotional development. Children with CHD have been noted to have a distinct neuropsychiatric profile, including deficits in executive control and cognitive performance, inattention, difficulties with social interaction, and impairment in pragmatic language (20).

Delays in cognitive development and psychosocial functioning are more likely to become evident as children grow and develop language skills. By school age, children with critical congenital heart disease (CCHD) have lower scores on intelligence and achievement subsets of psychological batteries, display impairments in fine and gross motor function, and have a higher likelihood of learning disabilities (21).

There are also cultural and environmental factors that come into play, such as living conditions, quality and quantity of medical care, perinatal risks, family and social interactions, and housing conditions that affect the functioning (22). The following factors have not been noted to be related to delays: age and education of the parents, number of children per family, care before and after delivery, breastfeeding, mother's health, and use of controlled medication or substances; however, future studies should continue to investigate these factors further.

In children with CCHD, neurocognitive development may be affected by hypoxic-ischemic injury to brian during brain development and impairments in progression and rate of early brain maturation (23, 24). The severity of the CHD also impacts the overall cognitive functioning of patients. Specifically, more severe patients exhibit lower verbal and performance IQ than same-age peers. There were also differences in cognitive ability based on the type of CHD present. Those with an atrial septal defect and ventricular septal defect had higher overall, verbal, and performance *intelligence quotient* (IQ) than the normative sample; on the other hand, those with hypoplastic left heart syndrome (HLHS) and TGA had lower IQs than the normative sample, especially in the area of perceptual reasoning ability.

Specific to treatment procedures for CHD patients, a relationship in the literature is emerging between deep hypothermic circulatory arrest and cognitive score. Some have found a relationship between the length of time of arrest and IQ; however, others have found IQ to be impacted not by the cooling itself, but by the length of the cooling period, with shorter cooling periods being linked to lower IQ (25, 26). Some studies have shown that even when children with CHD have a similar IQ to their healthy peers, they continue to demonstrate deficits in visual-spatial and visual-motor skills, speech-language impairments, and executive functioning (27).

There are also reports of inattention and hyperactivity in the complex CHD population in schools. In parent's reports, the most common school and cognitive concerns were related to memory and attention; however, these individuals also have impairment in behavioral regulation, lower working memory, and problems with organizational and planning skills (28-30). In some samples, the rate of students with attention and executive functioning concerns was three to four times as high as the general population (15). Cyanotic patients were more likely to exhibit more concerns with poor attention and executive functioning skills than acyanotic patients. Although the exact prevalence of ADHD as a diagnosis in this population cannot be conclusively stated, it is a significant risk factor to consider in managing these children.

Research has also noted larger than normal numbers of CHD patients receiving remedial services as compared to their same-age peers in school (15). In general, parents note more academic difficulties in their children than teachers. However, teachers may have a higher threshold for behavior and academic difficulties because they may also be comparing the cardiac patient to other children who are in a special education classroom, where there is a high prevalence of behavioral and developmental issues. In contrast, parents may be comparing their children to typically developing same-age peers. Therefore, the consistent and systematic identification of patients with CHD's need for support is imperative to improve their school functioning and, in turn, their social functioning; such is consequently linked to psychological adjustment and quality of life.

Quality of life in pediatric heart transplant patients

A cardiac transplant is a life-saving surgery, and in addition to the preservation of life, the majority of recipients do not have any limitations on physical activity. However, the need for a transplant is difficult to understand for anyone, and while growing up, cardiac transplant patients struggle with a slew of psychosocial problems. For adolescents who are developing the ability to build peer relationships, think in new ways and explore new thoughts, the idea of a significant surgery triggers fears, worries, and concerns about body image and the overall quality of life.

The children who have more psychosocial difficulties before the procedure continue to have numerous hospitalizations after the procedure (31). A significant number of patients (33%), have behavioral problems, 25% have emotional difficulties, 20-24% have psychological distress, and others have academic and school-related difficulties (32, 33). Other studies have identified concerns regarding the inability to keep up with peers and being teased. In a small study sample, more than 40% of the transplant recipients reported being teased and bullied because of their surgery scars and medication side effects, including hirsutism (34).

Few studies have noted resentment, anger, and difficulty talking to others regarding their fears, feelings, and worries about transplant rejection and life expectancy (17, 18, 35-37). Current research has not found any correlation between the psychological-psychosocial functioning and age and time since transplant and socioeconomic status (18); however, psychosocial functioning was noted to be significantly correlated with family and school functioning in multiple studies (17, 38).

Parental mental health

As noted above, the children's survival with CHD has improved considerably during the last decade; however, about 25% of the children with CHD have CCHD and require two or more surgeries in the first year of life with varied outcomes (39). These children undergo numerous hospitalizations and multiple surgeries and are at increased risk of medical complications, which poses a significant emotional and physical burden to the parents (40-43). These risks are further exacerbated, mainly when the medical procedures occur during the immediate postpartum period, in which mothers are already at risk of developing postpartum depression. Studies have noted an exponential increase in postpartum depression among mothers of children who spend time in the Intensive Care Unit (ICU) after birth (44). It is also well noted that impairment in maternal mental health leads to the dysfunctional parent-child relationship and results in long-term emotional, behavioral, and cognitive problems in children (45-47).

Different studies have evaluated the long-term psychological functioning of the parents of children with CHD and critical congenital heart disease (CCHD). They have focused on general distress, stress, trauma, and depression, as well as anxiety symptoms. Studies that specifically focused on trauma symptoms noted symptoms of acute stress disorder (ASD) and post-traumatic stress disorder (PTSD) among both parents. In a study of infants who underwent surgery before three months of age, 35% of the mothers and 18% of the fathers reported symptoms of ASD one month after discharge (48). In another study, 25% of the parents met the criteria for PTSD one month post-surgery, while 12% still met PTSD criteria six months after surgery (49).

Studies have also focused on the symptoms of depression and anxiety in parents. Research has noted an increased prevalence of depression among mothers of children undergoing two or more cardiac procedures (50). Symptoms of depression and anxiety were present within four weeks of cardiac procedures. They were also associated with impaired bonding and lower levels of maternal attachment with their infants (51). Surprisingly, in some cases, mood and anxiety symptoms persisted as long as five years post-surgery (52). There is considerable heterogeneity among the studies defining and measuring the global level of stress, distress, and overall quality of life of parents. However, most of the studies have noted elevated levels of stress/distress before surgery and improvement in the mood by two months post-surgery (53). In summary, parents of children with CCHD are at increased risk of mental health problems, with 80% experiencing symptoms of trauma, about 50% reporting mood and anxiety problems, and 30-80% experiencing psychological distress (54).

Psychopharmacological considerations in children with CHD/CVD

A variety of psychotropics are associated with cardiac side effects, including cardiac arrhythmias and sudden cardiac death. Different medications have different propensity to affect the heart. Antipsychotic medications used to manage behavioral problems in children with autism and intellectual disability, along with psychosis and treatment of mood disorders, warrant particular attention. In the literature, the most common cardiovascular adverse effects of typical and atypical antipsychotics in children were orthostatic hypotension, tachycardia, QTc interval prolongation, and arrhythmias. There are also reports of electrocardiographic (ECG) changes, myocarditis, and cerebrovascular events that further question the cardiovascular safety of these medications in children and adolescents (55-58).

In one study, the use of antipsychotics was associated with cardiomegaly, heart disease not otherwise specified (NOS), tachycardia, and arrhythmia NOS (59). In the same study, youth receiving typical (first generation, conventional) antipsychotics, multiple antipsychotics, and individuals with congenital heart defects were at increased risk of developing cardiovascular-related events. Children with pre-existing cardiac conditions are particularly at risk of developing these side effects; however, these risks need to be considered in the context of symptomatic relief that these medications can bring to debilitating mental health symptoms.

Hypotension, syncope, and rhythm disturbances

Orthostatic hypotension (decrease in systolic BP > 20 mm/Hg) is the most common side effect of antipsychotic medications and is reported to occur in more than 70% of these individuals. Low potency antipsychotics, including chlorpromazine and thioridazine, are more likely to cause postural hypotension than atypical antipsychotics. Among atypical antipsychotics, clozapine is associated with the most significant hypotension and benign sustained tachycardia (an average increase in the cardiac rate of 10-15 beats per minute). This effect is mediated via antagonism on the alpha one adrenergic receptor. Syncope is another side effect that is prevalent in individuals treated with clozapine (6%) as a comparison to the ones treated with risperidone (0.2%) and quetiapine (1%). Oral and intramuscular olanzapine is also associated with clinically significant bradycardia in 7.5% of the patients (58).

QTc prolongation and cardiac conduction delays

QTc prolongation is of particular importance while treating a patient with pre-existing cardiac conditions who already have prolonged or abnormal cardiac repolarization. Prolonged QTc leads to torsade de pointes with symptoms of palpitations, syncope, fibrillation, and sudden cardiac death. There is no direct correlation between the degree of QTc prolongation and the development of torsades; however, the risk appears to increase significantly with QTc prolongation of 500 ms. Several psychotropics are associated with QTc prolongation, including haloperidol, ziprasidone, citalopram, methadone, and lithium (list not exhaustive). Other than electrophysiological changes and direct effects on cardiac adrenoreceptors (antagonism), it is speculated that psychotropics treatment may have predisposed or exacerbated metabolic changes and ultimately led to cardiovascular events.

Stimulants and sudden cardiac death

Children with CHD suffer from impairment in numerous psychosocial domains, including impairment in cognition, speech and language difficulties, learning disabilities, inattention, impulsivity, and impairment in executive functioning (15, 20, 60). A higher prevalence of ADHD with elevated scores in inattention and hyperactivity at times warrants the use of stimulants for adequate behavioral control and to improve academic functioning (61, 62). Stimulant medications cause a slight increase in heart rate and blood pressure, and their cardiovascular safety has been hotly debated (63).

A study from South Korea published in 2016 found an increase in the risk of arrhythmias among children and adolescents who were prescribed methylphenidate for ADHD (64). The risk was substantially higher (a three-fold increase) in individuals with pre-existing heart disease, and the highest risk was observed during the initial three days of the treatment. A higher risk of hypertension was also noticed from day four to seven (64). This study is at odds with the United States studies of private and Medicaid insurance as those studies have not found elevated cardiac side effects among individuals with or without pre-existing heart disease who were started on methylphenidate (65-67). The average rate of sudden cardiac death in children with CHD ranges from 1/454 to 1/7157 cases. The above study results suggest that children with CHD are at three times more risk of suffering from sudden cardiac death than children of their peers (68).

Conclusion

Current research regarding the psychological, behavioral, and developmental impact of CHD on children provides important information to guide the management and care that they receive (1-3, 5, 17). However, the current body of literature on this topic presents its own limitations, which hinder the clinician's ability to integrate the findings and draw a meaningful conclusion for a variety of CHD patients. One limitation is that few studies have examined the psychological or cognitive effects longitudinally, which makes it difficult to plan the allocation of resources and document the benefits of early interventions. Another is the rapidly developing treatments in this area, which creates much variability in the patients' cohort to generalize the research results.

Future research should investigate more narrow-band psychological and cognitive functions as opposed to broader internalizing or externalizing behaviors and verbal or performance IQ. Including a psychologist as part of the patient's medical team could also offer a more proactive approach to treatment and interventions for psychological and cognitive deficits. There is little research on the impact of treatment and psychological interventions; therefore, research should also investigate the effectiveness of those interventions.

Finally, as about 20% of the adolescents with CHD struggle with some form of mental illness (i.e., developmental disorders, anxiety disorder, impulse control disorders, and mood disorder), it is imperative to screen individuals for these disorders. It is best to embed mental health professionals in CHD clinics, and if this is not possible, an early referral needs to be made to the appropriate child and adolescent mental health service. It is also essential to further examine the impact of a child's cardiovascular disease on families. With a better understanding of the impact on family dynamics, employment, and overall stress, appropriate advocacy and clinical services can be established to improve the overall wellbeing of the child and the family.

References

[1] Areias ME, Pinto CI, Vieira PF, Teixeira F, Coelho R, Freitas I, et al. Long term psychosocial outcomes of congenital heart disease (CHD) in adolescents and young adults. Transl Pediatr 2013;2(3):90-8.

[2] Lane DA, Millane TA, Lip GYH. Psychological interventions for depression in adolescent and adult congenital heart disease. Cochrane Database Syst Rev 2013;10: CD004372.

[3] Latal B, Helfricht S, Fischer JE, Bauersfeld U, Landolt MA. Psychological adjustment and quality of life in children and adolescents following open-heart surgery for congenital heart disease: a systematic review. BMC Pediatr 2009;9(1):6. doi: 10.1186/1471-2431-9-6.

[4] Bernier PL, Stefanescu A, Samoukovic G, Tchervenkov CI. The challenge of congenital heart disease worldwide: epidemiologic and demographic facts. Semin Thorac Cardiovasc Surg Pediatr Card Surg Annu 2010;13(1):26-34.

[5] Uzark K, Jones K, Slusher J, Limbers CA, Burwinkle TM, Varni JW. Quality of life in children with heart disease as perceived by children and parents. Pediatrics 2008; 121(5):e1060-e7.

[6] Karsdorp PA, Everaerd W, Kindt M, Mulder BJM. Psychological and cognitive functioning in children and adolescents with congenital heart disease: A meta-analysis. J Pediatr Psychol 2006;32(5):527-41.

[7] Johnson B. Behaviour problems in children with congenital heart disease. BMH Med J 2015;2(1):14-19.

[8] Moons P, Van Deyk K, De Bleser L, Marquet K, Raes E, De Geest S, et al. Quality of life and health status in adults with congenital heart disease: a direct comparison with healthy counterparts. Eur J Cardiovasc Prev Rehabil 2006;13(3):407-13.

[9] Marino BS, Shera D, Wernovsky G, Tomlinson RS, Aguirre A, Gallagher M, et al. The development of the pediatric cardiac quality of life inventory: a quality of life measure for children and adolescents with heart disease. Qual Life Res 2008;17(4): 613-26.

[10] Marino BS, Tomlinson RS, Wernovsky G, Drotar D, Newburger JW, Mahony L, et al. Validation of the pediatric cardiac quality of life inventory. Pediatrics 2010; 126(3):498-508.

[11] Utens E. Prediction of behavioural and emotional problems in children and adolescents with operated congenital heart disease. Eur Heart J 1998;19(5):801-7.

[12] Landolt MA, Valsangiacomo Buechel ER, Latal B. Health-related quality of life in children and adolescents after open-heart surgery. J Pediatr 2008;152(3):349-55.

[13] O'Connor AM, Wray J, Tomlinson RS, Cassedy A, Jacobs JP, Jenkins KJ, et al. Impact of surgical complexity on health-related quality of life in congenital heart disease surgical survivors. J Am Heart Assoc 2016;5(7). pii: e001234.

[14] Mari MA, Cascudo MM, Alchieri JC. Congenital heart disease and impacts on child development. Braz J Cardiovasc Surg 2016;31(1):31-7.

[15] Shillingford AJ, Glanzman MM, Ittenbach RF, Clancy RR, Gaynor JW, Wernovsky G. Inattention, hyperactivity, and school performance in a population of school-age children with complex congenital heart disease. Pediatrics 2008;121(4):e759-67.

[16] Brosig CL, Whitstone BN, Frommelt MA, Frisbee SJ, Leuthner SR. Psychological distress in parents of children with severe congenital heart disease: The impact of prenatal versus postnatal diagnosis. J Perinatol 2007;27(11):687-92.

[17] Uzark KC, Sauer SN, Lawrence KS, Miller J, Addonizio L, Crowley DC. The psychosocial impact of pediatric heart transplantation. J Heart Lung Transplant 1992; 11(6):1160-7.

[18] Brosig C, Hintermeyer M, Zlotocha J, Behrens D, Mao J. An exploratory study of the cognitive, academic, and behavioral functioning of pediatric cardiothoracic transplant recipients. Prog Transplant 2006;16(1):38-45.

[19] Mussatto KA, Hoffmann RG, Hoffman GM, Tweddell JS, Bear L, Cao Y, et al. Risk and prevalence of developmental delay in young children with congenital heart disease. Pediatrics 2014;133(3):e570-e7.

[20] Wernovsky G. Current insights regarding neurological and developmental abnormalities in children and young adults with complex congenital cardiac disease. Cardiol Young 2006;16 Suppl 1:92-104.

[21] Bellinger DC, Wypij D, Rivkin MJ, DeMaso DR, Robertson RL, Dunbar-Masterson C, et al. Adolescents with d-transposition of the great arteries corrected with the arterial switch procedure. Circulation 2011;124(12):1361-9.

[22] Newburger JW, Sleeper LA, Bellinger DC, Goldberg CS, Tabbutt S, Lu M, et al. Early developmental outcome in children with hypoplastic left heart syndrome and related anomalies. Circulation 2012;125(17):2081-91.

[23] Limperopoulos C, Tworetzky W, McElhinney DB, Newburger JW, Brown DW, Robertson RL, et al. Brain volume and metabolism in fetuses with congenital heart disease. Circulation 2010;121(1):26-33.

[24] von Rhein M, Buchmann A, Hagman n C, Huber R, Klaver P, Knirsch W, et al. Brain volumes predict neurodevelopment in adolescents after surgery for congenital heart disease. Brain 2013;137(1):268-76.

[25] Fuller S, Rajagopalan R, Jarvik GP, Gerdes M, Bernbaum J, Wernovsky G, et al. Deep hypothermic circulatory arrest does not impair neurodevelopmental outcome in school-age children after infant cardiac surgery. Ann Thorac Surg 2010;90(6):1985-95.

[26] Snookes SH, Gunn JK, Eldridge BJ, Donath SM, Hunt RW, Galea MP, et al. A systematic review of motor and cognitive outcomes after early surgery for congenital heart disease. Pediatrics 2010;125(4):e818-e27.

[27] Bellinger DC. Are children with congenital cardiac malformations at increased risk of deficits in social cognition? Cardiol Young 2008;18(1)3-9.

[28] Calderon J, Bellinger DC. Executive function deficits in congenital heart disease: why is intervention important? Cardiol Young 2015;25(7):1238-46.

[29] Cassidy AR, White MT, DeMaso DR, Newburger JW, Bellinger DC. Executive function in children and adolescents with critical cyanotic congenital heart disease. J Int Neuropsychol Soc 2015;21(1):34-49.

[30] Marelli A, Miller SP, Marino BS, Jefferson AL, Newburger JW. Brain in congenital heart disease across the lifespan. Circulation 2016;133(20):1951-62.

[31] DeMaso DR, Douglas Kelley S, Bastardi H, O'Brien P, Blume ED. The longitudinal impact of psychological functioning, medical severity, and family functioning in pediatric heart transplantation. J Heart Lung Transplant 2004;23(4):473-80.

[32] Todaro JF. Cognitive and psychological outcomes in pediatric heart transplantation. J Pediatr Psychol 2000;25(8):567-76.

[33] Wray J, Radley-Smith R. Longitudinal assessment of psychological functioning in children after heart or heart–lung transplantation. J Heart Lung Transplant 2006; 25(3):345-52.

[34] Green A, McSweeney J, Ainley K, Bryant J. In my shoes: Children's quality of life after heart transplantation. Prog Transplant 2007;17(3):199-208.

[35] Green A, Meaux J, Huett A, Ainley K. "It Has its Ups and Downs": Adolescents' quality of life after heart transplantation. ProgTransplant 2011;21(2):115-20.

[36] Mintzer LL. Traumatic stress symptoms in adolescent organ transplant recipients. Pediatrics 2005;115(6):1640-4.

[37] Wray J, Radley-Smith R. Depression in pediatric patients before and 1 year after heart or heart-lung transplantation. J Heart Lung Transplant 2004;23(9):1103-10.

[38] Hirshfeld AB, Kahle AL, Clark BJ, Bridges ND. Parent-reported health status after pediatric thoracic organ transplant. J Heart Lung Transplant 2004;23(9):1111-8.

[39] Centers for Disease Control and Prevention (CDC). Critical congenital heart defects, 2019. URL: https://www.cdc.gov/ncbddd/heartdefects/cchd-facts.html.

[40] Connor JA, Kline NE, Mott S, Harris SK, Jenkins KJ. The meaning of cost for families of children with congenital heart disease. J Pediatr Health Care 2010;24(5):318-25.

[41] Hopkins J, Marcus M, Campbell SB. Postpartum depression: A critical review. Psychol Bull 1984;95(3):498-515.

[42] Ross LE, McLean LM. Anxiety disorders during pregnancy and the postpartum period. J Clin Psychiatry 2006;67(8):1285-98.

[43] Vesga-López O, Blanco C, Keyes K, Olfson M, Grant BF, Hasin DS. Psychiatric disorders in pregnant and postpartum women in the United States. Arch Gen Psychiatry 2008;65(7):805-15.

[44] Lefkowitz DS, Baxt C, Evans JR. Prevalence and correlates of posttraumatic stress and postpartum depression in parents of infants in the neonatal intensive care unit (NICU). J Clin Psychol Med Settings 2010;17(3):230-7.

[45] Lyons-Ruth K, Wolfe R, Lyubchik A. Depression and the parenting of young children: Making the case for early preventive mental health services. Harv Rev Psychiatry 2000;8(3):148-53.

[46] McPeak KE, Sandrock D, Spector ND, Pattishall AE. Important determinants of newborn health. Curr Opin Pediatr 2015;27(1);138-44.

[47] Mirhosseini H, Moosavipoor SA, Nazari MA, Dehghan A, Mirhosseini S, Bidaki R, et al. Cognitive behavioral development in children following maternal postpartum depression: A review article. Electron Physician 2015;7(8):1673-9.

[48] Franich-Ray C, Bright MA, Anderson V, Northam E, Cochrane A, Menahem S, et al. Trauma reactions in mothers and fathers after their infant's cardiac surgery. J Pediatr Psychol 2013;38(5):494-505.

[49] Helfricht S, Latal B, Fischer JE, Tomaske M, Landolt MA. Surgery-related posttraumatic stress disorder in parents of children undergoing cardiopulmonary bypass surgery: A prospective cohort study. Pediatr Crit Care Med 2008;9(2):217-23.

[50] Hearps SJ, McCarthy MC, Muscara F, Hearps SJC, Burke K, Jones B, et al. Psychosocial risk in families of infants undergoing surgery for a serious congenital heart disease. Cardiol Young 2013;24(4):632-9.

[51] Jordan B, Franich-Ray C, Albert N, Anderson V, Northam E, Cochrane A, et al. Early mother-infant relationships after cardiac surgery in infancy. Arch Dis Child 2014; 99(7):641-5.

[52] Guan G, Liu H, Wang Y, Han B, Jin Y. Behavioural and emotional outcomes in school-aged children after surgery or transcatheter closure treatment for ventricular septal defect. Cardiol Young 2013;24(5):910-7.

[53] Wray J, Sensky T. Psychological functioning in parents of children undergoing elective cardiac surgery. Cardiol Young 2004;14(2):131-9.

[54] Woolf-King SE, Anger A, Arnold EA, Weiss SJ, Teitel D. Mental health among parents of children with critical congenital heart defects: A systematic review. J Am Heart Assoc 2017;6(2). pii: e004862.

[55] Cheng-Shannon J, McGough JJ, Pataki C, McCracken JT. Second-generation antipsychotic medications in children and adolescents. J Child Adolesc Psychopharmacol 2004;14(3):372-94.

[56] Correll CU, Penzner JB, Parikh UH, Mughal T, Javed T, Carbon M, et al. Recognizing and monitoring adverse events of second-generation antipsychotics in children and adolescents. Child Adolesc Psychiatr Clin N Am 2006;15(1):177-206.

[57] McIntyre RS, Konarski JZ. Tolerability profiles of atypical antipsychotics in the treatment of bipolar disorder. J Clin Psychiatry 2005;66(Suppl 3):28-36.

[58] Wagstaff AJ, Easton J, Scott LJ. Intramuscular olanzapine. CNS Drugs 2005;19(2): 147-64.

[59] McIntyre RS, Jerrell JM. Metabolic and cardiovascular adverse events associated with antipsychotic treatment in children and adolescents. Arch Pediatr Adolesc Med 2008;162(10):929-34.

[60] Hansen E, Poole TA, Nguyen V, Lerner M, Wigal T, Shannon K, et al. Prevalence of ADHD symptoms in patients with congenital heart disease. Pediatr Int 2012;54(6): 838-43.

[61] Marino BS, Lipkin PH, Newburger JW, Peacock G, Gerdes M, Gaynor JW, et al. Neurodevelopmental outcomes in children with congenital heart disease: Evaluation and management. Circulation 2012;126(9):1143-72.

[62] Sistino JJ, Atz AM, Simpson KN, Ellis C, Ikonomidis JS, Bradley SM. The prevalence of attention-deficit/hyperactivity disorder following neonatal aortic arch repair. Cardiol Young 2014;25(4):663-9.

[63] Martinez-Raga J, Knecht C, Szerman N, Martinez MI. Risk of serious cardiovascular problems with medications for zttention-deficit hyperactivity disorder. CNS Drugs 2012;27(1):15-30.

[64] Shin JY, Roughead EE, Park BJ, Pratt NL. Cardiovascular safety of methylphenidate among children and young people with attention-deficit/hyperactivity disorder (ADHD): nationwide self controlled case series study. BMJ 2016;353:i2550.

[65] Cooper WO, Habel LA, Sox CM, Chan KA, Arbogast PG, Cheetham TC, et al. ADHD drugs and serious cardiovascular events in children and young adults. N Engl J Med 2011;365(20):1896-904.

[66] Schelleman H, Bilker WB, Strom BL, Kimmel SE, Newcomb C, Guevara JP, et al. Cardiovascular events and death in children exposed and unexposed to ADHD agents. Pediatrics 2011;127(6):1102-10.

[67] Winterstein AG, Gerhard T, Kubilis P, Saidi A, Linden S, Crystal S, et al. Cardiovascular safety of central nervous system stimulants in children and adolescents: population based cohort study. BMJ 2012;345:e4627.

[68] Jackson JW. The cardiovascular safety of methylphenidate. BMJ 2016;353:i2874.

Chapter 5

Mental health considerations in renal disease

Salma Malik, MD, Stephanie Kuntz, DO, Sumayya Ayaz, MD and Ahsan Nazeer*, MD

Child and Adolescent Psychiatry, Department of Psychiatry, Institute of Living, Hartford, Connecticut, United States of America and Child and Adolescent Psychiatry, Department of Psychiatry, Sidra Medicine, Doha, Qatar

Abstract

Mental health issues of persons with renal disease are considered in this discussion and include factors seen in renal transplantation, dialysis, and end-stage renal disease. The potential negative impact on the pediatric patient and the family can be considerable. Psychopharmacological considerations are reviewed that are unique to those with chronic renal disease. Problems of treatment adherence and barriers to non-adherence are also considered. Healthcare professionals should be aware of the mental health impacts that may arise in their patients with chronic renal disease and seek to address them to optimize the overall outcomes for the patient and family.

Introduction

In this discussion, we focus on mental health considerations in renal disease. Mental health issues in renal transplantation, dialysis, and end-stage renal disease (ESRD) are explored; these include common psychiatric disorders, cognitive difficulties, and quality of life experience of the patient and the caregiver. Treatment considerations are reviewed, including patient and family-centered care, psychopharmacological considerations, and family support. Pharmacokinetic and pharmacodynamics factors are explored, which are essential to understand while managing patients with chronic renal diseases. Compliance and medical adherence are also assessed.

* ***Correspondence***: Ahsan Nazeer, Division Chief, Child and Adolescent Psychiatry, Department of Psychiatry, Sidra Medicine, Doha, Qatar. Email: anazeer@sidra.org.

In: Behavioral Pediatrics
Editors: Donald E. Greydanus, Dilip R. Patel, Ahsan Nazeer et al.
ISBN: 979-8-88697-060-9

Impact on quality of life for the adolescents and families

End-stage renal disease (ESRD) is a significant risk factor for developing mental health problems in children and adolescents. Patients' day-to-day lives are significantly affected when they undergo life-saving procedures, either peritoneal dialysis or hemodialysis, for ongoing care. One study assessed the quality of life of patients with ESRD based on the emotional impact of interactions with individual providers, the emotional impact of the health system encounters, and the emotional impact of meaning-making (1). *Meaning-making* was defined as making sense of their illness experience and managing how it has been affecting their lives. Patients described emotions of "alienation, mistrust, abandonment, and isolation." They endorsed challenges, including lack of knowledge and lack of autonomy in making their day-to-day decisions, including what to eat and what not to eat (1). As negative life experiences can negatively affect the patient's prognosis, researchers have highlighted the need for early identification and provision of empathic care to the patients during this time (2).

In the pediatric population, procedures involved in managing end-stage renal disease (ESRD) significantly restrict the patient's physical and social wellbeing. Frequent hospitalizations lead to irregular school attendance, restriction of activities, and disruptions in social networking. Because of the increased psychological vulnerability, poor coping skills, and increased stress levels, adolescents are at risk of developing mental health problems; these include depression, anxiety, poor self-esteem, and hopelessness (3, 4). One study described the adolescent patient with ESRD as viewing their situation as a "loss or challenge" when compared to the older population with a similar diagnosis (5). Another study focused on the difficulty of integrating academic expectations and peer social support in patients who are managing invasive procedures. Researchers have noted significantly low quality of life in dimensions of energy-vitality, physical wellbeing, relationships with friends, and leisure activities.

The adolescent population was also susceptible to negative coping skills such as "avoidant behavior," which negated their ability to process the significance of their diagnoses and the need to be adherent to the treatment recommendations. Avoidant behaviors tended to occur in patients already diagnosed with an "emotional disorder," making those with comorbid psychiatric disorders even more vulnerable to the decrease in quality of life compared to a control group.

The quality of life experience of the caregiver

Another vulnerable population in managing ESRD is the caregiver, who can be a friend, spouse, parent, or adult sibling; these persons may also experience psychological ramifications and frustrations of this disorder (6). While caring for ESRD patients, caregivers play different roles, including ensuring compliance with the treatments, being an advocate, and being a translator for the available treatment options. The chronic nature of the ESRD treatment with associated complications, hospitalization, and visits for outpatients' care causes a high level of care burden in the caregivers (7). In the scientific literature, care burden is described as a level of stress and distress that caregivers endure while taking care of their loved ones (8). Increased care burden leads to decreased quality of life, depression, caregiver's burnout, and numerous social and financial challenges (9).

Due to the chronicity of renal disease, additional research was done to determine the long-term effects on the quality of life in the patient's caregivers (10, 11). Life factors that were found to be affected included dietary restrictions, reduced social activities, economic concerns, marital conflicts, sexual dysfunction, emotional stress, and anxiety. Male caregivers usually displayed a higher degree of care burden in this instance. Family members are susceptible to numerous burdens while trying to comprehend the treatment that their loved ones are going through (12). Thus, further evaluation of the system of care, and its ability to support the fundamental aspects of the patient's and caregiver's psychosocial challenges is warranted.

Common psychiatric disorders in adolescents with renal disease

Adolescence is a time of significant physical, psychological, social, and cognitive change as part of healthy development. Chronic health conditions, including chronic kidney disease (CKD) and ERSD during adolescence, significantly increases the risk of psychological, emotional, and behavioral disorders. Depression, anxiety, loss, and pain management issues are more prevalent in patients with renal disease as compared to the normal cohort (13). The prevalence of psychiatric disorders in adolescence with renal disease is different among different studies, which is partly explained by the variation in the study population and study methods. Most studies, however, indicate a high prevalence of psychiatric symptoms in this patient population, with one study reporting a prevalence as high as 50% (14). The prevalence is higher in patients with invasive treatment (i.e., dialysis or transplant) than the ones on conservative treatment.

Depression and other mood symptoms

Depression is one of the most prevalent psychiatric disorders in this population, second only to adjustment disorders (3). Research has found depressive symptoms in 30-35% of pediatric patients with CKD (3, 15). One study that focused on the factors that were negatively associated with depression identified maternal education, shorter stature, prior psychiatric diagnosis, less advanced CKD, longer duration of the disease, and history of transplant (16).

Several factors lead to increased susceptibility to depression in this population, and surprisingly, the severity of depression does not appear to be associated with the intensity of CKD. Patients with CKD often report increased levels of stress, feelings of hopelessness about their health, limitations on multiple aspects of their lives, and being a burden on their families. These patients present with poor self-esteem, negative self-image, and feelings of inferiority in relation to their peers as well as isolation. Along with psychosocial issues contributing to depression, numerous metabolic and neurochemical abnormalities can also lead to irritability, restlessness, insomnia and depressive symptoms; these include uremia, low levels of brain-derived neurotrophic factor (BDNF), and serotonin (17).

Children and adolescents with CKD also have growth retardation due to osteodystrophy and delayed puberty due to uremia. Also, patients undergoing hemodialysis develop multiple scars as well as disfiguring fistula/shunt; these, along with other changes, create a negative image of self, being different from others and feelings of alienation from the peers. The presence of depression is associated with worse long-term outcomes due to poor treatment adherence, neurocognitive impairments, and social functioning difficulties (18).

Despite its high prevalence, depression in this population is underdiagnosed and undertreated. One study focused on possible barriers to diagnosis and treatment of depression; these included lack of time to screen for depression, misconceptions among patients, caregivers, and providers regarding the need for depression treatment, and concerns about using psychotropic medications in CKD patients (19).

Because of the long-term morbidity associated with depression and chronic illness, it is recommended that the treatment team should engage the family and the patients in actively screening for depression, discussing the importance of treatment, conducting structured interviews, and making an appropriate referral to mental health providers.

Anxiety disorders

While anxiety symptoms in pediatric patients with chronic medical illness range from 7 to 40%, anxiety disorders in pediatric renal disease have been understudied; however, a few authors have found elevated symptoms of separation anxiety disorder in the range of 22-65% (20, 21). One study focused on the level of anxiety in children with CKD using the State-Trait Anxiety Inventory (STAI) (22). Based on STAI, two levels of anxiety were reported; these were *state anxiety*, i.e., transitory emotional condition, and *trait anxiety*, defined as a personality trait with a disposition to perceive situations as threatening.

The study found a significantly higher level of anxiety-state among 8–12-year-old children undergoing hemodialysis (HD) (22). The increased level of anxiety among patients on hemodialysis could be due to the nature of the treatment as the process of going through the hemodialysis sessions can create acute feelings of anxiety (23). The level of anxiety among 13–18-year-old adolescents, both anxiety-state and anxiety-trait, was also significantly higher in patients undergoing hemodialysis. In adolescents undergoing hemodialysis, there was a correlation between the anxiety-state, duration of the disease, and the number of hospitalizations. Adolescents with peritoneal dialysis who were in mainstream education had higher anxiety-state and anxiety-trait levels than homeschooled patients (22).

Cognitive and learning difficulties

Another common finding in children with CKD is cognitive and learning difficulties. While most children with mild to moderate CKD have no major neurocognitive deficits, a significant percentage did show cognitive dysfunction; the most common was learning difficulties in reading, attention, memory, and inhibitory control (24). Also, ESDR has been identified as a risk factor for lower intelligence quotient (IQ) and poor academic performance. The prevalence of cognitive and learning difficulties is higher in younger children with longer duration of ESRD (25, 26).

Psychopharmacology considerations

Non-adherence is a significant concern in children and adolescents with chronic renal disease. According to the research data, only about 25-50% of the youth with chronic illness adhere to chronic treatment (27-31). Treatment of CKD/ERSD is complex and involves invasive procedures, lifestyle change, dietary modification, routine visits to the doctor's office, frequent hospitalizations and the need to take multiple classes of oral medications; these include immunosuppressive agents, corticosteroids, and other medications to treat comorbid medical conditions.

Adherence to such a complex treatment regimen can be challenging for the children and their families. For adolescents, adherence to treatment becomes more difficult as they begin to develop a sense of self, start seeking autonomy from caregivers, and focus on the physical appearance as well as peer relationships. Psychiatric disorders, particularly depression, also negatively impact treatment adherence. Another major factor that can impact treatment adherence is family dynamics and caretaker burdens. One study found that compliance was positively associated with the mother's education level and higher household income (32).

Non-adherence leads to serious medical consequences, and it is well established that non-adherence to immunosuppressant medications is a major contributing factor to graft rejection in young people (33). Hence, identifying adherence barriers and proper interventions is essential to better long-term outcomes. Some of the common barriers to adherence are simply forgetting to take the medication, time management, medication side effects, inconvenience of taking numerous doses of medications per day, limited understanding of the long-term consequences, and time management problems (34).

Pharmacodynamics and pharmacokinetics

CKD/ESDR and dialysis affect almost all aspects of pharmacokinetics and pharmacodynamics of most commonly used drugs, as listed in Table 1 (35-39). Special considerations should be taken when prescribing medications to CKD patients. Inappropriate dose adjustments may lead to sub- or supra-therapeutic concentrations predisposing the patient to either therapeutic failure or adverse drug reactions. Since the research is limited to the pediatric CKD population, prescribing an appropriate dose requires knowledge of specific pharmacokinetic alterations. In rare circumstances, in the absence of good options, dosing advice from the adult population can be extrapolated in the pediatric CKD population (40, 41).

Renal considerations for psychotropic agents

Managing the dosing of psychotropic medications is one of the main challenges while treating psychiatric disorders in individuals with CKD. For instance, in the setting of poor metabolism or excretion in advanced renal disease, the patient may require reduced dosing based on blood urea nitrogen (BUN) and creatinine measurements. Using the example of antidepressants, as depression is a highly prevalent comorbid disorder in renal disease, medications that are metabolized through the renal system are to be monitored in dosing based on the medication's half-life and its clearance after oral intake (42). Table 2 lists the medications that need close monitoring during their use in CKD.

Table 1. Drug absorption, distribution, metabolism and excretion (35-39)

Drug absorption and bioavailability	Increased gastric alkalinity, changes in gastrin level, nausea, vomiting, and delayed gastric emptying
	Uremia cause decrease gastrointestinal absorption of drugs and alters first-pass hepatic metabolism
	Changes in the first-pass metabolism can cause increased bioavailability leading to increase chances of drug toxicity
Drug distribution	Impaired kidney functions alter the volume of distribution
	Edema and ascites increase the volume of distribution of water-soluble drugs, which can lead to therapeutic failure due to low plasma level
	Dehydration and muscle wasting decrease the volume of distribution leading to high plasma levels and toxicity
	Renal failure may increase or decrease protein binding. Reduced plasma protein binding may result in freer drug available at the site of drug action/toxicity
Drug metabolism	Impaired kidney functions slow the rate of phase-I metabolism- reduction, oxidation, and hydrolysis
	In dialysis patients, drug metabolism is unpredictable
	Most drugs undergo hepatic metabolism to less active, compounds that require intact renal function for elimination. Impaired renal function may lead to accumulation of active or toxic metabolites from parent compounds
Drug excretion	In end-stage renal disease (ESRD), drugs may accumulate due to impaired glomerular filtration, decreased renal tubular secretion, and impaired renal epithelial cell metabolism. This can lead to increased toxicity.

Table 2. Psychotropics that must be monitored in the setting of impaired renal function

Class	Medications
Anticonvulsants	Gabapentin, Lamotrigine, Oxcarbazepine, Pregabalin, Topiramate, Lithium
Antidepressants	Bupropion, Desvenlafaxine, Duloxetine, Fluvoxamine, MAOIs, Mirtazapine, Paroxetine, TCAs, Venlafaxine
Benzodiazepines	All
Second Generation Antipsychotics (SGAs):	Brexpiprazole, Cariprazine, Lurasidone, Paliperidone, Risperidone
Others	Buspirone

Special considerations: Dialysis patients

Adjusting the medication dosages in patients on dialysis poses another set of challenges. A renal patient may undergo different forms of dialysis: hemodialysis, peritoneal dialysis, and continuous arteriovenous or venovenous hemofiltration; however, the type of dialysis used will also determine post-dialysis blood levels of a specific drug. For instance, hemodialysis is much more efficient than peritoneal dialysis in its ability to remove drugs from the body. Within each type of dialysis, dosing should consider the molecular weight of the drug being used, as well as identifying whether the type of filter being used affects different molecular weights in their filtration process (43).

The total volume of the fluid in the patient's body also affects the amount of the drug molecules that will be filtered out of the body. If the drug attaches itself to a serum protein, it is less likely to be filtered out of the body. Clinically, the three most important variables that influence the removal of the medication by continuous renal replacement therapies (CRRT) are the volume of distribution, binding to serum protein, and molecular size of the drug. For medications that are removed by dialysis, a marked lowering of blood levels of that medication will occur post-dialysis, in which case the need for a supplemental dose should be considered.

Conclusion

Patients suffering from chronic renal diseases have numerous implications on their psychosocial wellbeing. The presence of renal disease increases the risk of psychological, emotional, and behavioral disorders. In addition to the burdens on these individuals, there is an enormous emotional and financial impact on the family members. Combined, the above factors can result in numerous complications in family functioning and the possibility of poor long-term medical outcomes. As psychiatric illnesses are common in patients with chronic renal diseases, clinicians treating these patients have to consider the biopsychosocial approach while addressing medical illnesses. Additionally, there are psychopharmacological considerations such as pharmacokinetic and pharmacodynamic factors that are unique to patients who have a preexisting renal disease that must be kept in mind. Adherence to the treatment is of paramount importance for a good overall prognosis, and barriers to non-adherence also need to be considered.

References

[1] O'Hare AM, Richards C, Szarka J, McFarland LV, Showalter W, Vig EK, et al. Emotional impact of illness and care on patients with advanced kidney disease. Clin J Am Soc Nephrol 2018;13(7):1022-9.

[2] Kimmel PL, Patel SS. Quality of life in patients with chronic kidney disease: focus on end-stage renal disease treated with hemodialysis. Semin Nephrol 2006;26(1):68-79.

[3] Berney-Martinet S, Key F, Bell L, Lépine S, Clermont MJ, Fombonne E. Psychological profile of adolescents with a kidney transplant. Pediatr Transplant 2009;13(6):701-10.

[4] Kilicoglu AG, Bahali K, Canpolat N, Bilgic A, Mutlu C, Yalçın Ö, et al. Impact of end-stage renal disease on psychological status and quality of life. Pediatr Int 2016; 58(12):1316-21.

[5] Laudański K, Nowak Z, Niemczyk S. Age-related differences in the quality of life in end-stage renal disease in patients enrolled in hemodialysis or continuous peritoneal dialysis. Med Sci Monit 2013;19:378-85.

[6] Abbasi A, Asayesh H, Rahmani H, Shariati A, Hosseini S, Rouhi G. The burden on caregivers from hemodialysis patients and related factors. J Res Development Nurs Midwifery 2011;8(1):26-33.

[7] Suri RS, Larive B, Hall Y, Kimmel PL, Kliger AS, Levin N, et al. Effects of frequent hemodialysis on perceived caregiver burden in the Frequent Hemodialysis Network trials. Clin J Am Soc Nephrol 2014;9(5):936-42.

[8] Sajadi SAM, Ebadi AP, Moradian STP. Quality of life among family caregivers of patients on hemodialysis and its relevant factors: A systematic review. Int J Community Based Nurs Midwifery 2017;5(3):206-18.

[9] Nogueira PC, Rabeh SAN, Caliri MHL, Dantas RAS, Haas VJ. Burden of care and its impact on health-related quality of life of caregivers of individuals with spinal cord injury. Revista Latino-Americana de Enfermagem 2012;20(6):1048-56.

[10] Belasco AG, Sesso R. Burden and quality of life of caregivers for hemodialysis patients. Am J Kidney Dis 2002;39(4):805-12.

[11] Jafari H, Ebrahimi A, Aghaei A, Khatony A. The relationship between care burden and quality of life in caregivers of hemodialysis patients. BMC Nephrol 2018;19(1):321. doi: 10.1186/s12882-018-1120-1..

[12] Baek HS, Park KS, Ha IS, Kang HG, Cheong HI, Park YS, et al. impact of end-stage renal disease in children on their parents. Nephrology (Carlton) 2018;23(8):764-70.

[13] Palmer S, Vecchio M, Craig JC, Tonelli M, Johnson DW, Nicolucci A, et al. prevalence of depression in chronic kidney disease: Systematic review and meta-analysis of observational studies. Kidney Int 2013;84(1):179-91.

[14] Bakr A, Amr M, Sarhan A, Hammad A, Ragab M, El-Refaey A, et al. Psychiatric disorders in children with chronic renal failure. Pediatr Nephrol 2007;22(1):128-31.

[15] Kogon AJ, Vander Stoep A, Weiss NS, Smith J, Flynn JT, McCauley E. Depression and its associated factors in pediatric chronic kidney disease. Pediatr Nephrol 2013;28(9): 1855-61.

[16] Kraenbring MM, Zelikovsky N, Meyers KEC. Medication adherence in pediatric renal transplant patients: The role of family functioning and parent health locus of control. Pediatr Transplant 2019;23(2):e13346.

[17] Marciano RC, Soares CM, Diniz JS, Lima EM, Silva JM, Canhestro MR, et al. Mental disorders and quality of life in pediatric patients with chronic kidney disease. J Bras Nefrol 2010;32(3):316-22.

[18] Kogon AJ, Matheson MB, Flynn JT, Gerson AC, Warady BA, Furth SL, et al. Depressive symptoms in children with chronic kidney disease. J Pediatr 2016;168:164-70.

[19] Hedayati SS, Yalamanchili V, Finkelstein FO. A practical approach to the treatment of depression in patients with chronic kidney disease and end-stage renal disease. Kidney Int 2012;81(3):247-55.

[20] DeSousa DA, Salum GA, Isolan LR, Manfro GG. Sensitivity and specificity of the screen for child anxiety related emotional disorders (SCARED): A community-based study. Child Psychiatry Hum Dev 2013;44(3):391-9.

[21] Fukunishi I, Kudo H. Psychiatric problems of pediatric end-stage renal failure. Gen Hosp Psychiatry 1995;17(1):32-6.

[22] Kiliś-Pstrusińska K, Medyńska A, Adamczak P, Bałasz- Chmielewska I, Grenda R, Kluska-Jóźwiak A, et al. Anxiety in children and adolescents with chronic kidney disease - Multicenter National Study Results. Kidney Blood Press Res 2013;37(6):579-87.

[23] Moreira JM, Bouissou Morais Soares CM, Teixeira AL, Simoes ESAC, Kummer AM. Anxiety, depression, resilience and quality of life in children and adolescents with pre-dialysis chronic kidney disease. Pediatr Nephrol 2015;30(12):2153-62.

[24] Ruebner RL, Laney N, Kim JY, Hartung EA, Hooper SR, Radcliffe J, et al. Neurocognitive dysfunction in children, adolescents, and young adults With CKD. Am J Kidney Dis 2016; 67(4):567-75.

[25] Gipson DS, Wetherington CE, Duquette PJ, Hooper SR. The nervous system and chronic kidney disease in children. Pediatr Nephrol 2004;19(8):832-9.

[26] Gerson A, Butler R, Moxey-Mims M, Wentz A, Shinnar S, Lande M, et al. Neurocognitive outcomes in children with chronic kidney disease: Current findings and contemporary endeavors. Ment Retard Dev Disabil Res Rev 2006;12(3):208-15.

[27] Bender B, Wamboldt F, O'Connor SL, Rand C, Szefler S, Milgrom H, et al. Measurement of children's asthma medication adherence by self report, mother report, canister weight, and Doser CT. Ann Allergy Asthma Immunol 2000;85(5):416-21.

[28] Dean AJ, Walters J, Hall A. A systematic review of interventions to enhance medication adherence in children and adolescents with chronic illness. Arch Dis Child 2010;95(9): 717-23.

[29] McGrady ME, Hommel KA. Medication adherence and health care utilization in pediatric chronic illness: a systematic review. Pediatrics 2013;132(4):730-40.

[30] Murphy DA, Wilson CM, Durako SJ, Muenz LR, Belzer M. Antiretroviral medication adherence among the REACH HIV-infected adolescent cohort in the USA. AIDS Care 2001;13(1):27-40.

[31] Robin DiMatteo M, Giordani PJ, Lepper HS, Croghan TW. Patient adherence and medical treatment outcomes. Med Care 2002;40(9):794-811.

[32] Ramay BM, Cerón A, Méndez-Alburez LP, Lou-Meda R. Factors associated to acceptable treatment adherence among children with chronic kidney disease in Guatemala. PloS One 2017;12(10):e01866 44-e.

[33] Rianthavorn P, Ettenger RB. Medication non-adherence in the adolescent renal transplant recipient: A clinician's viewpoint. Pediatr Transplant 2005;9(3):398-407.

[34] Simons LE, McCormick ML, Mee LL, Blount RL. Parent and patient perspectives on barriers to medication adherence in adolescent transplant recipients. Pediatr Transplantat 2009;13(3):338-47.

[35] Cohen LM, Tessier EG, Germain MJ, Levy NB. Update on psychotropic medication use in renal disease. Psychosomatics 2004;45(1):34-48.

[36] Matzke GR, Frye RF. Drug administration in patients with renal insufficiency minimising renal and extrarenal toxicity. Drug Saf 1997;16(3):205-31.

[37] Naud J, Michaud J, Boisvert C, Desbiens K, Leblond FA, Mitchell A, et al. Down-regulation of intestinal drug transporters in chronic renal failure in rats. J Pharmacol Exp Ther 2007;320(3):978-85.

[38] Sun H, Frassetto L, Benet LZ. Effects of renal failure on drug transport and metabolism. Pharmacol Ther 2006;109(1-2):1-11.

[39] Wilde MI, Benfield P. Tianeptine. A review of its pharmacodynamic and pharmacokinetic properties, and therapeutic efficacy in depression and coexisting anxiety and depression. Drugs 1995;49(3):411-39.

[40] Vasylyeva TL, Singh R, Sheehan C, Chennasamudram SP, Hernandez AP. Self-reported adherence to medications in a pediatric renal clinic: psychological aspects. PLoS One 2013; 8(7):e69060-e.

[41] Schijvens AM, de Wildt SN, Schreuder MF. Pharmacokinetics in children with chronic kidney disease. Pediatr Nephrol 2020;35(7):1153-72.

[42] Nagler EV, Webster AC, Vanholder R, Zoccali C. Antidepressants for depression in stage 3–5 chronic kidney disease: a systematic review of pharmacokinetics, efficacy and safety with recommendations by European Renal Best Practice (ERBP). Nephrol Dial Transplant 2012;27(10):3736-45.

[43] McIntyre RS, Baghdady NT, Banik S, Swartz SA. The use of psychotropic drugs in patients with impaired renal function. Prim Psychiatry 2008;15(1):73-88.

Chapter 6

The pediatric liver: Mental health considerations

Christina Helen Vlahos*, PhD
and Muhammad Waqar Azeem, MD
Department of Psychiatry, Weil Cornell Medical School, Doha, Qatar

Abstract

Mental health issues regarding pediatric persons with liver disease are discussed. Considerable research has been accomplished with respect to liver transplantation that includes the key issue of medical adherence; considerations in this regard include psychological factors influencing adherence, identifying barriers to adherence, interventions to improve adherence, transition of care and adherence, measuring medical adherence, and the importance of pre-operative psychological screening. Issues of post-operative neuropsychological outcomes and hepatic encephalopathy are also reviewed. Cognitive dysfunction in those with liver disease and liver transplantation is also considered as well as such concerns as medical trauma and post-traumatic stress disorder. Finally, mental health issues are also presented regarding children with Wilson's disease and hepatitis C virus infection as well as metabolic side-effects of psychotropic medications.

Introduction

The liver is a vital, complicated organ with many different functions. As a result, liver disease can have a profound impact on health, with liver failure potentially being fatal. Infants, children, and adolescents are unlikely to suffer from certain types of liver disease that are common in adults such as those resulting from chronic alcohol abuse, cancer or viruses that are frequently transmitted through behaviors uncommon to children; however, there remains a wide range of factors that result in childhood liver disease. In many cases, the underlying cause is the result of an interplay between inherited, genetic and environmental factors. Examples include but are not limited to Alagille syndrome, alpha -1 antitrypsin deficiency, Gilbert's syndrome, and Wilson's disease.

* ***Correspondence***: Christina Helen Vlahos PhD, Assistant Professor, Department of Psychiatry, Weil Cornell Medical School, Doha, Qatar. Email: cvlahos@sidra.org.

In: Behavioral Pediatrics
Editors: Donald E. Greydanus, Dilip R. Patel, Ahsan Nazeer et al.
ISBN: 979-8-88697-060-9

The non-alcoholic fatty liver disease is a condition in which genetic and environmental factors interact resulting in fat building up around the liver. Other times, the liver may be impacted by autoimmune or chronic conditions, such as cystic fibrosis, lupus erythematosus or autoimmune liver disease. The liver can also be impacted by problems in the functioning of other systems or organs, such as poor blood supply or obstruction of bile flowing out of the liver. In some cases, the cause is due to an environmental factor, such as toxic levels of drugs or chemical substances. Liver disease can also be the result of a viral infection and subsequent acute or chronic complications and inflammation (hepatitis A, B, or C virus), although, as mentioned above, these are less common in children (1).

Given how heterogeneous the causes and manifestations of liver disease can be, all conditions impacting the liver cannot be grouped and examined together. In the case of some conditions, the consequences for mental health have been researched, whereas, in the case of other, rare conditions, the scientific literature is lacking. Liver disease can directly impact the brain and thus behavior, resulting in a neurocognitive or psychiatric condition. However, mental health can also be indirectly impacted as is often the case with both acute medical problems and chronic illness. Pediatric patients with liver disease share all of the common challenges documented in children with chronic health problems; these include negatively impacted health-related quality of life, need for psychological support, and a need for a smooth transition to adult care. On the flip side, liver disease may also be the result rather than the cause of mental health problems, when the liver is impacted by psychotropic medication prescribed to treat mental illness.

Large-scale meta-analytic studies have been conducted on pediatric patients with a wide range of chronic health problems ranging from cancer, cerebral palsy, diabetes and asthma to inflammatory bowel disease, HIV infection, sickle cell disease and spinal bifida. They found that, overall, these children have lower levels of physical, academic, and social functioning, with physical functioning impacted the most, and social functioning impacted the least. Notably, there was considerable variability in these findings when comparing different diseases (2). Elevated behavior problems were also found, mainly for internalizing problems, social problems, attention problems, and thought problems, rather than externalizing problems (3).

These children were also found to have lower rates of finishing higher education and achieving adult milestones – such as finding employment, leaving the parental home, marrying and becoming parents in comparison to healthy and nondisabled peers. This was particularly the case for individuals with neurological illness and sensory impairment (4). This line of research can prove useful when identifying areas in need of intervention and support in children with liver disease. Although these studies were conducted with large, mixed samples that did not include patients with liver disease, there are several studies that have replicated these findings in children and adolescents who present with various liver conditions.

Chronic liver conditions can sometimes result in cirrhosis of the liver, in which case the liver does not function properly due to long-term damage. A liver transplant may be considered necessary with an average 5-year survival rate of 85% in cases in which a chronic liver disease has not responded to treatment and is negatively impacting the child's quality of life, or in cases of acute liver failure. These children will require medication and monitoring for the rest of their lives to prevent them from rejecting the transplanted organ (1).

Mental health issues in liver transplantation

Children who have been subjected to liver transplantation are one of the most widely studied populations of pediatric liver disease with regard to mental health research. One of the main reasons for this is certain unique challenges that are of particular importance. Also, liver transplantations are a last resort, indicating a chronic and most likely deteriorating experience with the illness. Modern developments in medicine have allowed for the option of a live donor, increasing the frequency of these procedures. Adherence to post-operative medication regimens as well as medical advice are crucial in these cases, as poor adherence can lead to the organ being rejected and the patient being in need of a new one. Further, there is research to suggest that liver transplantations can impact the child's cognitive abilities, both acutely, as in hepatic encephalopathy, or in the long-run.

Medical Adherence in Pediatric Liver Transplant Recipients

Following discharge, patients who have undergone a liver transplantation surgical procedure are required to take medications and follow medical guidelines for care. Medications are mainly immunosuppressants, such as azathioprine and tacrolimus, to prevent the immune system from rejecting the transplant. Medical guidelines include keeping up with physician visits, where liver enzymes and markers of inflammatory activity in the liver, such as alanine transaminase, can be routinely monitored. This allows for medication and dosage adjustment. Other medical guidelines include living a healthy lifestyle, and avoiding medications, food and drink that burden the liver.

Adherence to prescribed medications and medical guidelines for care following the transplant are imperative for maintaining the organ; failure to adhere can result in organ failure at any point in the patient's lifetime. However, adherence is not as much a medical challenge, as it is a behavioral one; thus, this falls within the scope of practice of mental health professionals, specializing in behavioral medicine. The issue of medical adherence has been extensively researched and continues to be a top challenge for both children and adults to date. However, in the case of organ transplantation, non-adherence can have especially severe consequences, as non-adherence is the leading cause of morbidity in this population.

Researchers have investigated several different aspects of the adherence challenge in an effort to identify common barriers to adherence, effective interventions to improve adherence, the ideal age to transfer responsibility for taking medication from the parent to the child, developmental milestones at which vulnerability for non-adherence increases, and best practices for measuring adherence to identify children with poor adherence.

Various issues regarding adherence are now considered: psychological factors influencing adherence, identifying barriers to adherence, interventions to improve adherence, transition of care and adherence, measuring medical adherence, and the importance of pre-operative psychological screening.

Psychological factors influencing adherence

Unfortunately, post – operative poor adherence is a common problem, with prevalence estimates of pediatric transplant patients being non-adherent at some point in time ranging from 25% to 70%, depending on the operational definition of non-adherence and method of measurement. Several studies have identified problems in psychosocial functioning that are related to adherence issues; these include symptoms of depression and anxiety, poor quality of life, and behavior problems. This finding has been replicated across all populations of children with chronic illnesses, but also has been found to be specific to pediatric liver transplant recipients.

However, as this research is correlational, there is bidirectional ambiguity and it is difficult to determine whether poor adherence is the result or the cause of poor psychosocial adjustment. Indeed, a child with a poorly managed disease who is actively symptomatic is likely to experience symptoms of depression and anxiety, or poor quality of life, that potentially leads to a vicious cycle of further non-adherence (6, 7). Interestingly, one study found depressive symptoms and adherence to be mediated by hope and illness-related uncertainty (8).

Identifying barriers to adherence

One study aimed to prospectively validate the Parent and Adolescent Medication Barrier Scales (PMBS and AMBS) in a group of adolescents who had received organ transplantations (including kidney, liver, heart and lungs transplantations) and their parents (9). These researchers administered the measure once at least four months post-operatively for the purpose of identifying barriers (Time 1), and a second time after 18 months, for the purpose of examining barrier stability over time (Time 2). This study compared perceived barriers, perceived adherence, and clinical outcomes (i.e., rejection episodes, hospitalizations, and mortality) (9).

Interestingly, they found an association between clinical outcomes and reported ingestion issues, according to both the parents and the adolescents. According to the parents and adolescents, respectively, the study examined which perceived barriers identified at Time 1 were significantly correlated with perceived poor adherence or poor clinical outcomes at Time 2. For the parents, they identified (9):

1. "My child does not like other people to notice him/her taking the medication," "My child believes the medication has too many side effects;"
2. "My child is forgetful and doesn't remember to take his/her medication every time;"
3. "My child is not very organized about when and how s/he takes his/her medication;"
4. "I am not always there to remind my child to take his/her medication;"
5. "My child has a hard time swallowing the medicine;"
6. "My child does not like how the medication tastes;"
7. "My child relies on me to remind him/her when to take his/her medication."

For the adolescents, they identified (9):

1. "I don't want to take medicine at school;"
2. "I do not want other people to notice me taking the medicine;"
3. "I do not like what the medicine does to my appearance;"
4. "I am tired of taking medicine;"
5. "I am tired of living with a medical condition;"
6. "Sometimes I don't realize when I run out of pills;"
7. "I believe that the medicine is hard to swallow;"
8. "I believe that I have too many pills to take;"
9. "I believe the medicine has too many side effects."

Another study found that adolescents with specific barriers to adherence will continue to experience similar levels of those barriers in the absence of targeted intervention (10).

Interventions for improving adherence

In studies using the PMBS and AMBS with this population, the "*cognitive issues*" subscale were among the most frequently endorsed barriers at both time points; also, many of the identified barriers seem to be subject to interventions involving behavioral management. Thus, cognitive behavioral therapy (CBT) is indicated with this population. However, evidence-based manualized intervention strategies have not been developed and adequately tested with pediatric solid organ transplant recipients; thus, current clinical practice, in the absence of empirically supported treatments, is for nonadherence in pediatric solid organ recipients (10). Research has shown that transition of responsibility for medication taking is commonly shifted to the child around the age of 12 in the pediatric liver population, and interventions should target the child's increasing role beginning in early adolescence (11).

The transition of care and medical adherence

One developmental milestone that seems to result in vulnerability to compromised adherence practices is the period of transition of adolescents followed in specialized pediatric clinics to adult hepatology care. Common practice is for patients to be transferred to adult care at the age of 18 if stable; patients who are not stable may sometimes remain in pediatric care until stabilized. Vulnerability for poor adherence and an increase in drop-out rates during this period is well-established across the pediatric chronic illness literature in general; however, studies have also examined this in the pediatric liver recipient population (12).

In this population, it was found that medical outcomes deteriorated when patients transitioned. For example, the mortality rates were found to be significantly higher among patients who were in the process of transition in comparison to those cared for exclusively in pediatric or adult care. However, these findings must be interpreted with caution. Patients who died in the pediatric service would not have been included in the study. Further, such findings could be because the transition coincides with adolescence, and adolescents have repeatedly been found to be less adherent than children. Another explanation may be the fact that non-adherence is treated more aggressively in pediatrics. Several checklists for determining patient readiness for transition have been developed and can be utilized for early detection of problems or weaknesses for improvement.

Measuring medication adherence

A standard objective measure for medication adherence in this population is to combine the consecutive measurements of tacrolimus blood levels performed in clinic visits and calculate the standard deviation (SD) of these measurements. A larger SD is indicative of variations in blood levels, showing lack of consistency in taking the medication.

Other studies have used MEMS™ caps, an electronic monitoring system inserted into the medication bottle's cap via microchip which records bottle opening. However, there are several limitations to this approach, as patients might open the bottle but not take the medication as prescribed, lose or fail to mail in their empty bottles, or the device's batteries might fail.

Finally, studies often also make use of subjective measures of adherence, such as medication logs or self-report questionnaires; however, these measures have been found to fail to predict medical outcomes, including a number of transplant-related hospitalizations and number of inpatient days, as well as number of biopsies or number of biopsy-proven rejection episodes (11).

The importance of pre-operative psychological screening

An increasing number of studies argue for the need of pre-operative screening to predict post-transplant outcomes. Psychosocial screening can contribute to early identification of barriers to adherence, allowing for individually tailored interventions to improve the likelihood of adherence. More importantly, however, psychological screening can be used to ensure appropriate organ allocation. Supply of organs is limited, and some argue that allocation of organs from cadaver donors should take into consideration the likelihood of future organ rejection – thus, turning appropriate pre-operative screening into an issue with ethical, apart from practical, ramifications.

However, the utility of psychological and neurocognitive factors as predictors of post-operative outcome remains unclear. and despite the fact that decisions for organ allocation take into consideration psychosocial evaluations, guidelines for these are loosely defined, with no absolute contraindications (13). Based on statistical analysis, some studies have recommended specific cutoff scores for providers to screen for patients at risk for a poor medication outcome (14).

Post-operative neuropsychological outcomes and hepatic encephalopathy

A significant concern in children and adolescents undergoing liver transplant surgery is the body of evidence suggesting chronic liver disease and liver transplantation can have a negative impact on the child's cognitive functioning. Hepatic encephalopathy post-surgery is also a common concern and is difficult to evaluate when mild, even when clinically suspected. Neuropsychological assessment and biomarkers, such as relationships between brain magnetic resonance (MR) spectroscopy metabolites and biochemical markers of encephalopathy, have been suggested for diagnosis in this arena (15).

One study compared a sample of children who were at least two years post-liver transplantation to a matched sample of children with cystic fibrosis on their performance on a neuropsychological battery; this included widely used measures of intellectual functioning, academic achievement, language, visual-motor perception, and learning as well as memory (16). Pediatric liver transplant patients were found to have a significantly lower performance on measures of verbal intelligence quotient (IQ), a measure of language, word memory, and visual memory (16). Therefore, a negative effect of liver disease on cognitive development was found above and beyond the effect of having a chronic, life-threatening disease (16).

It is important to note, however, that most of the children in this sample had undergone the transplant before the age of two, which might result in a more significantly impacted cognitive development (16). This study was a replication of an earlier study, which found similar results (17). There were, however, slight differences, as the previous study found liver transplant patients to have lower non-verbal intelligence and visual-spatial performance, a finding that was not replicated in the second study.

Another study reviewed 19 eligible studies on post-operative cognitive deficits (POCD) in adults who had been subjected to liver transplantations (18). It is important to note that these results cannot be generalized to the pediatric population; this is because pediatric liver disease is often of a different etiology, progression, as well as manifestation, and they are going through cognitive development at the same time (18). However, this study identified certain signs of POCD that may be useful to detect in children; these included postoperative delirium, fine motor skills impairment, a deficit of selective attention, visuospatial short- and long-term memory, language impairment, sleep disturbance, and somnolence that is not due to drug effects (18). Identifying and reversing, if possible, mild hepatic encephalopathy before surgery is indicated for a better postoperative outcome.

Executive functions are a group of cognitive abilities including organizing, sequencing, planning, inhibiting inappropriate responses, and remembering tasks that must be done in the future. These functions are grouped together as they are interdependent and mainly localized in the prefrontal cortex. By default, medication adherence is largely dependent on these skills, and patients who suffer from deficits in executive functioning are also found to struggle with adherence. Adolescents and young adults who are solid organ transplant recipients have been found to present with significant executive dysfunction when compared on an executive functioning checklist (i.e., Behavior Rating Inventory of Executive Function - BRIEF) to a normative sample; also, these patients with lower scores have been found to identify tasks with a high cognitive demand as barriers to adherence (19).

The emotional well-being of the pediatric transplant patient: Trauma, family stress, health-related quality of life, and the importance of psychological support

Liver disease leading up to the need for liver transplantation is a serious, life-threatening condition that profoundly impacts these patients and his or her family. Either the condition is chronic or acute, the experience is most times traumatic, and, as such, can result in post-traumatic stress disorder (PTSD). As psychological trauma and interventions for PTSD is a well-research topic in the mental health literature, one can turn to a plethora of studies to gain a better understanding. However, children who suffer from acute or chronic medical conditions are vulnerable to special, associated trauma and its psychological effects collectively termed *medical traumatic stress*. According to the National Child Traumatic Stress Network, "pediatric, medical traumatic stress refers to a set of psychological and physiological responses of children and their families to pain, injury, serious illness, medical procedures, and invasive or frightening treatment experiences (20)."

In a study examining PTSD in pediatric liver transplant patients, a group of children and adolescents 7-16 years old who had undergone liver transplantation were interviewed using the Child Post-Traumatic Stress Reaction Index (21). Scores were compared to a pediatric sample with a chronic, life-threatening illness, and also with a pediatric group who had undergone a surgical procedure. Transplant patients were found to score significantly higher on post-traumatic stress symptoms intensity in comparison to both groups (21).

Unfortunately, the pediatric patient is not the only one who suffers emotionally as a result of liver disease and transplantation. A longitudinal, descriptive study evaluated mothers of children undergoing transplants at the time of the surgery (both at hospital admission, and at discharge), and then again at least five years post-transplantation (22). The mothers were asked to complete measures of family stress, personal stress, coping, and adaptation; parent uncertainty was also measured pre-transplantation. Maternal stress levels were found to go down, particularly confusion, anger, anxiety, and vigor. Medical coping improved, as there was an improvement in understanding medical communication; maintaining social support also improved. Pre-transplantation family stress, anger, and confusion were related to poorer family adaptation in this study (22).

Multidisciplinary team

A single liver transplantation center in Hanover, Germany, set the stage for assembling a multidisciplinary team and supporting children undergoing liver transplantation procedure and their families (23). After 20 years of experience with liver transplants, they published a qualitative, descriptive paper detailing the evolution of this professional network that consisted of a hospital chaplain and nursery teacher in the early stages, until a social worker and clinical psychologist were recruited for this team (23).

The published paper provides information on the services provided, including evaluation and preparation of the family, support during the acute and intensive care period as well as the rehabilitation period. Factors contributing to a good psychological adaptation were identified as:

1. "The transplantation is foreseeable for the parents;"
2. "the child knows at least that a "surgery" will be done;"
3. "the child feels secure with the parents;"
4. "the parents were able to cope with feelings of guilt and anxiety;"
5. "there is good support from spouse and family;"
6. "there are a stable family and housing background;" and
7. "experienced staff, who are not continuously overworked, are available" (23).

Health-related quality of life (HRQoL)

Another important factor to consider when reviewing the well-being of this population is health-related quality of life. "Health-related quality of life (HRQoL) is a multi-dimensional concept reflecting the influence of the disease and its treatment on an individual's subjective assessment of his or her psychological functioning and emotional well-being" (7). HRQoL can be broken down into components, such as physical, psychological, social, family, or general well-being; these can be impacted by different factors and to different degrees by symptoms as well as severity of liver disease.

One study found that after controlling for other effects, persons with a higher pre-transplant severity score (Model for End-stage Liver Disease or MELD score) had better post-transplant physical HRQoL (24). However, the MELD score was not correlated with postoperative mental HRQoL (24). Another study examined prospective predictors for three important HRQoL domains in adolescents undergoing liver transplant surgery, namely physical functioning, mental health, and general health perceptions (25). They found modifiable factors predicted future HRQoL; these included adherence behaviors, income, and family conflict (25). The study concluded, "Thus, while medical issues are likely to influence HRQOL and should be addressed, behavioral characteristics may be better indicators of risk for poor future HRQOL and should also be targeted for intervention (25)."

A critical review of the 11 published research studies assessing HRQoL in children and adolescents after liver transplantation found that while there was a trend for poorer HRQoL compared to the healthy population, HRQoL was better post-transplantation compared to other chronic illness populations (26). Several methodological limitations were identified in these studies, one major one being that they relied exclusively on self –report (26). HRQoL is, by default, a subjective concept, which relates to individual factors such as personality, expectations, and interpretations. Even more of concern is that fact that such studies sometimes rely on self-report of the parent, rather than the child, potentially resulting in poor construct validity (26).

These final topics are considered: Wilson's disease, hepatitis C disease and metabolic side-effects of psychotropic medications.

Wilson's disease

Wilson's disease is an inherited condition in which there is a toxic buildup of copper in the liver and brain, due to the body not handling copper properly. Although quite rare (estimated to present in 1 in 30,000 children), it is more commonly seen in certain geographical areas, such as Sardinia and Eastern European countries. Wilson's disease has been studied in the mental health literature, as it is a condition that impacts both the liver and the brain. In some cases, it can cause acute liver failure (1). It has been noted in the literature that the most common psychiatric symptoms in this population seem to have an organic basis (5).

One study examined a large group of one hundred and twenty – nine children with Wilson's disease for the purpose of exploring the frequency of psychiatric, neuropsychiatric and neurological symptoms in this population (27). They found that the most common psychiatric symptoms were incongruous behavior, irritability, depression, and cognitive impairment (27). In a recent review study, it was found that psychiatric symptoms can even precede the diagnosis of Wilson's disease, with many patients having sought psychiatric care and treatment in the absence of a known etiology (28). In these cases, it took an average of 2.5 years for the children to be diagnosed with Wilson's disease. Psychiatric symptoms were found to be quite common in this population, estimated to present in as many as 30%-40%, with major depressive disorder being the most common, and psychotic symptoms occurring in only a small percentage of the population (estimated at approximately 1-10%) (28).

One of the studies reviewed found that more than half of the sample reported symptoms of anxiety when examined with the Structured Clinical Interview for DSM-IV Axis I Disorders, followed by depression, irritability, disinhibition, and apathy (29). Even among long-term, treated patients, psychiatric symptoms were reported in as many as 70% (29). Mental health providers are therefore cautioned to entertain this possibility, as psychiatric symptoms may be occurring in the absence of hepatic or neurological involvement, leading to misdiagnosis.

Hepatitis C

The hepatitis C virus is most frequently transmitted through the shared needle when practicing drug use, tattooing, or medical as well as dental treatment where equipment has not been properly sterilized. Less frequently, it can be sexually transmitted, or the result of workplace accidents (e.g., needlestick injuries). As these behaviors or incidents are less likely in children, children testing positive for hepatitis C have usually contracted the virus from mothers during childbirth. Chronic hepatitis C virus (HCV) infection in children is thought to be clinically mild; however, there has been an interest in how HCV in children can impact their HRQoL.

In one study conducted in Australia, despite being "asymptomatic," children who had early acquired HCV had a significantly poorer health status than a community control group (30). They score significantly lower on several scales of the Child Health Questionnaire mental health and the psychosocial summary score (30). Another study examined QoL, behavioral, emotional, and cognitive functioning in 114 treatment-naïve children with HCV who had been enrolled in a placebo – controlled, randomized, multi-site clinical drug trial in the United States (31). The study concluded that HCV infection in the early stages does not lead to global impairment in these areas; however, it is associated with increased caregiver stress as well as an increased strain on the family and can lead to some mild cognitive deficits or changes in the children (31).

Finally, a study conducted in Egypt compared a group of children with chronic hepatitis who were not receiving treatment, a group of children receiving treatment, and a control group of 60 health, matched controls on variables of HRQoL, behavioral/emotional functioning, as well as cognitive status (32). They found HRQoL and depression to be elevated in both groups of children with HCV, with both scores being higher in the group receiving treatment (32).

Metabolic side-effects of psychotropic medications

Pediatric liver disease and mental health is a two-way street. Although the effects of liver disease on the brain and mental health, in general, have been reviewed in this review thus far, one should not neglect also to examine the effects of medications used to treat psychiatric conditions on the liver. Indeed, metabolic side effects are a significant concern when treating children. In the adult population, certain psychiatric disorders have been associated with a significantly higher incident of liver disease. For example, in the case of bipolar disease, there is a higher incidence and prevalence of chronic liver disease associated with second-generation antipsychotic or antidepressant use, and hyperlipidemia (33).

Hepatotoxicity is a known side-effect of nefazodone, pemoline, and tacrine; also, carbamazepine and valproate products (such as divalproex) should be avoided in patients prone to liver disorders (34). One case report described an 8-year-old girl who was treated with atomoxetine hydrochloride for attention-deficit/hyperactivity disorder (ADHD) who was diagnosed with drug-induced hepatitis (35). It is important that providers are familiar with this literature and closely monitor patients receiving these drugs. Risks versus benefits should be continuously assessed, and patients should be educated on the "early warnings of liver injury" (34, 36).

Conclusion

Liver disease can impact brain and behavior directly, and mental health indirectly. The population that has been most widely studied are children who have undergone liver transplantation. This population faces the same challenges identified in children with various acute or chronic medical conditions. However, certain issues are of particular importance in pediatric liver recipients. Adherence to medication regimens and medical advice post-operative can determine clinical outcomes of the organ transplantation, including mortality.

Providers and parents should be alert for possible short-term or long-term cognitive effects of liver disease and liver transplantation. Children who suffer from liver disease and receive organ transplantations are vulnerable to medical trauma and PTSD. They and their family require long-term support from a multi-disciplinary team, and psychological health-related quality of life is not directly related to the physical condition.

Health care providers should understand that pediatric persons with Wilson's disease can present with psychiatric symptoms before any hepatic or neurological symptoms are noted. Children with chronic, early-acquired hepatitis C virus have a poorer quality of life compared to controls, even in the absence of symptoms. Metabolic side-effects of psychotropic medications are well-known and should be taken into consideration when using these drugs in a pediatric population.

References

[1] Children's Live Disease Foundation. Information on liver diseases. URL: https://www.childliver disease.org/Information/Medical-stuff/Information-on-liver-diseases.

[2] Pinquart M, Teubert D. Academic, physical, and social functioning of children and adolescents with chronic physical illness: A meta-analysis. J Pediatr Psychol 2012;37(4):376-89.

[3] Pinquart M, Shen Y. Behavior problems in children and adolescents with chronic physical illness: A meta-analysis. J Pediatr Psychol 2011;36(9):1003–16.

[4] Pinquart M. Achievement of developmental milestones in emerging and young adults with and without pediatric illness: A meta-analysis. J Pediatr Psychol 2014;39(6):577-87.

[5] O'Carroll R. Psychological aspects of liver disease and its treatment. Health Psychol Rev 2013; 7(1):111-28.

[6] Wu YP, Aylward BS, Steele RG. Associations between internalizing symptoms and trajectories of medication adherence among pediatric renal and liver transplant recipients. J Pediatr Psychol 2010; 35(9):1016-27.

[7] Fredericks EM, Lopez MJ, Magee JC, Shieck V, Opipari-Arrigan L. Psychological functioning, nonadherence, and health outcomes after pediatric liver transplantation. Am J Transplant 2007; 7(8):1974-83.

[8] Maikranz JM, Steele RG, Dreyer ML, Stratman AC, Bovaird JA. The relationship of hope and illness-related uncertainty to emotional adjustment and adherence among pediatric renal and liver transplant recipients. J Pediatr Psychol 2007;32(5):571-81.

[9] Simons LE, McCormick ML, Devine K Blount RL. Medication barriers predict adolescent transplant recipients' adherence and clinical outcomes at 18-month follow-up. J Pediatr Psychol 2010;35(9):1038-48.

[10] Lee JL, Eaton C, Gutierrez-Colina AM, Devine K, Simons LE, Mee L, et al. Longitudinal stability of specific barriers to medication adherence. J Pediatr Psychol 2014;39(7):667-76.

[11] Shemesh E, Shneider BL, Savitzky JK, Arnott L, Gondolesi GE, Krieger NR, et al. Medication adherence in pediatric and adolescent liver transplant recipients. Pediatrics 2004;113(4):825-32.

[12] Annunziato RA, Emre S, Shneider BL, Barton C, Dugan CA, Shemesh E. Adherence and medical outcomes in pediatric liver transplant recipients who transition to adult services. Pediatr Transplant 2007;11(6):608–14.

[13] Fineberg SK, West A, Na PJ, Oldham M, Schilsky M, Hawkins KA et al. Utility of pretransplant psychological measures to predict posttransplant outcomes in liver transplant patients: a systematic review. Gen Hosp Psychiatry 2016;40:4-11.

[14] Eaton CK, Lee JL, Simons LE, Devine KA, Mee LL, Blount RL. Clinical cutoffs for adherence barriers in solid organ transplant recipients: How many is too many? J Pediatr Psychol 2014;40(4):431-41.

[15] Foerster BR, Conklin LS, Petrou M, Barker PB, Schwartz KB. Minimal hepatic encephalopathy in children: Evaluation with proton MR spectroscopy. AJNR Am J Neuroradiol 2009;30(8):1610-3.

[16] Krull K, Fuchs C, Yurk H, Boone P, Alonso E. Neurocognitive outcome in pediatric liver transplant recipients. Pediatr Transplant 2003;7(2):111–8.

[17] Stewart SM, Hiltebeitel C, Nici, J, Waller DA, Uauy R, Andrews WS. Neuropsychological outcome of pediatric liver transplantation. Pediatrics 1991;87(3):367-76.

[18] Aceto P, Perilli V, Lai C, Ciocchetti P, Vitale F, Sollazzi L. Postoperative cognitive dysfunction after liver transplantation. Gen Hosp Psychiatr 2015;37:109–15.

[19] Gutierrez-Colina AM, Eaton CK, Lee JL, Reed-Knight B, Loiselle K, Mee LL, et al. Executive functioning, barriers to adherence, and nonadherence in adolescent and young adult transplant recipients. J Pediatr Psychol 2016;41(7):759-67.

[20] National Child Traumatic Stress Network. Information on liver diseases. URL: http://www.nctsn.org/trauma-types/medical-trauma.

[21] Walker AM, Harris G, Baker A, Kelly D, Houghton J. Post-traumatic stress responses following liver transplantation in older children. J Child Psychol Psychiatry 1999;40(3):363-74.

[22] LoBiondo-Wood G, Williams L, McGhee C. Liver transplantation in children: Maternal and family stress, coping, and adaptation. J Spec Pediatr Nurs 2004;9(2):59-66.

[23] Ullrich G, Meyke A, Haase H, Erzfeld C, Beckmann C, Schmidt-schaller S, et al. Psychological support of children undergoing liver transplantation and their parents: A single-centre experience. Pediatr Rehabilitation 1997;1(1):19-24.

[24] Castaldo ET, Feurer ID, Russell RT, Wright Pinson C. Correlation of health-related quality of life after liver transplant with the model for end-stage liver disease score. Arch Surg 2009;144(2):167-72.

[25] Devine KA, Reed-Knight B, Loiselle KA, Simons LE, Mee LL, Blount RL. Predictors of long-term health-related quality of life in adolescent solid organ transplant recipients. J Pediatr Psychol 2011; 36(8):891–901.

[26] Taylor R, Franck LS, Gibson F, Dhawan A. A critical review of the health-related quality of life of children and adolescents after liver transplantation. Liver Transpl 2005;11(1):51–60.

[27] Dening TR, Berrios GE. Wilson's disease: A longitudinal study of psychiatric symptoms. Biol Psychiatry 1990;28(3):255-65.

[28] Zimbrean PC, Schilsky ML. Psychiatric aspects of Wilson disease: A review. Gen Hosp Psychiatry 2014;36(1):53-62.

[29] Svetel, M, Potrebic A, Pekmezovic T, Tomic A, Kresojevic N, Jesic R, et al. Neuropsychiatric aspects of treated Wilson's disease. Parkinsonism Relat Disord 2009;15(10):772-5.

[30] Nydegger A, Srivastava A, Wake M, Smith AL, Hardikar W. Health-related quality of life in children with hepatitis C acquired in the first year of life. J Gastroenterol Hepatol 2008;23(2): 226–30.

[31] Rodrigue JR, Balistreri W, Haber B, Jonas MM, Mohan P, Molleston JP, et al. Impact of hepatitis C virus infection on children and their caregiver: Quality of life, cognitive and emotional outcomes. J Pediatr Gastroenterol Nutr 2009;48(3):341–7.

[32] Galal O, Behairy A. Health-related quality of life in children with chronic hepatitis C. Egyptian Pediatr Assoc Gaz 2016;64(3):120-5. URL: http://dx.doi.org/10.1016/j.epag.2016.08.001.

[33] Hsu JH, Chien IC, Lin CH. Increased risk of chronic liver disease in patients with bipolar disorder: A population-based study. Gen Hosp Psychiatry 2016;42:54-9.

[34] Sedky K, Nazir R, Joshi A, Kaur G, Lippmann S. Which psychotropic medications induce hepatotoxicity? Gen Hosp Psychiatry 2012;34(1):53-61.

[35] Stojanovski SD, Casavant MJ, Mousa HM, Baker P, Nahata MC. Atomoxetine-induced hepatitis in a child. Clin Toxicol (Phila) 2007;45(1):51-5.

[36] Correll CU, Carlson HE. Endocrine and metabolic adverse effects of psychotropic medications in children and adolescents. J Am Acad Child Adolesc Psychiatry 2006;45(7):771-91.

Chapter 7

Behavioral/emotional effects of COVID-19 on children and teens

Prasanth Narahari[1], MD, Myrtha Gregoire-Bottex[2,*], MD, Meredith Bishop[3], MA, Cristina Matheus[1], MD and Monica Dowling[4], PhD

[1]Holtz Children's Hospital/Jackson Memorial Hospital, Miami, Florida, [2]Pediatric Cystic Fibrosis Program, Pediatric Pulmonology, Department of Pediatrics. University of Miami Miller School of Medicine, Miami, Florida, [3]University of Miami Miller School of Medicine, Mailman Center for Child Development, Miami, Florida and
[4]Pediatrics, University of Miami Miller School of Medicine. Mailman Center for Child Development, Miami, Florida, United States of America

Abstract

A pediatrician's role is constantly evolving and involves keeping up to date with advances in technology including electronic health records and prescriptions. The current pandemic has taken their role into another dimension with telehealth for interacting with a patient who lives far away from the healthcare facility. The effects of the COVID-19 pandemic include rising rates of anxiety, depression, and behavioral issues in the general population of children and adolescents worldwide; also new challenges and stressors have arisen for families. Although everyone has been impacted by the COVID-19 pandemic, studies demonstrate that specific populations may be particularly vulnerable to negative outcomes; these include those with pre-existing conditions, neurodevelopmental or psychological disorders, and racial as well as ethnic minorities. This discussion provides a summary of preliminary information on how COVID-19 has impacted the lives of children, particularly their mental health. The pandemic has presented new challenges for children and families, and specific populations may be particularly vulnerable to negative outcomes. It is recommended that primary care physicians regularly screen their pediatric patients for mental health conditions and consider referrals for supportive intervention for those needing management of these issues.

---

* ***Correspondence:*** Email: mxg1809@med.miami.edu.

In: Behavioral Pediatrics
Editors: Donald E. Greydanus, Dilip R. Patel, Ahsan Nazeer et al.
ISBN: 979-8-88697-060-9

Introduction

One hundred years after the Spanish flu, the COVID-19 pandemic has taken the world by storm. The COVID-19 virus has changed the lives of families from working and learning from home, to feeling trapped indoors and to a constant fear of getting sick. It has forced us to adjust the way we learn, develop, communicate, and interact with each other. Wearing a mask that covers our smile, staying at home, avoiding parties as well as crowds, along with washing and sanitizing our hands frequently have become the "new normal." Although the research is preliminary, there is emerging evidence that these changes have presented significant challenges to the mental health of children, and exacerbated mental health conditions, leading to an increased demand for mental health services. At the same time, health systems around the world are challenged, leading to a disruption of essential services, especially for the most vulnerable populations. The focus of this review is how the pandemic has taken a toll on the behavior and emotions of children as well as teens and how primary care physicians can play a crucial role in mitigating the impact of the COVID-19 pandemic and future public health emergencies.

COVID-19 in children

An 11-year-old male passed away in July 2020 from COVID-19 complications, becoming Florida's youngest victim of the virus. He was African American and had several underlying health conditions linked to poverty as well as developmental disabilities. His case highlights limitations in existing services and supports the increased vulnerability of racial as well as ethnic minorities to the disease.

The severe acute respiratory syndrome coronavirus 2 (SARS-CoV-2), also known as coronavirus disease-2019 (COVID 2019), was initially identified in China in December 2019 (1). The first non-travel related case in the United States was reported in February 2020 in the state of California and by March, a pandemic had been declared (2). "Lockdowns" started to be the go-to-strategy by public health officials in an attempt to decrease the mobility of the population, control the spread of the virus, and reduce the strain on hospital resources (3).

From March 2020, the number of COVID – 19 cases have been rising but fortunately fewer cases and hospitalizations have been reported in children (age 0-17 years) compared with adults. This may be due to school closures, which has led to children staying at home.

Looking at the virus as a double-edged sword, this confinement has led to many mental health effects on children as we will look into in further sections (4). According to the American Academy of Pediatrics (AAP) report as of Feb 2021, children constitute 12% of all the cases that amounts to 3,899 per 100,000 children (5). Children constitute up to 0.25% of all deaths related to the virus (5). Non-Hispanic blacks and Hispanic children had the highest rates of infection (6).

The most common symptoms of the virus are fever and/or cough and 16% of the children with the virus are asymptomatic. Children are less likely to develop severe complications as compared to adults. However, those who do develop the severe illness are usually less than 1 year of age and have a pre-existing medical condition (4). Some children who have the virus develop "multi-system inflammatory syndrome (MIS-C)" which can lead to multi-organ failure and shock (1). In short, the U.S. Centers for Disease Control and Prevention (CDC) definition for MIS-C is anyone less than 21 years of age who is positive or has been recently positive for COVID-19 and presents with a fever, laboratory evidence of inflammation, and clinically severe illness requiring hospitalization with greater than two organ systems being involved (7).

A growing body of research evidence suggests that there are a wide range of direct neurocognitive and neuropsychiatric consequences. Multiple clinical neurological and neuropsychological manifestations have been observed, including both short-term and long-term sequelae (8, 9). Data from the Centers for Medicare & Medicaid Services (CMS) highlighted a decline in services used by children covered by Medicaid and the Children's Health Insurance Program (CHIP) in March through May 2020 compared to the same period in 2019 (10). This included fewer screening services that assess physical and cognitive development, outpatient mental health services, and vaccinations up to the age of two (10).

Changes for families

During the current COVID-19 pandemic, children and families have experienced significant changes to daily life, increased exposure to stressors, and decreased access to support and services. The pandemic has disrupted the traditional ways in which people interact with one another in daily life. According to the CDC, physical restrictions such as socially distancing and avoiding physical contact are an important part of mitigating the spread of the COVID-19 virus (11). However, these essential practices, by nature, may contribute to social isolation and feelings of loneliness. Children have experienced a prolonged state of separation from their usual sources of interaction (e.g., peers, teachers, extended family) and the contexts in which those interactions typically occur (e.g., childcare centers, schools, after-school programs), understandably contribute to children's feelings of loneliness and social isolation. This is especially concerning given evidence from a recent systematic review reporting that social isolation and loneliness are associated with an increased risk of depression in children (12).

Especially during times of crisis, social connectedness and support are protective against inevitable stressors and promote well-being as well as adjustment. The American Academy of Pediatrics (AAP) is able to stratify risk of COVID-19 spread per activity and states that avoidance of in-person playdates and use of virtual interactions is the best way to reduce children's risk. Given the current physical restrictions, children and families are relying on technology (e.g., video chatting, online gaming) for staying connected and accessing social support more than ever. However, concerns regarding prolonged screen time have arisen. For parents, this may mean loosening restrictions on the amount of screen time their children are allowed daily to maintain contact with peers and other family members. Encouraging and facilitating social connection and support for children may be especially important during this unique time in modern history in which the practices that prevent the spread of the virus may also be increasing the risk for social isolation, loneliness, and negative mental health outcomes.

During the pandemic, family stressors have increased, and new challenges have arisen for parents. Many families have experienced financial hardship and changes or uncertainty regarding employment. Compared to households without children, households with children have been more likely to be negatively impacted financially during the pandemic (13). This includes greater temporary or permanent loss of employment, decreases in income, and loss of health insurance. In contrast to households without children, households with children have also been more likely to experience food insecurity, rely on government aid (e.g., unemployment or supplemental nutrition assistance program [SNAP] benefits), or miss rent or mortgage payments. These disparities are even greater for single-parent households.

In addition to financial losses, many families are grieving the loss of family members or friends. For many children, this may be their first experience with death, and given the nature of the COVID-19 virus and the necessity of quarantining, opportunities to prepare and say goodbye to loved ones may be limited. Although parents or caregivers may want to protect children from experiencing the pain associated with the death of a family member, child and adolescent psychologists indicate that providing children with age-appropriate information about death, including its permanence, is important for helping children grieve and cope with death. Parents may encourage children to talk about their feelings and share memories of the person they lost. It is important to note that there is no "right" way to grieve, and even children of the same age or from the same family may have significantly different responses to death. Parents should seek to validate children's individual experiences and provide reassurance that children are safe and loved. Family routines should be maintained as much as possible to re-establish structure for children, and engagement in other positive or fun activities should be encouraged. Although grief does tend to fade with time, children may experience waves of grief especially at significant events such as birthdays or graduation when the absence of their loved one is especially noticeable.

As COVID-19 cases increase and uncertainty lingers, children's fears related to the illness need to be addressed by parents and caregivers. The Centers for Disease Control and Prevention (CDC) recommends that parents and caregivers provide simple, factual information about the virus (14). Parents can help children learn behaviors to help prevent the spread of COVID-19 (e.g., hand sanitation, physical distancing) by demonstrating and reinforcing these preventative behaviors. Parents may discuss the importance of these safety behaviors and the impact they can have on others who are at high risk of contracting the virus.

In addition to the increase in family stressors, many systems on which families previously relied for structure and support (e.g., childcare, schools) became unavailable or modified during the pandemic. The U.S. Department of Agriculture (USDA) National School Lunch Program, School Breakfast Program, as well as Child and Adult Care Food Program serve meals to approximately 35 million children daily (**15**). Without these programs, children and families who relied on school breakfasts and lunches are at a higher risk for household food insecurity. Evidence shows that even brief periods of food insecurity during childhood can have a negative impact on children's development, academic performance, and mental health (16). Additionally, parents working in essential industries (i.e., healthcare, food service) without the opportunity to work remotely have scrambled to find alternative childcare as many daycare centers, schools, and after school programs closed.

The transition from in-person to virtual learning has presented several challenges for children and families. With children no longer in the classroom, many parents are logistically challenged with the task of working from home while helping their child engage in virtual learning. Many parents report that behavioral management is challenging during virtual learning. The American Psychological Association (APA) recommends that parents promote structure, set clear expectations, and focus on praising their child's positive behaviors. Parents can help promote structure for children learning virtually by implementing many strategies used in classroom settings, such as maintaining a schedule and creating a specific environment for their child to work without distractions. Parents should set clear expectations for the school day and focus on praising children's on-task behaviors (17).

As traditional learning was suddenly interrupted during the pandemic, parents and teachers have expressed concern about children falling behind academically. The transition to remote services presented challenges both in terms of access and the quality of education. Surveys suggest that typical learners have continued to perform at the same level in reading as in the fall of 2019, but showed lower than average mathematics gains (18). However, lower levels of performance were noted for Black and Hispanic students, suggesting increased vulnerability and need for connecting with these families. Black and Hispanic students are less likely to have computers and Internet access, though wide gaps seen in the spring on this point have narrowed. In the spring, 79 percent of Black students had a device for school; by the fall, the census found this reached 89 percent, but that was still short of the nearly 93 percent of White students who had devices in the fall.

Mental health-general population

Months into the COVID-19 pandemic, rates of anxiety, depression, and behavioral issues were rising in the general population of children and adolescents worldwide. Beginning in April 2020, the proportion of children's mental health–related ED visits among all pediatric ED visits increased and remained elevated through October 2020. Compared with 2019, the proportion of mental health–related visits for children aged 5–11 and 12–17 years increased approximately 24% and 31%, respectively (19) Prior to the pandemic, the international prevalence of child and adolescent mental illness, across all disorders was 13.4% (20).

The number of studies examining the prevalence of mental illness during the COVID-19 pandemic is limited, but the few existing studies do indicate an increase in depressive and anxiety symptoms. One study from China involving more than 2000 children found 22.6% reported depressive symptoms on the Children's Depression Inventory (short form) and 18.9% endorsed anxiety symptoms on the Screen for Anxiety Related Disorders (SCARED) (21).

Another even larger study (>8,000) conducted in China found the prevalence of depressive and anxiety symptoms in adolescents was 43.7% and 37.4% respectively (22). Interestingly, the high prevalence of psychological health problems among adolescents was negatively associated with the level of awareness of COVID-19.

A third study investigating somatic complaints found only 2.4% of children endorsing concerns (23). However, parent report of mental health concerns included clinginess (37%), inattention (33%), irritability (32%), worry (28%), obsessive requests (27%), fear of death of relatives (22%), sleep disorders (22%), poor appetite (18%), fatigue (17%), nightmares (14%) and agitation (13%) in a sample of 320 children and adolescents (24). A second survey in the U.S. found that 40.1% of parents noted signs of distress in their children (25).

A systematic review of twelve studies with individuals $\leq$ 18 years of aged (n = 12,262) found that COVID-19 has an impact on youth mental health and was particularly associated with depression and anxiety in adolescent cohorts (26). COVID-19 longitudinal studies have been ongoing internationally and a catalog of longitudinal studies on mental health during COVID-19 is maintained by the University College of London and updated weekly (https://www.covidminds.org) (27). Open access materials, including the most widely recommended scales and newly validated COVID-19 mental health measures, are available in multiple languages.

Research also provides information as to how to improve coping and well-being. In the period between April 1 and April 10, 2020, 306 adolescents aged 15-21 filled out an online survey consisting of 33 questions investigating socio-demographic characteristics, lifestyle behaviors, coping strategies, and subjective well-being (28).

Most adolescents planned their daily routine (57.8%), engaging in structured activities (17.6-67.3%) and developing new interests (54.6%) (28). They reported a positive outlook for the time period (57.8%), thus revealing adaptive coping strategies. Family wise, even though it was hard to stay at home (66%) and difficulties emerged, including self-isolation (50.7%) and quarrels (31.7%), a relevant proportion of adolescents shared their feelings (40.5%) and re-evaluated their family relationships (29.4-39.7%) (28). In terms of social and school engagement, almost all adolescents kept contacts with their partner, friends, and teachers (90.2-93.5%).

School commitments at home were sufficiently preserved (63.1%); however, adolescents expressed preoccupations about their educational path (56.2%) (28). A change in subjective well-being (49.3%) and symptoms of anxiety (39.9%) were frequently reported. A number of factors predicted a change in subjective well-being, including adaptive coping strategies (physical activity; engaging in different activities than before), family issues (finding it hard to stay at home; having quarrels), school-related behaviors (fearing a negative educational outcome), and female gender. The research suggests that both personal and environmental coping resources are relevant to subjective wellbeing in adolescence and should be taken into account for prevention and early intervention in youth mental health concerns (28). The CDC's COVID-19 Parental Resource Kit can help support parents, caregivers, and other adults serving children and young people in recognizing children as well as young people's social, emotional, and mental challenges along with helping to ensure their well-being (29).

Disproportionately negative impact

Although everyone has been impacted by the COVID-19 pandemic, specific populations may be particularly vulnerable to negative outcomes; these include those with pre-existing health conditions, neurodevelopmental or psychological disorders, and racial as well as ethnic minorities. Parents of children with disabilities and complex care needs are struggling to make difficult decisions about how to keep their children safe and engaged in learning. Individuals with intellectual and developmental disabilities (IDD) have a higher prevalence of specific comorbidities associated with poorer COVID-19 outcomes (30). Distinct age-related differences in COVID-19 trends have been noted among those with IDD, with a higher concentration of COVID-19 cases at younger ages and greater fatality (ages < 17 with IDD 1.6%, without IDD < 0.01%).

An analysis of individuals with Down syndrome (DS) who were hospitalized with COVID-19 in New York City found that patients with DS are at an 8.9-fold higher risk of hospitalization with COVID-19 when compared to non-DS patients. Hospitalized DS individuals are on average 10 years younger than non-DS patients with COVID-19. Moreover, type 2 diabetes mellitus appears to be an important driver of this susceptibility to COVID-19. Finally, patients with DS have more severe outcomes than controls, and are more likely to progress to sepsis in particular (31).

Individuals with autism spectrum disorder (ASD) have a greater likelihood of allergy or autoimmune diseases than the general population placing them at greater risk of requiring hospitalization and poor outcomes (32). One study investigated whether any pre-pandemic sociodemographic or clinical characteristics would predict a negative outcome (33). Parents and guardians of individuals with ASD completed an online survey of socio-demographic and clinical characteristics of their children, the impact of the COVID-19 outbreak on their wellbeing and their needs to deal with the emergency. The COVID-19 emergency resulted in a challenging period for 93.9% of 527 families with increased difficulties in managing daily activities, especially free time (78.1%) as well as structured activities (75.7%); also, children presented with more intense (35.5% and more frequent (41.5%) behavior problems (33).

Behavior problems predating the COVID-19 outbreak predicted a higher risk of more intense and more frequent disruptive behavior. Even though ASD children were receiving different types of support, a number of needs emerged, including receiving more healthcare support (47.4%), especially in-home support (29.9%), as well as interventions to tackle a potentially disruptive quarantine (16.8%) (33). In a survey from the Georgia State University School of Public Health, people with IDD and the professionals who support them reported significantly reduced quality of life during the COVID-19 pandemic, contributing to heightened feelings of emotional distress (34).

Evidence suggests that ethnic and racial minorities are disproportionately affected by the COVID-19 virus. Systemic inequities in social determinants of health such as type of occupation, housing, and healthcare access have put racial and ethnic minorities at higher risk for contracting the virus. Higher rates of COVID-19 cases, hospitalizations, and COVID-19-related deaths have been reported for racial and ethnic minorities (35, 36). Racial and ethnic minorities are more likely to work in settings that are considered essential (e.g., grocery stores, healthcare facilities; *United States Bureau of Labor Statistics, 2020*), limiting their ability to work remotely and increasing their vulnerability to COVID-19 exposure. Additionally, higher rates of medical conditions (e.g., heart disease, diabetes) that increased risk for severe COVID-19 are found in racial and ethnic minorities compared to non-Hispanic white individuals (37).

The disproportionate number of cases of COVID-19 in racial and ethnic minorities may increase risk for negative mental health outcomes. In a CDC survey published in August 2021, researchers found that Latinos reported higher prevalence of anxiety, depression, increased substance abuse, and suicidal ideation (38). Many who responded to the survey were also exhibiting symptoms of trauma- and stressor-related disorders related to COVID-19 (38).

Disruption of critical mental health services

In addition, the COVID-19 virus has interrupted mental health and/or developmental services for children at risk or diagnosed with psychological concerns. The COVID-19 pandemic has disrupted or halted critical mental health services in 93% of countries worldwide while the demand for mental health is increasing, according to a WHO survey conducted from June to August 2020 (39). The survey of 130 countries provided the first global data showing the devastating impact of COVID-19 on access to mental health services and underscored the urgent need for increased funding in this regard. Countries reported widespread disruption of many kinds of critical mental health services while less than 30% of countries reported no disruption to children's and adolescent mental health services. Almost 60% of all psychotherapy and counselling services were reported as being partially disrupted. Also, over 60% of countries reported disruptions to mental health services for vulnerable people, including children and adolescents (72%), older adults (70%), and women requiring antenatal or postnatal services (61%) (39). Around three-quarter of the surveyed countries reported at least partial disruptions to school and workplace mental health services (78% and 75% respectively).

Pediatrics in pandemia

A pediatrician's role is constantly evolving and requires keeping up to date with advances in technology including electronic health records and electronic prescriptions. The pandemic has taken their role into another dimension with telehealth, the many applications that are used for it, and having to interact with patients who are miles away (40). The effects of the pandemic on the behavior and emotions of children and adolescents are multifold as mentioned in the previous sections. What we know now are the acute effects, and we are learning more about such effects as every day passes. Our aim at the end of this section is for the pediatrician to be well equipped to deal with the mental health needs of children as well as adolescents during a pandemic and provide the necessary anticipatory guidance. There may be a few topics that overlap with the general management of the pandemic in the following section, but we feel it is essential as the mental health of a child depends on the overall well-being of the child. Further, this would help children and families through natural disasters and other public health emergencies in the future. Pediatricians, clinicians, and other practitioners must work together to ensure people with developmental disorders have access to tailored and culturally appropriate mental health supports during and following the pandemic period.

Psychological screening and referral

During a well child visit, as pediatricians have been doing historically, it is important to screen for behavioral/mood changes and developmental delays in children as well as adolescents, and ensure timely referral to a specialist as needed. We can start off by asking parents/families what they need and how we may be able to help. In many cases, the needs may not be treating mental health symptoms at all, but rather priorities such as housing, health, safety, and access to food.

The HEADSS assessment is a psychosocial assessment tool that includes screening for suicide and depression (41). The PROMIS (Parent-Reported Outcomes Measurement Information System) Global Health measures assess an individual's physical, mental, and social health. The measures are generic, rather than disease-specific, and often use an "In General" item context as it is intended to globally reflect individuals' assessments of their health. The PROMIS Pediatric and PROMIS Parent Proxy Global Health measures assess a child's overall evaluations of his or her physical, mental, and social health (42).

As soon as concerns are noted/reported, referrals to appropriate community and/or mental health specialists should be made. If unsure the clinician can contact local mental health/infant mental health associations or local/state psychological associations, telehealth consults, parent training such as parent child interaction therapy (PCIT), and/or community-based intervention programs (i.e., Healthy Start or Children's Trust in the state of Florida). Moreover with telehealth, this process becomes easier, and a team consisting of the physician, psychologist, psychiatrist, and social worker can be involved in the management, all at the same time by just the click of a button (43).

In developing children, a thorough developmental assessment is crucial, especially given the potential impact of quarantine and social isolation. Children have been experiencing regression of milestones (i.e., bed wetting, thumb sucking) and from our experience, developmental delays (e.g., delays in speech) from the lack of social interaction (44). The modified checklist for autism in toddlers (M-CHAT) can be used for children 16-30 months to assist ruling out autism (45). If any delay is identified, prompt referral to behavioral and development specialists should be done.

Management of chronic conditions

With disruption in health care services, it is essential to ensure that children with chronic medical conditions continue to receive their prescription medications and have continued follow-up whether in-person or through telehealth (46). As there may be changes in weight which may not be recorded during multiple telehealth visits, it is essential for parents to weigh their child at home so dose adjustments can be made according to weight if necessary. For children who require speech therapy, occupational therapy, or physical therapy, we also need to make sure that these therapies are continued online. With disruption of in-person school, children loose access to peer support groups and guidance counselors (47). We need to identify this and suggest alternative channels for them to have continued support.

While managing children who have a diagnosis of autism spectrum disorder (ASD) or an intellectual disability (ID), it is important to understand that a disruption in their regular routine is extremely difficult for them. Under normal circumstances, the rate of developing a psychiatric disorder (primarily anxiety and mood disorders) is higher in people with an ID/ASD diagnosis compared to the general population, which may be exacerbated by the pandemic and quarantine. While we communicate with children diagnosed with ASD in our clinic, we need to make sure that we refrain from metaphors and abstractions and clearly explain things to them (with respect to the personal safety measures as well as social distancing). Further in children with ID who have language and comprehension difficulty, nonverbal communication can be used (48). Specific measures are discussed below.

Guidance specific to mental health + general COVID

At the end of a clinic visit, in addition to the usual anticipatory guidance we provide children and their parents, we need to make it a routine to ask about how they are dealing with the pandemic; for example, we ask them about school, learning from home, if they get enough fresh air and sunlight. We will divide the following into general COVID precautions and specific guidance for the mental and behavioral health of a child.

General guidance during a pandemic

Such guidance includes these concepts:

- Continue routine immunizations and developmental screening.
- Information on handwashing and social distancing measures can be distributed in the form of hand- outs.
- Hand hygiene (i.e., hand washing and sanitizer use). The hand sanitizer must have at least 60% alcohol and as there is a chance of accidental ingestion, adult supervision is required during the process (49, 50).
- The following is a summary combining the American Academy of Pediatrics' (AAP) and CDC's guidance for childcare centers. As a parent who is sending their child to daycare or school, they should keep in mind that the facility they send their child to should screen children upon arrival (>100.4 degrees F or 38 degrees C, should not be allowed inside), practice social distancing measures (6 feet apart), ensure a mask is worn (not for kids < 2 years old), student-teacher ratio should be low, same group every day and modified pick up as well as drop-off procedures (so that there is not crowding) and toys as well as equipment are regularly cleaned. Schools need to have guidelines on what to do if a child becomes sick at school or is found to be COVID positive (49, 50).
- Using personal protective equipment (PPE) (for children above the age of 2).
- In a child with ASD or ID who may have difficulty in using and understanding the function of PPE, gradual introduction of it along with positive reinforcement can be beneficial. Children can be routinely trained on hygiene practices with the help of visual communication (48).
- If children attend in person school, it is important that parents are aware of their school's policies and that they are in line with the local and state guidelines.
- As discussed in the previous sections, it is important to reinforce to parents to explain the current situation to their children using age-appropriate terms and allow children to voice their concerns. Children should also be reassured of their safety (if they are indeed safe) and parents can take part in recreational activities with them (playing outdoor and indoor games) (24, 49). Parents can also be encouraged to listen to music and sing with their children as a form of music therapy (24).
- The basic safety measures (washing hands, mask usage, and social distancing) have to be reinforced. The importance of safety measures and the impact that they have on the others who are at high risk can be included in the discussion.

Specific guidance for mental and behavioral wellness

Such guidance includes these concepts:

- Providers and parents should look out for the following signs that their kids/teens need more support, such as problems with sleep patterns, eating and play.

- Maintaining a routine is important when children stay at home for so long. Parents can help kids create a schedule to reduce anxiety and uncertainty (45, 47). Waking up, sleeping and having meals at regular times could be a part of the process. Large calendars can be used with pictures and drawings. Alarm clocks can be used and children can be involved in the planning process (48).
- Since the children are confined to their homes for a long period of time, it is important to have areas designated for a specific activity, such as reading, sleeping, and eating (48).
- For children specifically with ASD and ID, the present and near future should be made predictable by telling them what will happen in advance (48). This could be applicable to all children.
- Encourage children to play and socialize. It is okay to go out to parks and take walks outdoors if adequate social distancing measures are taken (51).
- Find positive ways for children to express their feelings of sadness by channelizing them to something creative, such as drawing or playing (51).
- Limit screen time. This is a complex topic as children are forced to use a computer as a means of schooling. However, parents can supervise and limit their access to social and mass media with time restrictions, which has the potential to give them misinformation, aggravate their mental distress, increased vulnerability to online predators and cyber bullying (44, 51). However, watching age-appropriate television with the family can serve as a means on bonding, as well as video chats with relatives who are far away or in isolation (48). For gathering news, parents and children can refer to official resources such as the World Health Organization (WHO) (51).
- Screen for neglect, exploitation and child abuse. Children may be witness to domestic violence as well (44).
- Parents should be aware of the mental health facilities a school is capable of providing and ensure that their child has access to it.
- If a parent were to be separated from a child in an event of hospitalization, social workers can be used to seek alternative care arrangements and regular communication with the parent has to be ensured (51). Organization and community leaders can be partnered with to support those separated from their families (48).
- Parents should pay attention to any sleep difficulties or nightmares their child develops over time. Good sleep hygiene can be encouraged, by avoiding screens before bed, and avoiding daytime naps (24).
- Parents can take their children out for walks and encourage them to exercise (48). If they prefer not to go outdoors, they can be encouraged to get sunlight exposure in their balconies or exercise in their backyards or watch exercise videos to exercise at home. Children can be taken on car rides as a method of relaxation (47).
- Personal hygiene should be continued to be maintained such as taking a bath, brushing ones teeth and combing ones hair (48).
- Children and families can be encouraged to maintain any routine spiritual activities, such as prayer, meditation and celebrate festivals as well as anniversaries (48).
- Children can be encouraged to water their plants and appreciate art.
- Support should be provided to families who are dealing with grief (48).
- Coloring books can be distributed to children.

Identifying parental anxiety

Children mirror their parents, as for example, anxiety in a parent would lead to anxiety in children (52). As a primary care physician (PCP) who would screen for postpartum depression in a new parent, we also need to be on the look-out for mood disorders in parents during a visit, even by a simple question of " how are you coping with the pandemic" and suggest them to get help if necessary.

Conclusion

Children's mental health during public health emergencies can have both short- and long-term consequences to their overall health and well-being. This discussion highlights some of the changes associated with the COVID-19 pandemic. At the end of the reference section are 5 resources that are available to the general public at no cost.

The importance of what has been learned during the COVID-19 pandemic cannot be overstated. Implementation of technology-based, remote mental health services and prevention activities to enhance healthy coping and resilience in children might effectively support their well-being throughout response and recovery periods. The CDC supports efforts to promote the emotional well-being of children as well as families and provides developmentally appropriate resources for families to reduce stressors that might contribute to children's mental health-related emergency department (ED) visits.

We could be the shepherds of change, including the importance of transition, transformation and telehealth in clinical practice (maybe the most lasting positive impact) and use of social platforms to share advice and reach a broader audience than pre-COVID-19. Mental health apps are leading more people to therapy rather than replacing it.

The American Psychological Association's (APA's) 2020 Stress in America survey released in October 2021 revealed that Americans have been profoundly affected by COVID-19 and the survey sounds "the alarm on a growing mental health crisis that could yield serious health and social consequences for years to come (17)." The full report can be found at www.stressinamerica.org.

Disclaimer

This subject is rapidly evolving and hence we are capturing it at a point in time. We expect more change to occur and we do not yet know all of the long-term health consequences of the COVID-19 pandemic; however, we do know that the implications are significant. Patients (children and families) those who contract COVID or experience the secondary effects could feel the impact for years to come. Measures that are critical during the COVID-19 pandemic include monitoring indicators of children's mental health, promoting coping as well as resilience, and expanding access to services to support children's mental health.

Additional resources:

No-cost materials for families and children

- Guide: Living with worry and anxiety amidst global uncertainty. Psychologytools.com 2020.
- URL: https://www.psychologytools.com/resource/living-with-worry-and-anxiety-amidst-global-uncertainty
- Helping children and families cope with the COVID-19 pandemic -7-dippity. 7-Dippity.com
- URL: https://7-dippity.com/helping-children-and-families-cope-with-the-covid-19-pandemic/
- R Growe, J Martin Burch. A kid's guide to coronavirus. Washington, DC: Magination Press, American Psychological Association. URL: https://www.apa.org/pubs/magination/kids-guide-coronavirus-ebook.pdf.
- COVIBOOK. Mindheart.co. URL: https://www.mindheart.co/descargables.
- The Coronavirus explained & what you should do. Youtube; 2020. URL: https://www.youtube.com/watch?v=BtN-gov9VOY.

References

[1] Wu Y, Ho W, Huang Y, Jin DY, Li S, Liu SL, et al. SARS-CoV-2 is an appropriate name for the new coronavirus. Lancet 2020;395(10228):949-50.

[2] CDC COVID-19 Response Team, Jorden MA, Rudman SL, Villarino E, Hoferka S, Patel MT, Bemis K, et al. Evidence for limited early spread of COVID-19 within the United States, January-February 2020. MMWR 2020;69(22):680-4.

[3] Vinceti M, Filippini T, Rothman KJ, Ferrari F, Goffi A, Maffeis G, et al. Lockdown timing and efficacy in controlling COVID-19 using mobile phone tracking. EClinicalMedicine 2020;25:100457.

[4] CDC. Information for pediatric healthcare providers. URL: https://www.cdc.gov/coronavirus/2019-ncov/hcp/pediatric-hcp.html.

[5] Children and COVID-19. State-level data report. Aap.org. URL: https://services.aap.org/en/pages/2019-novel-coronavirus-covid-19-infections/children-and-covid-19-state-level:data-report/

[6] CDC COVID-19 Response Team. Coronavirus disease 2019 in children - United States, February 12-April 2, 2020. MMWR Morb Mortal Wkly Rep 2020;69(14):422-6.

[7] CDC. Information for healthcare providers about multisystem inflammatory syndrome in children (MIS-C). URL: stacks.cdc.gov/view/cdc/88595.

[8] Mukaetova-Ladinska EB, Kronenberg G, Raha-Chowdhury R. COVID-19 and neurocognitive disorders. Curr Opin Psychiatry 2021;34(2):149-56.

[9] Hassett CE, Gedansky A, Migdady I, Bhimraj A, Uchino K, Cho SM. Neurologic complications of COVID-19. Cleve Clin J Med 2020;87(12):729-34.

[10] Wyckoff AS. Delayed care: AAP responds to report on drop in pediatric visits in Medicaid, CHIP. AAP News, 2021. URL: https://www.aappublications.org/news/2020/09/28/delayedcare092820.

[11] CDC. COVID-19 Archived Webpage. CDC.gov.2021. URL: https://www.cdc.gov/coronavirus/2019-ncov/prevent-getting-sick/cloth-face-cover-guidance.html

[12] Loades ME, Chatburn E, Higson-Sweeney N, Reynolds S, Shafran R, Brigden A, et al. Rapid systematic review: The impact of social isolation and loneliness on the mental health of children and adolescents in the context of COVID-19. J Am Acad Child Adolesc Psychiatry 2020;59(11):1218-39.

[13] The disproportionate effects of COVID-19 on households with children. Newyorkfed.org. 2020. URL: https://libertystreeteconomics.newyorkfed.org/2020/08/the-disproportionate-effects-of-covid-19-on-households-with-children/.

[14] CDC. Families and COVID-19. Cdc.gov.2021. URL: https://www.cdc.gov/coronavirus/2019-ncov/groups/families-covid-19.html.

[15] Dunn CG, Kenney E, Fleischhacker SE, Bleich SN. Feeding low-income children during the Covid-19 pandemic. N Engl J Med 2020;382(18):e40.

[16] Gallegos D, Eivers A, Sondergeld P, Pattinson C. Food insecurity and child development: A state-of-the-art review. Int J Environ Res Public Health 2021;18(17):8990.

[17] Apa.org. URL: https://www.apa.org/monitor/2020/09/distance-learning-accomplish.

[18] Minnich C. Learning during COVID-19: Initial findings on students' reading and math achievement and growth-NWEA. Nwea.org. 2020. URL: https://www.nwea.org/research/publication/learning-during-covid-19-initial-findings-on-students-reading-and-math-achievement-and-growth/.

[19] Leeb RT, Bitsko RH, Radhakrishnan L, Martinez P, Njai R, Holland KM. Mental health- related emergency department visits among children aged <18 years during the COVID-19 pandemic - United States, January 1-October 17, 2020. MMWR 2020;69(45):1675-80.

[20] Polanczyk GV, Salum GA, Sugaya LS, Caye A, Rohde LA. Annual research review: A meta-analysis of the worldwide prevalence of mental disorders in children and adolescents. J Child Psychol Psychiatry 2015;56(3):345-65.

[21] Xie X, Xue Q, Zhou Y, Zhu K, Liu Q, Zhang J, et al. Mental health status among children in home confinement during the coronavirus disease 2019 outbreak in Hubei Province, China. JAMA Pediatr 2020;174(9):898-900.

[22] Zhou SJ, Zhang LG, Wang LL, Guo ZC, Wang JQ, Chen JC, et al. Prevalence and socio- demographic correlates of psychological health problems in Chinese adolescents during the outbreak of COVID-19. Eur Child Adolesc Psychiatry 2020;29(6):749-58.

[23] Liu S, Liu Y, Liu Y. Somatic symptoms and concern regarding COVID-19 among Chinese college and primary school students: A cross-sectional survey. Psychiatry Res 2020;289: 113070.

[24] Jiao WY, Wang LN, Liu J, Fang SF, Jiao FY, Pettoello-Mantovani M, et al. Behavioral and emotional disorders in children during the COVID-19 epidemic. J Pediatr 2020;221:264-6.

[25] Rosen Z, Weinberger-Litman SL, Rosenzweig C. Rosmarin DH, Muennig P, Carmody ER, et al. Anxiety and distress among the first community quarantined in the US due to COVID-19: Psychological implications for the unfolding crisis. PsyArXiv 2020:1-18. http://dx.doi.org/10.31234/osf.io/7eq8c.

[26] Nearchou F, Flinn C, Niland R, Subramaniam SS, Hennessy E. Exploring the impact of COVID-19 on mental health outcomes in children and adolescents: A systematic review. Int J Environ Res Public Health 2020;17(22):8479.

[27] Home. Covidminds.org. URL: https://www.covidminds.org.

[28] Pigaiani Y, Zoccante L, Zocca A, Arzenton A, Menegolli M, Fadel S, et al. Adolescent lifestyle behaviors, coping strategies and subjective wellbeing during the COVID-19 pandemic: An online student survey. Healthcare (Basel). 2020;8(4):472.

[29] No title. Cdc.gov. URL: https://www.cdc.gov/coronavirus/2019-ncov/daily-life-coping/parental-resource-kit/.

[30] Turk MA, Landes SD, Formica MK, Goss KD. Intellectual and developmental disability and COVID-19 case-fatality trends: TriNetX analysis. Disabil Health J 2020;13(3):100942.

[31] Malle L, Gao C, Bouvier N, Percha B, Bogunovic D. COVID-10 hospitalization is more frequent and severe in Downs syndrome and affects patients a decade younger. MedRxiv 2020;5(26):20112748.

[32] Chen M-H, Su T-P, Chen Y-S, Hsu J-W, Huang K-L, Chang W-H, et al. Comorbidity of allergic and autoimmune diseases in patients with autism spectrum disorder: A nationwide population-based study. Res Autism Spectr Disord 2013;7(2):205–12.

[33] Colizzi M, Sironi E, Antonini F, Ciceri ML, Bovo C, Zoccante L. Psychosocial and behavioral impact of COVID-19 in autism spectrum disorder: An online parent survey. Brain Sci 2020;10(6):341.

[34] Quality of life during COVID-19. Colorado.edu. URL: https://hazards.colorado.edu/quick-response-report/quality-of-life-during-covid-19.

[35] Price-Haywood EG, Burton J, Fort D, Seoane L. Hospitalization and mortality among Black patients and white patients with Covid-19. N Engl J Med 2020;382(26):2534-43.

[36] Kim SJ, Bostwick W. Social vulnerability and racial inequality in COVID-19 deaths in Chicago. Health Educ Behav 2020;47(4):509-13.

[37] Disease ED in. Health, United States. CDC.gov. URL: https://www.cdc.gov/nchs/hus/spotlight/HeartDiseaseSpotlight_2019_0404.pdf.

[38] Czeisler MÉ, Lane RI, Petrosky E, Wiley JF, Christensen A, Njai R, et al. Mental health, substance use, and suicidal ideation during the COVID-19 pandemic - United States, June 24-30, 2020. MMWR 2020;69(32):1049-57.

[39] COVID-19 disrupting mental health services in most countries, WHO survey. Who.int. URL: https://www.who.int/news/item/05-10-2020-covid-19-disrupting-mental-health-services-in-most-countries-who-survey.

[40] Olson CA, McSwain SD, Curfman AL, Chuo J. The current pediatric telehealth landscape. Pediatrics 2018;141(3):e20172334.

[41] Dryer B. Child and adolescent depression. Aap.org. URL: https://brightfutures.aap.org/Bright%20Futures%20Documents/History,%20Observation,%20and%20Surveillance.pdf.

[42] Hays RD, Spritzer KL, Schalet BD, Cella D. PROMIS®-29 v2.0 profile physical and mental health summary scores. Qual Life Res 2018;27(7):1885-91.

[43] Lima CKT, Carvalho PMM, Lima IAAS, Nunes JVAO, Saraiva JS, de Souza RI, et al. The emotional impact of Coronavirus 2019-nCoV (new Coronavirus disease). Psychiatry Res 2020;287:112915.

[44] Imran N, Zeshan M, Pervaiz Z. Mental health considerations for children and adolescents in COVID-19 Pandemic. Pak J Med Sci 2020;36(COVID19-S4):S67-72.

[45] Dumont-Mathieu T, Fein D. Screening for autism in young children: The Modified Checklist for Autism in Toddlers (M-CHAT) and other measures. Ment Retard Dev Disabil Res Rev 2005;11(3):253-62.

[46] Rath B, Donato J, Duggan A, Perrin K, Bronfin DR, Ratard R, et al. Adverse health outcomes after Hurricane Katrina among children and adolescents with chronic conditions. J Health Care Poor Underserved 2007;18(2):405-17.

[47] Lee J. Mental health effects of school closures during COVID-19. Lancet Child Adolesc Health 2020;4(6):421. doi: 10.1016/S2352-4642(20)30109-7.

[48] Koman R. Advices for managing the COVID-19 outbreak and the associated factors of mental distress for people with intellectual disability and autism spectrum disorder with high and very high support needs. World Psychiatry Association website. URL: https://3ba346de-fde6-473f-b1da-536498661f9c.filesusr.com/ugd/e172f3_c427b7464ef84ec2bfaf2eba061a4e59.pdf.

[49] nctsnadmin. PFA: Parent tips for helping school-age children after disasters. Nctsn.org. 2018. URL: https://3ba346de-fde6-473f-b1da-536498661f9c.filesusr.com/ugd/e172f3_c427b7464ef84ec2bfaf2eba061a4e59.pdf.

[50] CDC. Guidance for operating child care programs during COVID-19. Cdc.gov. URL: https://www.cdc.gov/coronavirus/2019-ncov/community/schools-childcare/guidance-for-childcare.html.

[51] WHO. Mental health and psychosocial considerations during the COVID-19 outbreak. URL: https://www.who.int/docs/default-source/coronaviruse/mental-health-considerations.pdf.

Section two: Perspectives of substance use disorders

Chapter 8

Neurobiology of substance use disorders

Nehdia Hashemi[1], MD, Nazish Imran[2], MRCPsych, Muhammad Waqar Azeem[3], MD and Ahsan Nazeer[3,*], MD

[1]Western Michigan University, Homer Stryker MD School of Medicine, Kalamazoo, Michigan, United States of America, [2]Department of Psychiatry, King Edward Medical University, Lahore, Pakistan and [3]Department of Psychiatry, Division of Child and Adolescent Psychiatry, Sidra Medicine, Doha, Qatar

Abstract

While substance use disorders have an onset in childhood or adolescence, untreated substance use disorders typically progress into adulthood, growing in severity and becoming chronic, relapsing, and potentially fatal disorders. These behaviors that were traditionally viewed as stemming from poor "choices" appear to have strong neurobiological and genetic underpinnings. Understanding the causes of addiction and underlying neurobiological processes is an active area of research. Most of the current knowledge is derived from preclinical studies and animal models of addiction, and the following is a brief review of the neurobiological basis of substance use disorders.

Introduction

The "Diagnostic and statistical manual of mental disorders, Fifth Edition (DSM-5)" has replaced the terms substance abuse and substance dependence in favor of a single category of "substance use disorder" and classifying them as mild, moderate, or severe to indicate the level of severity. These levels of severity can be determined by the number of diagnostic criteria that an individual can meet. The symptoms associated with substance use disorder can be summarized under four major groupings: impaired control, social impairment, risky use, and tolerance/withdrawal (1).

Substance use disorders are characterized by chronic remitting and relapsing course. Psychoactive substances act on the neuronal structures and processes that are important for regulating mood, behavior, and motivation. Most of our current understanding of the neurobiology of substance use disorders is derived from animal models of addiction. Some of

* ***Correspondence:*** Email: anazeer@sidra.org.

In: Behavioral Pediatrics
Editors: Donald E. Greydanus, Dilip R. Patel, Ahsan Nazeer et al.
ISBN: 979-8-88697-060-9

these models include the following: models of chronic drug preference, self-administration, reward, cravings, tolerance development, and withdrawal.

These models have been beneficial to understand mechanisms at the neuronal and synaptic levels during the acute phase of drug intake. With a better understanding of the role of genes and the interactions of receptors with neuronal circuits, our understanding of how addictive drugs work in the brain has advanced. Recent positron emission tomography (PET) and functional magnetic resonance imaging (fMRI) techniques have provided critical insights into this highly complex neuro-cognitive loop. Progress in neurobiological research is so rapid and findings at times so contradictory that authors suggest a continued review of literature for up-to-date information.

General concepts

In the majority of cases, substance use starts either as a recreational activity or as a means to gain some perceived benefits from a particular drug (e.g., pain relief from prescription opioids, increased energy, augmented attention, and/or control anxiety, way to deal with anger and depression). With repeated intake, a maladaptive pattern of behavior occurs that is characterized by loss of control and leads to drug dependence. Some of the factors that lead to chronic use include those listed in Table 1. In the face of chronic use, the pattern becomes more habitual and continues despite ongoing adverse effects and deterioration in psychosocial functioning.

Table 1. Factors leading to chronic drug use and dependence

Seeking faster routes of administration
Escalating doses
Repeated use of the drug
Limited social network
Ease of access to drugs
Emotional stress
Ignorance or disregard of danger warnings
Lack of access to treatment facilities

From a clinical point of view, this use results in the emergence of complex behavioral problems that probably result from substance-induced neurochemical changes in the nervous system. Abuse of illicit drugs costs more than $740 billion a year in increased health care costs, crime, and lost productivity in the United States alone (2). These disorders also contribute to the death of more than 90,000 Americans, while tobacco alone is linked to an estimated 480,000 deaths per year.

The development of drug addiction is a complex and insufficiently understood process at this phase of research. Among the factors favoring the development of drug dependence, those of particular interest include pharmacodynamic and pharmacokinetic characteristics, the amount consumed, the frequency of use, and the route of administration. Research regarding the mechanisms of action of drugs of abuse indicates that their reinforcing properties may be due to actions on a common neural circuit. With repeated administration of drugs of abuse, a neuro-adaptation response occurs. Some of the neuro-adaptation responses include long-term alterations in gene expression and protein regulation that cause a change in the neural circuits governing reward and motivation – leading to a maladaptive pattern of behavior.

During the early days of addiction research, the brain reward system was considered the final common pathway in addiction. Recent research, however, has shown that the addiction models are more complicated than can be explained by the reward model alone (3). Numerous brain structures are involved in the circuitry of learning, motivation, reward, and pleasure. The basal ganglia consist of the caudate, putamen, globus pallidus, and amygdala; the caudate and putamen together are called the striatum. The nucleus accumbens (NAc) is associated with reward, motivation, and learning. The hippocampus in the limbic system has widely dispersed neuronal connections and plays a role in developing dependence. Other anatomical areas of interest include the orbitofrontal cortex (inhibitory control), prefrontal cortex (executive control), and hypothalamic-pituitary-adrenal axis (associated with stress).

Given the importance of these areas in regulating behavior and emotion, it is no surprise that the above structures have been the focus of substance abuse research. Dense connections between the above areas and the forebrain – including mesolimbic and mesocortical dopaminergic pathways – are of particular interest in understanding the positive reinforcing effects of drugs. However, with ongoing research, researchers also understand the role of non-dopaminergic systems in the development and persistence of substance use disorders.

Dopamine

Drugs of abuse are heterogeneous in their mechanism of action and target receptors. Table 2 provides a classification based upon the mechanism of illicit drugs directly responsible for the increase in dopamine concentration (4).

Table 2. Classification of illicit drug mechanisms based on dopamine concentration increase (see text)

I.	Substances that activate the receptors coupled to G-proteins-GPCRs (opiates, cannabinoids, gamma-hydroxybutyrate)
II.	Substances that bind to the ionotropic receptors and ion channels (nicotine, benzodiazepines, alcohol)
III.	Substances that bind to the biogenic amine transporters (cocaine, amphetamine, MDMA)

Dopamine (DA) was discovered by Swedish neuropharmacologist and Nobel laureate Arvid Carlsson (1923-2018); also, along with serotonin and epinephrine, dopamine (DA) is one of the most widely studied and researched neurotransmitters in the nervous system. Dopamine is also involved in numerous essential brain functions, including regulating fine motor movements, learning, motivation, and cognitive functioning. Numerous stimuli (including food, sex, and addictive drugs) increase intrasynaptic DA levels in the nucleus accumbens (NAc) and prefrontal cortex (PFC) via their effects on the ventral tegmental area (VTA). The precise role of dopamine in the modulation of reward-related behavior remains controversial.

Most experts agree that some aspects of reward, including euphoria and pleasure, are dopamine-independent (5). Research also suggests that once compulsive use is established, the progression of addictive behaviors is mostly dopamine-independent. These observations come from the fact that many noxious and novel stimuli can increase DA within the brain without causing a reward or an addiction potential and that dopamine blockers do not stop drug-induced highs. In addition, acute DA release in the NAc does not fully explain the desire and compulsions that arise when individuals are exposed to drug use places, persons, and paraphernalia (i.e., triggers, cues). Other evidence comes from animal models with a hypodopaminergic genetic trait that, despite the DA signal blockage, show pleasurable responses to sweet fluids (6, 7).

It is worth noting that animal models of addiction have shown a variable pattern of DA neuronal firing that depends on cues to reward and the reward itself. In these models, a reward causes firing in DA neurons, but as the animals learn the signals, the response to reward habituates and firing occurs in response to the cues themselves (8, 9). This pattern suggests extensive input from the cerebral cortex and interactions between the hippocampus, amygdala, and striatum, implicating complex pathways in this neuro-circuitry of reward, craving, and habituation. A homeostatic state is reached with repeated stimuli, which is indicated by decreased DA response to such stimuli, a condition synonymous with tolerance in humans.

Numerous studies also have converged on the hypothesis that the above-mentioned cue-based neuronal firing is the cause of persistent drug use. This hypothesis is supported by the fact that most drug use and relapses follow exposure to environmental cues, including places of drug use, drug-using peers, and drug-related paraphernalia. These processes gradually lead to long-term changes and reorganization of neuronal circuitry. The candidate mechanisms underlying this neuronal reorganization are long-term potentiation (LTP) and long-term depression (LTD), the same processes involved in long-term memory and learning.

So far, five DA receptors (D1-D5) have been identified and are categorized into two different families: D1, D5 receptors, and D2, D3 receptors.

D1, D5 receptors

These receptors are G protein-linked and stimulate cyclic AMP. They are located postsynaptically and are associated with reward and behavioral inhibition. Research indicates that D1 receptor activation plays a crucial role in psychostimulant-induced behaviors, including locomotor activation, sensitization, conditioned place preference (CPP), and self-administration (SA) (10). This activation causes numerous extracellular and intracellular changes at a molecular level, including induction of Fos in the NAc and caudate-putamen regions. In experimental studies, inhibition of D1 receptors attenuates locomotor activation and CPP for cocaine; however, cocaine sensitization is not significantly affected by D1 antagonists.

Research is ongoing to identify the exact role of D1 receptors in the addiction process. In preclinical studies, an increased pattern of cocaine self-administration is found among animals exposed to a DA antagonist (11). The super-sensitivity of DA receptors can explain this behavioral change in the NAc, an observation that suggests the role of D1 receptors in the addiction process. D1 receptors are also involved in the relapse following abstinence. For example, cue-induced use of nicotine and MDMA seeking is prevented by D_1 antagonists. Stress-induced opioid seeking is partially reduced by both D_1 and D_2 antagonists, with a more significant effect of a non-selective DA receptor antagonist. In contrast, stress-induced cocaine-seeking is only prevented by a D_1 antagonist.

D2 and D3 receptors

These receptors also play a significant role in the signaling of DA neurons. Studies using animal models have yielded complex results. Pharmacological blockade of D2 receptors leads to a decreased response to morphine and ethanol (12). D2 receptors have two isoforms: D2L, which has postsynaptic effects, and D2S, which acts as a presynaptic autoreceptor. Because of its inhibitory function as a presynaptic autoreceptor in genetically modified D2-negative mice, the administration of cocaine causes significant elevations in the striatum (13). PET and SPECT studies have shown decreased D2 density in infrequent users of cocaine, heroin, and methamphetamine (14).

Other studies have found an inverse correlation between the D2 receptor density and self-administration of cocaine (15). In human studies of ethanol and methylphenidate, individuals with fewer D2 receptors required higher doses of these drugs to get the same response compared to individuals with higher D2 density in the NAc (16). Whether the decrease in D2 receptors is a predisposing event that causes drug addiction is an area of ongoing research (17).

D3 receptors are mainly localized in the limbic region and are structurally similar to D2 receptors. In animal studies, pharmacological blockage of these receptors was found to reduce the ethanol-seeking behavior, self-administration of ethanol, and reinstatement of cocaine and nicotine-seeking behaviors (18-20).

Serotonin and norepinephrine

Serotonin (5-HT) is a neurotransmitter involved in numerous bodily functions, including impulse control, sleep, appetite, sexual behaviors, and pain modulation. There are several serotonin receptors, with some being excitatory and some inhibitory in their function. Most important among these in addiction research is 5-HT1B, which is widely distributed across the central nervous system (CNS) and present in the terminal regions of DA and GABA neurons. Stimulation of this receptor inhibits GABA release, which removes the inhibitory influence of GABAergic effects on the DA system. In genetically modified 5-HT1B negative mice, the reinforcing effects of cocaine were markedly reduced (21).

Norepinephrine (NE) is another neurotransmitter present in abundance in the CNS. NE has widespread projections from the locus coeruleus, pons, and medulla to the hippocampus, hypothalamus, and amygdala. It plays a role in stress and arousal responses by its actions on α- and β-adrenergic receptors. During the early 1980s, animal models of self-administration (reward) failed to show a role for NE in addiction research.

However, in the 1990s, numerous other animal models emerged. Among them, the model of drug-induced locomotion proved critical to our understanding of the neurobiology of drug addiction. Most drugs of abuse induce locomotor activity, which suggests sensitization that, in turn, is a sign of craving. By using different models of NE antagonism (prazosin, lesions of locus ceruleus), studies have shown NE to play an essential role in psychostimulant-induced locomotion (22). On the other hand, increasing extracellular NE also increases the locomotor response to psychostimulants (23).

Cannabinoid (CB1) receptors

Endocannabinoids (eCBs) are lipid metabolites that act as modulators throughout the nervous system. Within the brain, eCBs activate CB1 receptors mostly located in presynaptic terminals and are also the primary target for Δ^9-tetrahydrocannabinol (Δ^9THC). CB1 receptors show widespread expression throughout the nervous system and are involved in the presynaptic depression of neurotransmitter release, possibly by inhibiting voltage-gated calcium and certain potassium channels (24). This synaptic depression is both short- and long-term. Short-term depression persists only as long as eCBs occupy CB1 receptors, while long-term depression outlasts receptor occupancy.

Cannabinoids are partial agonists at CB1 and mimic the effects of eCBs on CB1 receptors. Presynaptic CB1 receptors are also present on GABAergic terminals in the midbrain and reduce inhibition of dopaminergic neurons. This mechanism is thought to account for the rewarding effects of cannabinoid drugs; however, chronic exposure to cannabinoids produces tolerance to many of the behavioral effects seen during initial exposure.

γ-Aminobutyric acid (GABA)

GABA is the main inhibitory neurotransmitter in the nervous system and exerts its inhibitory effects by hyperpolarizing neurons. Three types of GABA receptors have been identified: GABA A, B, and C. GABA-A receptors also bind benzodiazepines and barbiturates. These are transmembrane ligand-gated ion channels that are mostly present in the postsynaptic membranes. Type A receptors play a vital role in ethanol's immediate and long-term effects. Ethanol increases the ion influx by increasing the amount of time ion channels are in the open state and decreasing their time in the closed state. GABA-A receptor antagonists reduce self-administration of ethanol and cocaine. On the other hand, agents that potentiate the effects of GABA-A receptors increase the self-administration of ethanol (25, 26).

Glutamate receptors

Glutamate is an excitatory neurotransmitter in the central nervous system (CNS), and glutamate receptors are divided into three subgroups. So far, two glutamate receptors, group III mGlu ($mGlu_7$) and group II mGlu receptors ($mGlu_{2/3}$), have received attention in the addiction field because they modulated the actions of drugs of abuse and representing possible therapeutic targets for the treatment of substance use disorders. Group II mGlu receptors are postsynaptic receptors and are widely distributed in the CNS. They function by inhibiting glutamate release in critical brain areas, including the prefrontal cortex, dorsal striatum, and nucleus accumbens (27). The effort to understand the exact role of these receptors in the neurobiology of substance use disorder has come up with conflicting results (28).

Magnetic resonance imaging (MRI)

Recent use of MRI has opened new opportunities for a better understanding of neurobiology and linking these findings to behaviors. It is well known that cortical and subcortical structures play an important role in emotions, compulsive seeking, and excessive use of substances during different phases of intoxication or withdrawals. MRI research has consistently shown the reduction in the gray matter of frontal lobes along with reductions in the insula, prefrontal cortex, and pregenual anterior cingulate. At the same time, a corresponding increase in the volumes of subcortical structures is associated with dependency on stimulants and cocaine (29, 30).

While the reduction in grey matter in frontal lobes has been associated with duration independency, it has proven to be challenging to find corresponding white matter volumetric changes in individuals with substance use disorders by using traditional MRI techniques. However, with the advent of diffusion tensor imaging, an MRI technique that probes brain structures by imaging the diffusion of water, a reduction in supratentorial and infratentorial white matter bundles has been noticed in chronic alcoholics. Functional MRI (fMRI) has helped researchers identify brain structures associated with specific cognitive processes, including cue-reactivity, in which exposure to stimuli induces cravings. Literature has reported increased activation in prefrontal and orbitofrontal cortex regions (31).

Another meta-analysis has reported increased amygdala, anterior cingulate cortex, and ventral striatum activity in individuals with alcohol, nicotine, and cocaine abuse (32). Another MRI technique, measurement of blood perfusion with arterial spin labeling (ASL), has identified significantly lower perfusion in frontal and parietal gray matter in individuals with chronic heart disease and alcoholism. Similarly, decreased perfusion is noted in the insula, anterior cingulate, and parietal gray matter in individuals with chronic opioid use (33).

Overall, studies that have used fMRI to predict relapse and treatment response are scarce. One such study conducted on individuals with stimulant abuse (methamphetamines) during a decision-making task identified 90-94% certainty of the individuals who will and will not relapse. Researchers achieved this by identifying the activation patterns in the insular, posterior cingulate, and temporal cortex (34). Although MRI studies in the addiction area are somewhat scarce and contradictory, a certain pattern is still emerging, making it worthwhile for researchers to further pursue this line of research.

Neuropharmacology of specific drugs

In the following text, we review the mechanism of action of various common drugs of abuse: stimulants, alcohol, opioids, nicotine/tobacco, and cannabinoids.

Stimulants

This category of drugs includes cocaine, amphetamines, and methylphenidate; these drugs produce many of their psychoactive effects by interacting with the dopamine transporter (DAT). DAT is a plasma membrane protein that actively translocates the released transmitter from the extracellular space into the presynaptic neuron, thus modulating dopamine availability in the nervous system. Chronic use of stimulants leads to long-term changes in DAT activities by mechanisms that are not well understood (35). Such changes, however, indicate that these compounds act by making both pharmacological and physiological alterations that lead to long-term transporter adaptations during the phases of addiction or treatment.

It is also known that stimulants prolong the time course and increase the extracellular concentration of DA following vesicular release with a net effect of producing longer lasting and widespread activation of DA receptors. As DAT is mostly expressed in the striatum, the effects of stimulants on DAT and dopamine are also largest in this area, with lesser effects in cortical regions and even in the midbrain itself.

Cocaine administration increases DA concentration and D1 receptor density in the striatum. This increased concentration in mesolimbic and mesocortical pathways is postulated to be responsible for the behavioral actions after cocaine administration. In animal studies, D1 receptor blockade in the NAc and the VTA reduces cocaine self-administration. In human studies, the acute "high" response to cocaine is correlated with DAT occupancy and DA release in the NAc (36).

It is important to note that dopamine antagonists do not block the rewarding effects of DA or other stimulants. One possible explanation for this lack of effect is that stimulants (including cocaine) also exert their effects by acting on the norepinephrine neurons. This point is validated from animal studies in which DAT deficient strains of mice appear to experience the rewarding effects of cocaine; this effect suggests an essential role of other neurotransmitters in the neurobiology of reward and addiction (37).

Norepinephrine, serotonin, and glutamate are other major neurotransmitter systems that are involved in the neurobiology of stimulant addiction. Cocaine administration increases norepinephrine activity by its action on the norepinephrine transporter. This increased plasma concentration of norepinephrine is correlated with the psychological effects of cocaine. Cocaine administration also increases extracellular serotonin concentration in the striatum and VTA by its effects on the serotonin transporter.

The exact role of serotonin in the reward pathway is unclear. Cocaine exerts its rewarding effects in serotonin transporter deficient strains of mice, whereas mice who are missing both DAT and serotonin transporters do not find cocaine rewarding (38). Human studies have failed to conceptualize the persistent role of serotonin in this pathway. Research reports that serotonin agonists (SSRIs), antagonists, or partial agonists all reduce the "high" cravings for cocaine (37).

Also, glutamate appears to play a role in relapse to cocaine (39). Acutely administered low-dose cocaine increases glutaminergic neuronal firing in the cortex and NAc, whereas higher doses inhibit this phenomenon. Cocaine also upregulates N-methyl-D-aspartate (NMDA) receptors binding in the striatum and amygdala.

Alcohol

All drugs of abuse, including alcohol, enhance the release of DA within the mesolimbic and mesocortical pathways of the brain. Alcohol intake causes a release of β-endorphins from the arcuate nucleus, which along with its effects on GABA and DA, is thought to cause pleasurable effects after alcohol intake. Acute intake of alcohol appears to increase the firing rate of midbrain DA neurons, while chronic exposure leads to the decreased excitability of these neurons. Decreased density in striatal dopamine receptors, as commonly seen in alcohol dependence, attenuates the effects of the reward circuit and leads to increased alcohol consumption.

Besides DA, it is widely accepted that alcohol also increases inhibitory neurotransmission at GABA receptors and reduces excitatory transmission at glutamate neurons. Alcohol acts on presynaptic glutamate receptors and calcium channels to inhibit glutamate release. These initial effects on neurotransmitters and ion channels lead to a cascade of events that involve glycine, serotonin, and opioid systems.

Glutamate is a major excitatory neurotransmitter in the nervous system. AMPA and NMDA receptors are two ion channels associated with the glutamate system and are responsible for excitatory neurotransmission in the mechanisms of learning and memory. NMDA receptors are sensitive to alcohol, while AMPA receptors show insensitivity. Inhibition of NMDA receptors in the prefrontal cortex may explain some of the sedative effects and cognitive deficits are seen after alcohol use. These receptors also play a critical role in regulating DA in the nucleus accumbens. NMDA receptor antagonists increase the DA level in the NAc, and this antagonism by alcohol can be one reason for its rewarding properties. These receptors also increase density in glutamatergic synapses after chronic alcohol consumption.

As noted above, alcohol increases the blood level of certain opioids, including β-endorphins. There is evidence that competitive inhibition of acetaldehyde, the first oxidative metabolite of ethanol, can interfere with removing monoamine neurotransmitter aldehydes in the brain, leading to the persistence of monoamine neurotransmitter aldehydes from the cerebrospinal fluid (CSF). It has been demonstrated that mixing these monoamine aldehydes with monoamines facilitates chemical combinations known as tetrahydroisoquinolines, which are opioid agonists that can be blocked by opioid receptor antagonists (39, 40).

Naltrexone also blocks the rewarding effects of ethanol while increasing its sedative effects but not its neurological effects (41). These findings explain why the opioid antagonist naltrexone is effective for treating alcoholism.

Table 3. List of opioids (partial)

Heroin
Morphine
Codeine
Methadone
Hydrocodone
Oxycodone
Fentanyl
Tramadol
Pentazocine
Others

Opioids

Opioids are natural and synthetic compounds related to natural opium and include those listed in table 3. So far, three different types of opioid receptors have been identified: mu, kappa, and delta. These receptors are abundant in the central nervous system and are found in the amygdala, caudate, cortex, putamen, and thalamus. These are Gi-coupled transmembrane receptors and have different affinities for endogenous peptides. β-endorphins are more selective for mu receptors, while dynorphins (Dyn) have more selectivity for kappa receptors. In opioid addiction, mu receptors are at the forefront of the research.

Numerous drugs (including heroin, morphine, and other opioid analgesics) are agonists of these receptors. Mu receptor agonists cause various effects, as noted in table 4. Kappa receptor agonists may reverse the mu receptor actions and cause dysphoria, delirium, dissociation, hallucinations, and seizures. These receptors are quite sensitive to stress. Delta opioid receptors may produce mild analgesia, respiratory depression, and seizures in high doses.

Table 4. Effects of Mu receptor agonists

Euphoria
Analgesia
Sedation
Constipation
Hypotension
Respiratory depression
Itching
Nausea
Meiosis

Most of what we know about the neurobiology of opioid addiction has been derived from animal models. Different approaches have been used in these models, including self-administration of opioids, use of opioid antagonists to disrupt the reward pathway, and lesions in the critical areas that are thought to be involved in the addiction pathway. In mice models of opioid self-administration, numerous areas of interest have been identified, including the ventral striatum, lateral septum, VTA, hippocampus, and periaqueductal gray (42, 43).

An increase in self-administration has been noticed after the injection of an opioid antagonist into the NAc and lateral hypothalamus. However, it is worth noting that the administration of an opioid antagonist into the VTA– a site that is considered one of the central areas in the reward pathway– failed to disrupt self-administration (44).

The role of the mesolimbic dopaminergic system is also suggested, but more research is needed in this area. DA antagonists do not influence the self-administration of opioids. However, opioids exert their reinforcing effects by increasing DA in the NAc, an effect that is thought to be the result of opioid-induced GABA inhibition (45).

Nicotine/tobacco

Tobacco continues to be the single most significant cause of preventable morbidity and mortality in the Western world (46). In the United States, tobacco-related health problems cost about 75 billion dollars per year in treatment expenditures. Despite this awareness, tobacco use continues to increase all over the world.

Nicotine is a psychoactive substance that affects numerous neuronal pathways and neurotransmitter systems. Nicotine acts on neuronal nicotinic-subtype acetylcholine receptors (nAChR) that are widely distributed in the nervous system. These are ligand-gated ion channels that, in the open stage, permit cations to pass through the channel pores. Evidence suggests a role of the VTA and DA pathways in nicotine addiction. VTA contains various nAChR receptors, and nicotine administration has been shown to activate DA signaling in the mesolimbic and mesocortical pathways and increase DA release in the nucleus accumbens. Continued activation of nAChR receptors leads to desensitization, which partially explains the decreased rewarding effects of nicotine that a smoker experiences later in the day (47).

Besides acting on the DA system in the VTA, nicotine also affects the GABA system in various ways. During the early phases of nicotine administration, it activates GABA neurons that are inhibitory on the DA system. However, nAChRs of the GABA system desensitize rather quickly, removing this inhibitory influence on the DA system. GABA agonists have been shown to decrease the self-administration of nicotine. This also corresponds to the activation of nAChRs on presynaptic glutamatergic neurons leading to increased excitatory glutamatergic transmission to the dopaminergic system.

The VTA receives excitatory glutamatergic projections from the prefrontal cortex that modulate the activity of DA and GABA. The tegmental pedunculo-pontine nucleus (TPP) is a brain region that receives descending GABA projections from the VTA and sends ascending glutamatergic and cholinergic projections to the VTA. This area is associated with a non-DA-related reward system that plays an essential role in the acute rewarding effects of opioids and nicotine (48).

It is essential to recognize that the reward characteristics of tobacco products as nicotine delivery systems vary depending on the mode of entry into the body and whether or not acetaldehyde is combined with the nicotine. Smoking delivers both acetaldehyde and nicotine to the brain within seconds of inhalation of a puff of smoke. Acetaldehyde is also involved in the alcohol reward process (see above) and has been shown to enhance the addictive properties of smoking (49).

Most heavy smokers (i.e., one to two packs a day) consume 200 to 400 rewarding puffs per day, the largest number of rewards of any known drug of abuse, accounting for the difficulty most smokers have in quitting. It should also be mentioned that most lifelong smokers begin smoking as adolescents, and 75% of those who smoke three cigarettes (30 puffs) will become committed lifelong smokers. Other forms of tobacco products such as snuff and chewing tobacco do not deliver acetaldehyde, yet many of the harmful constituents of tobacco are still present.

Smoking provides the most dangerous set of toxins, many resulting from combustion, as listed in table 5. The reward pathways reinforce the persistent ingestions despite noxious signals from the body to the contrary. Blockade of the alpha-4-beta-2 nicotinic cholinergic receptors by the partial agonist/antagonist varenicline removes the reward and lets the dysphoric effects of smoking speak for themselves (50).

Table 5. Toxins from smoking combustion (partial list)

Carbon monoxide
Cyanide
Formaldehyde
Hydrogen sulfide
Carcinogenic long-chain hydrocarbons (tar)
Ashes
Others

Nicotine delivery systems (such as the gum, patch, and lozenge) provide a slow nicotine delivery system devoid of acetaldehyde and the other 35,000 dangerous chemicals in tobacco smoke. The reduction in the reward, both by eliminating the acetaldehyde and by spreading out and delaying the reward, reduces its ability to reinforce self-administration behavior and permits extinction. By diminishing the extent of the withdrawal syndrome, persons trying to quit smoking find greater self-efficacy. If a smoking slip occurs, the occupancy of the nicotinic cholinergic receptors reduces the potency of the reward. Inhaled forms of nicotine delivery, such as e-cigarettes and nicotine spray inhalers, do provide harm avoidance but do not delay the nicotine reward—hence keeping the enslavement of the smoker active (51).

Bupropion helps reduce craving and response to smoking by its tendency to inhibit the reuptake of DA and norepinephrine from synapses; this causes enhanced and prolonged dopaminergic and noradrenergic activity and reduced reward strength of nicotine and acetaldehyde-mediated opioids. Smokers may worry about weight gain, depression, and decreased concentration—symptoms commonly seen in withdrawal. Bupropion may help reduce these symptoms, especially if started several weeks before the quit date (52).

Many smokers evoke the stress-reducing anxiolytic properties of smoking as a reason why they cannot quit smoking right now. However, studies of stress in smokers revealed that the only stress that smoking relieves is the stress of nicotine withdrawal that is additive with any other stress they might be experiencing (53). Smokers smoke to maintain a steady nicotine level in the blood and cerebral spinal fluid (CSF). Stress can increase adrenergic tone, thereby increasing heart rate, renal glomerular filtration, and excretion of nicotine. Every time the nicotine concentration drops below a certain level, craving surfaces causing an urge to smoke; this increases during stress causing increased consumption of cigarettes. Smokers increase their overall stress by adding recurrent nicotine withdrawal to their underlying anxiety by continuing to smoke.

Cannabinoids

Alcohol, nicotine, and marijuana are the most commonly used illicit drugs worldwide. Marijuana has a rich history and has been used as a legitimate medicine in some civilizations across the centuries. In Western medicine, its role in appetite stimulation, pain management, and the management of chemotherapy-induced nausea has been appreciated for some time.

So far, two cannabinoid receptors, CB1 and CB2, have been identified; both are G protein-coupled receptors. CB1 is predominantly found in the central and peripheral nervous system, including the VTA, NAc, hippocampus, and amygdala, while CB2 is predominantly found in immune cells. It is interesting to note that other than modulating the abuse potential of marijuana, cannabinoid receptors also are involved in the rewarding potential of other drugs, including alcohol, cocaine, and nicotine (54, 55). CB1 receptors play a significant role in addiction to marijuana; CB1 antagonists reduce drug-seeking behavior in animal models (56).

Administration of tetrahydrocannabinol (THC) increases DA in the reward center, including the NAc, striatum, and prefrontal cortex. This effect is considered a result of indirect action on glutamatergic and GABAergic neurons that modulate the DA system. Another interesting finding in this sequence has been the role of opioid receptors. It is shown that DA release after THC administration is not solely the result of CB1 receptor stimulation but that the opioid receptors also are involved in this cascade of events. Administration of the opioid antagonist naloxone blocks this effect, a finding that leads to the complex interaction of numerous neurotransmitters in the final pathway of the effect of the cannabinoids.

Conclusion

Current research has advanced our knowledge of the basic concept of the DA reward system to a more complex understanding of intracellular signal transduction and the harmonious interactions of different areas of the nervous system. Much remains unknown, with more questions arising with every discovery. With passing years, models of addiction will be further refined that, in turn, will help to find successful treatment modalities for this population in need.

References

[1] American Psychiatric Association. Diagnostic and Statistical Manual of Mental Disorders. 5th ed. Arlington, VA: American Psychiatric Publishing, 2013.

[2] National Institute on Drug Abuse (NIDA). Trends and statistics 2017. URL: https://www.drugabuse.gov/related-topics/trends-statistics.

[3] Koob GF, Le Moal M. Drug abuse: hedonic homeostatic dysregulation. Science 1997; 278(5335):52-8.

[4] Luscher C, Ungless MA. The mechanistic classification of addictive drugs. PLoS Med 2006;3(11):e437.

[5] Bechara A, Nader K, van der Kooy D. A two-separate-motivational-systems hypothesis of opioid addiction. Pharmacol Biochem Behav 1998;59(1):1-17.

[6] Pettit HO, Justice JB, Jr. Effect of dose on cocaine self-administration behavior and dopamine levels in the nucleus accumbens. Brain Res 1991;539(1):94-102.

[7] Robinson S, Sandstrom SM, Denenberg VH, Palmiter RD. Distinguishing whether dopamine regulates liking, wanting, and/or learning about rewards. Behav Neurosci 2005; 119(1):336-41.

[8] Hyman SE. Addiction: a disease of learning and memory. Am J Psychiatry 2005;162(8): 1414-22.

[9] Hyman SE, Malenka RC. Addiction and the brain: the neurobiology of compulsion and its persistence. Nat Rev Neurosci 2001;2(10):695-703.

[10] Baik JH. Dopamine signaling in reward-related behaviors. Front Neural Circuits 2013; 7:152.

[11] Goodman A. Neurobiology of addiction. An integrative review. Biochem Pharmacol 2008;75(1):266-322.

[12] Barone P, Tucci I, Parashos SA, Chase TN. Supersensitivity to a D-1 dopamine receptor agonist and subsensitivity to a D-2 receptor agonist following chronic D-1 receptor blockade. Eur J Pharmacol 1988;149(3):225-32.

[13] Risinger FO, Freeman PA, Rubinstein M, Low MJ, Grandy DK. Lack of operant ethanol self-administration in dopamine D2 receptor knockout mice. Psychopharmacology (Berl) 2000;152(3):343-50.

[14] Welter M, Vallone D, Samad TA, Meziane H, Usiello A, Borrelli E. Absence of dopamine D2 receptors unmasks an inhibitory control over the brain circuitries activated by cocaine. Proc Natl Acad Sci U S A 2007;104(16):6840-5.

[15] Volkow ND, Chang L, Wang GJ, Fowler JS, Ding YS, Sedler M, et al. Low level of brain dopamine D2 receptors in methamphetamine abusers: association with metabolism in the orbitofrontal cortex. Am J Psychiatry 2001;158(12):2015-21.

[16] Nader MA, Morgan D, Gage HD, Nader SH, Calhoun TL, Buchheimer N, et al. PET imaging of dopamine D2 receptors during chronic cocaine self-administration in monkeys. Nat Neurosci 2006;9(8):1050-6.

[17] Yoder KK, Kareken DA, Seyoum RA, O'Connor SJ, Wang C, Zheng QH, et al. Dopamine D2 receptor availability is associated with subjective responses to alcohol. Alcohol Clin Exp Res 2005;29(6):965-70.

[18] Volkow ND, Wang GJ, Fowler JS, Logan J, Gatley SJ, Wong C, et al. Reinforcing effects of psychostimulants in humans are associated with increases in brain dopamine and occupancy of D(2) receptors. J Pharmacol Exp Ther 1999;291(1):409-15.

[19] Heidbreder CA, Andreoli M, Marcon C, Hutcheson DM, Gardner EL, Ashby CR, Jr. Evidence for the role of dopamine D3 receptors in oral operant alcohol self-administration and reinstatement of alcohol-seeking behavior in mice. Addict Biol 2007; 12(1):35-50.

[20] Cervo L, Cocco A, Petrella C, Heidbreder CA. Selective antagonism at dopamine D3 receptors attenuates cocaine-seeking behaviour in the rat. Int J Neuropsychopharmacol 2007;10(2):167-81.

[21] Barot SK, Ferguson SM, Neumaier JF. 5-HT1B receptors in nucleus accumbens efferents enhance both rewarding and aversive effects of cocaine. Eur J Neurosci 2007;25(10):3125-31.

[22] Weinshenker D, Schroeder JP. There and back again: a tale of norepinephrine and drug addiction. Neuropsychopharmacology 2007;32(7):1433-51.

[23] Salomon L, Lanteri C, Glowinski J, Tassin J-P. Behavioral sensitization to amphetamine results from an uncoupling between noradrenergic and serotonergic neurons. Proc Natl Acad Sci U S A 2006;103(19):7476-81.

[24] Wiskerke J, Pattij T, Schoffelmeer AN, De Vries TJ. The role of CB1 receptors in psychostimulant addiction. Addict Biol 2008;13(2):225-38.

[25] Nowak K, McBride W, Lumeng L, Li TK, Murphy J. Blocking GABAA receptors in the anterior ventral tegmental area attenuates ethanol intake of the alcohol-preferring P rat. Psychopharmacol 1998;139(1-2):108-16.

[26] Boyle AE, Segal R, Smith BR, Amit Z. Bidirectional effects of GABAergic agonists and antagonists on maintenance of voluntary ethanol intake in rats. Pharmacol Biochem Behav 1993;46(1):179-82.

[27] Walker AG, Wenthur CJ, Xiang Z, Rook JM, Emmitte KA, Niswender CM, et al. Metabotropic glutamate receptor 3 activation is required for long-term depression in medial prefrontal cortex and fear extinction. Proc Natl Acad Sci USA 2015;112(4):1196-201.

[28] Johnson KA, Lovinger DM. Presynaptic G protein-coupled receptors: Gatekeepers of addiction? Front Cell Neurosci 2016;10:264.

[29] Fowler JS, Volkow ND, Kassed CA, Chang L. Imaging the addicted human brain. Sci Pract Perspect 2007;3(2):4-16.

[30] Ersche KD, Williams GB, Robbins TW, Bullmore ET. Meta-analysis of structural brain abnormalities associated with stimulant drug dependence and neuroimaging of addiction vulnerability and resilience. Curr Opin Neurobiol 2013;23(4):615-24.

[31] Wilson SJ, Sayette MA, Fiez JA. Prefrontal responses to drug cues: a neurocognitive analysis. Nat Neurosci 2004;7(3):211-4.

[32] Kuhn S, Gallinat J. Common biology of craving across legal and illegal drugs - a quantitative meta-analysis of cue-reactivity brain response. Eur J Neurosci 2011;33(7): 1318-26.

[33] Mon A, Durazzo TC, Gazdzinski S, Meyerhoff DJ. The impact of chronic cigarette smoking on recovery from cortical gray matter perfusion deficits in alcohol dependence: longitudinal arterial spin labeling MRI. Alcohol Clin Exp Res 2009;33(8):1314-21.

[34] Paulus MP, Tapert SF, Schuckit MA. Neural activation patterns of methamphetamine-dependent subjects during decision making predict relapse. Arch Gen Psychiatry 2005; 62(7):761-8.

[35] Mash DC, Pablo J, Ouyang Q, Hearn WL, Izenwasser S. Dopamine transport function is elevated in cocaine users. J Neurochem 2002;81(2):292-300.

[36] Kimmel HL, O'Connor JA, Carroll FI, Howell LL. Faster onset and dopamine transporter selectivity predict stimulant and reinforcing effects of cocaine analogs in squirrel monkeys. Pharmacol Biochem Behav 2007;86(1):45-54.

[37] Volkow ND, Fowler JS, Wang GJ, Baler R, Telang F. Imaging dopamine's role in drug abuse and addiction. Neuropharmacology 2009;56(Suppl 1):3-8.

[38] Filip M, Frankowska M, Zaniewska M, Golda A, Przegalinski E. The serotonergic system and its role in cocaine addiction. Pharmacol Rep 2005;57(6):685-700.

[39] Collins MA, Bigdeli MG. Tetrahydroisoquinolines in vivo. I. Rat brain formation of salsolinol, a condensation product of dopamine and acetaldehyde, under certain conditions during ethanol intoxication. Life Sci 1975;16(4):585-601.

[40] Yamanaka Y, Walsh MJ, Davis VE. Salsolinol, an alkaloid derivative of dopamine formed in vitro during alcohol metabolism. Nature 1970;227(5263):1143-4.

[41] Swift RM, Whelihan W, Kuznetsov O, Buongiorno G, Hsuing H. Naltrexone-induced alterations in human ethanol intoxication. Am J Psychiatry 1994;151(10):1463-7.

[42] David V, Cazala P. Anatomical and pharmacological specificity of the rewarding effect elicited by microinjections of morphine into the nucleus accumbens of mice. Psychopharmacology 2000;150(1):24-34.

[43] Le Merrer J, Gavello-Baudy S, Galey D, Cazala P. Morphine self-administration into the lateral septum depends on dopaminergic mechanisms: Evidence from pharmacology and Fos neuroimaging. Behav Brain Res 2007;180(2):203-17.

[44] Vaccarino FJ, Pettit HO, Bloom FE, Koob GF. Effects of intracerebroventricular administration of methyl naloxonium chloride on heroin self-administration in the rat. Pharmacol Biochem Behav 1985;23(3):495-8.

[45] Johnson SW, North RA. Opioids excite dopamine neurons by hyperpolarization of local interneurons. J Neurosci 1992;12(2):483-8.

[46] Centers for Disease Control and Prevention (CDC). Annual smoking-attributable mortality, years of potential life lost, and economic costs–United States, 1995-1999. MMWR 2002;51(14):300-3.

[47] Laviolette SR, Van Der Kooy D. The neurobiology of nicotine addiction: bridging the gap from molecules to behaviour. Nat Rev Neurosci 2004;5(1):55-65.

[48] Mansvelder HD, McGehee DS. Cellular and synaptic mechanisms of nicotine addiction. J Neurobiol 2002;53(4):606-17.

[49] Belluzzi JD, Wang R, Leslie FM. Acetaldehyde enhances acquisition of nicotine self-administration in adolescent rats. Neuropsychopharmacology 2005;30(4):705-12.

[50] Jorenby DE, Hays JT, Rigotti NA, Azoulay S, Watsky EJ, Williams KE, et al. Efficacy of varenicline, an alpha4beta2 nicotinic acetylcholine receptor partial agonist, vs. placebo or sustained-release bupropion for smoking cessation: a randomized controlled trial. JAMA 2006;296(1):56-63.

[51] Benowitz NL. Neurobiology of nicotine addiction: implications for smoking cessation treatment. Am J Med 2008;121(4 Suppl 1):S3-10.

[52] Hurt RD, Sachs DP, Glover ED, Offord KP, Johnston JA, Dale LC, et al. A comparison of sustained-release bupropion and placebo for smoking cessation. N Engl J Med 1997; 337(17):1195-202.

[53] Schachter S, Silverstein B, Kozlowski LT, Perlick D, Herman CP, Liebling B. Studies of the interaction of psychological and pharmacological determinants of smoking. J Exp Psychol Gen 1977;106(1):3-12.

[54] Mechoulam R, Parker L. Cannabis and alcohol–a close friendship. Trends Pharmacol Sci 2003;24(6):266-8.

[55] Forget B, Barthelemy S, Saurini F, Hamon M, Thiebot MH. Differential involvement of the endocannabinoid system in short- and long-term expression of incentive learning supported by nicotine in rats. Psychopharmacology (Berl) 2006;189(1):59-69.

[56] Economidou D, Mattioli L, Cifani C, Perfumi M, Massi M, Cuomo V, et al. Effect of the cannabinoid CB 1 receptor antagonist SR-141716A on ethanol self-administration and ethanol-seeking behaviour in rats. Psychopharmacology 2006;183(4):394-403.

Chapter 9

Substance use and abuse in adolescents: An overview

Donald E Greydanus[1,*], MD, DrHC(Athens), Prerna Kukreti[2], MD and Harish K Pemde[3], MD

[1]Department of Pediatric and Adolescent Medicine, Western Michigan University Homer Stryker MD School of Medicine, Kalamazoo, Michigan, United States of America
[2]Department of Psychiatry,
[3]Department of Pediatrics, Lady Hardinge Medical College, New Delhi, India

Abstract

Substance use and abuse remains a major public health issue of adolescents throughout the world, including the United States. Encouragement by the media, peers, and many adults along with easy access to drugs of all types continues to lure countless millions of youth into use and abuse of many drugs. Results of the 2019 US Centers for Disease Control and Prevention Youth Risk Behavior Surveillance notes that there is significant abuse of drugs including illicit drugs but also prescription medications including stimulants, synthetic narcotics, and "recreational" cough syrups and several more emerging as we write. This discussion considers various drugs, including tobacco, alcohol, marijuana, cocaine, heroin, hallucinogens, inhalants, and some of the designer drugs.

Introduction

The United States SAMHSA (Substance Abuse and Mental Health Services Administration) directs a survey every year of the US population (non-military, non-institutionalized) who are 12 years of age and older (NSDUH SAMHSA, 2018). The publications is called NSDUH (National Survey of Drug Use and Health) and its 2018 report noted that 164.8 million people aged 12 or older in the United States (60.2 percent) were past month substance users (i.e., tobacco, alcohol, or illicit drugs) in the month prior to the survey (1). Racial disparities in illicit drug use have already been identified by various studies (2, 3).

* ***Correspondence:*** Professor Donald E Greydanus, MD, DrHC (Athens), Founding Chair, Department of Pediatric and Adolescent Medicine, Western Michigan University Homer Stryker MD School of Medicine, Oakland Drive Campus, 1000 Oakland Drive, Kalamazoo, MI 49008-1284, United States. Email: donald.greydanus@med.wmich.edu.

In: Behavioral Pediatrics
Editors: Donald E. Greydanus, Dilip R. Patel, Ahsan Nazeer et al.
ISBN: 979-8-88697-060-9

It is important that clinicians caring for adolescents be directly involved in teaching their patients how to prevent the use and abuse of drugs (see Table 1); clinicians can also remain active in the management of substance abuse disorders, if it develops in their patient. Adolescent exposure to illicit drugs can lead to a lifetime of medical and psychiatric effects (4). The impact of illicit drugs when taken during pregnancy can be devastating to the fetus and child (5). Drug addiction involves mesocorticolimbic circuitry dysfunction and can be a lifelong problem especially from cannabis, cocaine, nicotine, alcohol, and ecstasy (6). A number of factors are involved in drug addiction including the role of serotonin, ghrelin, and other factors that are under study (7, 8). Death from use of illicit drugs continues as seen with use of heroin, amphetamines, inhalants and others (9).

Table 1. Drugs of abuse

- Tobacco
- Marijuana (Cannabis)
- Alcohol
- Cocaine
- Heroin
- Amphetamine
- Methamphetamine
- MDMA [*Ecstasy]*
- flunitrazepam [Rohypnol]
- Gamma-hydroxybutyrate [*GHB*]
- Ketamine [Ketalar]
- LSD {*lysergic acid diethylamide}*
- *PCP {phencyclidine}*
- *Tryptamines*
- Barbiturates
- Designer drugs
- *Sports Doping and Performance Enhancing Drugs*

Screening for substance abuse is critical because the neuro-psychiatric changes caused by some drugs (i.e., 3,4-methylenedioxy-methamphetamine [MDMA]; *ecstasy*) may be irreversible and there have been reports of acute psychosis following marijuana (cannabis) and phencyclidine (PCP) (8, 10). One should also consider the likelihood of co-morbid conditions (see Table 2) in any adolescent or young adult with a history of continuing or repeated substance abuse; these conditions include attention-deficit/hyperactivity disorder (ADHD), especially when associated with or secondary to a learning disorder where treatment is protective. Risk factors for drug abuse are reviewed in Table 3, while Table 4 considers non-specific indicators of drug abuse and Table 5 outlines protective factors for drug abuse (4, 11). Small screening tests may be helpful, such as the CRAFFT questions for alcohol use and Problem Oriented Screening Instrument for Teenagers (POSIT) (8). The role of prescription medication dependence must be considered also by clinicians (12).

Table 2. Co-morbid disorders of substance abuse disorder

- ADHD
- Oppositional Defiant Disorder
- Conduct Disorder
- Personality Disorders (antisocial, borderline, narcissistic)
- Mood Disorders
- Anxiety Disorders
- Evolving Psychosis
- Post-traumatic Stress Disorder
- Eating disorders

Table 3. Risk factors for substance abuse in adolescents*

Genetics	**Alcoholism among 1st or 2nd degree relatives** **Male gender**
Self/Individual/Personal	Abuse Early onset of drug use Early sexual activity / homosexuality Attention deficit disorders Antisocial behavior Aggressive temperament Depression Poor self image Learning disorders Parental rejection Lack of self control Low self-esteem Euphoric/mood altering effects of drugs Body modification (as cutting)
Family	Dysfunctional family dynamics Permissiveness Authoritarianism Parental conflict, divorce, separation Poor supervision, lack of supervision Poor parental role modeling
Community/Environmental/Societal	Easy availability of drugs and alcohol Acceptance of drug use behavior Poor general quality of life in the neighborhood Media influence Criminal activities in neighborhood Cultural and religious sanction Low religiosity Employment Increased use of drugs and alcohol in certain ethnic groups
Peer Group Influence	Substance using peers Rebellion Rites of passage of puberty Risk-taking behavior Curiosity Desire to belong Independence Early tobacco use
School/Academic	Poor school performance Poor school environment Truancy

*Modified with permission: Patel DR, Greydanus DE. Substance abuse: A pediatric concern. Indian J Pediatrics 1999;66:557-67 (11).

Treatment needs of adolescents are different as they often present with polydrug use, do not report withdrawal symptoms and sometimes the pattern of use is not able to fulfill diagnostic criteria for SUD (diagnostic orphan). Also, voluntary help seeking is less because of poor insight due to lack of maturity and peer approval for drug use practices that normalize this behavior (8). Additionally, concerns about lack of confidentiality and concern about parents being informed deter adolescents to inform clinicians about substance use problems. A major contribution that the primary care clinician can provide is to screen, provide brief intervention, refer appropriately and to establish a medical home for all youth including those with substance use (13).

Table 4. Non-specific indicators of substance abuse*

Physical indicators	Academic indicators	Behavioral and psychological indicators
Unexplained weight loss	Deterioration of short-term memory	Risk taking behavior
Hypertension		Mood swings
Red eyes	Poor judgment	Depression, withdrawal
Nasal irritation	Falling grades	Panic reaction
Frequent "colds" or "allergies"	Frequent absences	Acute psychosis
Hoarseness	Truancy	Paranoia
Chronic cough	Conflicts with teachers	Lying
Hemoptysis	Suspensions	Stealing
Chest pain	Expulsion	Promiscuity
Wheezing		Conflict with authorities and family members
Frequent unexplained injuries		Runaway behavior
Needle tracks		Altered sleep pattern
Blank stares into space		Altered appetite
Scratch marks		Poor hygiene
Tattoos		Loss of interest in extracurricular activities
Excessive acne		Drug using peers
Testicular atrophy		Preferences for dress, music, movies, identifying with drug using culture
Malaise		drug paraphernalia

*Used with permission: Patel DR, Greydanus DE. Substance abuse: Apediatric concern. Indian J Pediatrics 1999;66:557-67 (11).

Table 5. Factors protective of substance abuse in adolescents*

- Nurturing home environment
- Good communication within family
- Supportive parents, intact family, appropriate adult supervision
- Positive self-esteem
- Assertiveness
- Social competence
- Academic success
- Good schools
- Good general health
- High intelligence
- Positive adult role models
- Peer group with positive personal attributes
- Religious involvement
- A personal sense of morality

*Used with permission: Patel DR, Greydanus DE. Substance abuse: A pediatric concern. Indian J Pediatrics 1999;66:557-67 (11).

The success of management is partially based on the underling genetics of addiction for a person, especially with opioid, alcohol, and cocaine dependence (14). Straightforward talk with teens about drug use is important in the screening process, though the teenager's estimates are often lower than the actual use. The clinician can work with the community in supporting community-based drug abuse prevention programs. Models of treatment are available ranging from brief to intensive management (15). Attention to improving sleep dysfunction in those with substance dependence and depression is an important goal in overall management of these persons (16, 17).

Adolescents generally progress from initial drug use to more serious drug use behavior in a pattern that is recognizable (see Table 6). At first, there is curiosity about drugs, though no drug use may be occurring. A need for acceptance by some peer group along with a low self-esteem may lead to experimentation with some drugs—often the "gateway" drugs— tobacco, alcohol and/or marijuana (cannabis).

Table 6. MacDonald's stages of substance abuse*

Stage	**1. Learning the mood swing**	**2. Seeking the mood swing**	**3. Preoccupation with the mood swing**	**4. Using drugs to feel normal**
Mood Alteration	Euphoria Normal	Euphoria Normal Some pain	Euphoria Normal Definite pain	Euphoria Normal Marked pain
Feelings	Feels good; few consequences	Excitement; early guilt	Euphoric highs; doubts, including severe shame and guilt; depression, suicidal thoughts	Chronic guilt; shame, remorse, depression
Drugs	Tobacco Marijuana Alcohol	All of the above plus inhalants, hashish, depressants, methamphetamine, prescription drugs	All listed plus psilocybin, PCP, LSD, cocaine	Whatever is available
Sources	Peers	Buying	Selling	Any way possible
Behavior	Little detectable change; moderate after-the-fact lying	Dropping extracurricular activities and hobbies; mixed friends (straight and drug users); dress changing; erratic school performance and truancy; unpredictable mood and attitude swings; manipulative behavior	"Cool" appearance; straight friends dropped; family fights (verbal or physical); stealing (police incidents); pathological lying; school failure; truancy, expulsion, jobs lost	Physical deterioration (weight loss, chronic cough); severe mental deterioration (memory loss and flashbacks); paranoia, volcanic anger; school dropout; frequent overdosing
Frequency	Progress to weekend use	Weekend use progressing to four to five times per week; some solo use	Daily; frequent solo use	All day every day

PCP = phencyclidine; LSD = lysersic acid diethylamide.

*Used with permission: Patel DR, Greydanus DE. Substance abuse: Apediatric concern. Indian J Pediatrics 1999;66:557-67 (11).

At some point the euphoria some drugs deliver is felt by the adolescent, typically at weekend parties or when combined with other substances. In some youth, there develops a state of actively seeking out the euphoria of drug use with widening of the types of drugs used (i.e., cocaine, ecstasy, heroin, others), using personal drug paraphernalia, buying and/or stealing drugs on a regular basis, and becoming more dependent on one or more drugs. There is often a drop in grades, change of clothes, switching of peer group, and a strong denial of using/abusing any drugs. Seeking the euphoric state becomes the center piece of the individual's life which becomes out of control as the menu of drugs tried increases in scope. There may also be evidence of depression, worsening mood swings, acting out behaviors, suicide, violence, malaise, and lethargy. At this stage, the abuser seeks the euphoric state to feel "normal." This progression from experimenting with drugs to abuse and burnout can be seen over months to years (8).

DSM-5

The American Psychiatric Association published its 5th edition of the "Diagnostic and statistical manual of mental disorders (DSM-5)" in 2013 (18). Some changes were seen in this 5th edition in contrast to the 4th Edition. The DSM-5 provided changes in the diagnostic criteria of substance related disorders (SRD). In the previous edition (DSM-IV-TR, 2000), SRDs were classified as substance use disorders (SUD) and substance induced disorders (SID). SUD was also identified as "abuse" and "dependence" disorders according to specific substances (i.e., opioid abuse and dependence, alcohol abuse and dependence, and so forth) (19). SID included such classifications as intoxication, withdrawal, delirium, anxiety and others as induced by specific substances (i.e., opioids, alcohol, others). The diagnoses of "abuse" and "dependence" categories needed their own specific criteria. Abuse could be diagnosed by meeting only one of those criteria while dependence needed at least three of those criteria.

In the DSM-5 SUD and SID terms remain but in SUD the previous diagnostic distinction between abuse and dependence was removed and a single category was developed called "substance use disorder" that ranged from mild to severe. A mild disorder is defined as meeting 2-3 of the SUD criteria versus 4-5 for moderate and 6 or more for a severe disorder (18).

In the DSM-5 there was an increase in the diagnostic threshold in that at least two criteria (versus 1) are required for an SUD. "Craving" is added as a new criterion and refers to an intense desire or urge for a drug. Also, the criteria, "problems with law enforcement" was removed since laws vary from country to country and over time.

YRBS 2019

A variety of illicit drugs are reviewed in this review with prevalence mainly based on the US Centers for Disease and Prevention (CDC) 2019 Youth Risk Behavioral Surveillance Survey (YRBSS) (20). The reader is encouraged to review this document. Several new categories have been added such as prescription opioid misuse and synthetic cannabinoids.

The report also notes that 14% of students had taken prescription opioid drugs without a doctor's prescription one or more times during their life; these drugs included oxycontin, Percocet, Vicodin, codeine, Adderall, Ritalin, or Xanax (20). The prevalence was 17.8% in 2013. Also, 1.6% of students had used a needle to inject any illegal drug into their body one or more times during their life; this prevalence was 2.3% in 2011 (2, 17). The 2013 survey had noted that 22.1% of students had been offered, sold, or given an illegal drug by someone on school property during the 12 months prior to the survey; this prevalence was 24.0% in 1993 (2, 17).

Energy drinks

The negative effects of energy drinks often containing large amounts of caffeine is becoming an increasing problem in adolescents and young adults; cardiovascular and neurological adverse effects are particularly seen (21). The DSM-5 lists four caffeine-related disorders: caffeine intoxication, caffeine withdrawal, other caffeine-induced disorders, and unspecified caffeine-related disorders (18).

Designer drugs

Clandestine chemists and surreptitious laboratories are developing a wide variety of designer drugs or "legal highs" which are analogs of such drugs as opioids, cannabinoids, phencyclidine, amphetamine, and others (8, 22-27). Their development can be traced to the 1960s but their production has escalated since 2008. They are used to mimic the effects of these drugs such as synthetic cannabinoids which mimic the psychoactive effects of cannabis and have been called spice drugs or K2 drugs. Cathinone is a natural occurring amphetamine analogue that is found in the *Cathaedulis* plant leaves and synthetic cathinones (such as mephedrone or 3,4-methylenedioxypyrovalerone [MDPV]) are derivatives of phenylalkylamines which has amphetamine-like effects. Some are piperazine derivatives. Designer psychostimulants have been developed to mimic the effects of amphetamines, cocaine, or ecstasy (8). Methoxydine and methoxetamine are designer drugs with phencyclidine effects (8, 17).

They may be sold on the internet or elsewhere as "bath salts" or "plant foods" and marked as "not for human consumption" in order to escape legal prosecution. Many adverse side effects may result depending on the exact product, its doses, what impurities it contains and other factors. Their use can lead to negative effects that are cardiovascular, neurological, renal, psychotic and others including death. Management of adverse reactions can be difficult and complicated by lack of knowledge by the patient and clinician what was taken (8). Management of negative reactions to synthetic cathinones ("bath salts") for example, focus on lowing the agitation and psychosis that are seen along with supporting renal perfusion; benzodiazepines and antipsychotics are used (28). Persons seeking euphoric experiences, including adolescents and young adults, should be educated about these designer drugs that are increasingly becoming available outside local laws.

Tobacco

Tobacco remains a widely used and abused drug that enjoys a high level of acceptance by society, including governments that allow it to be grown for profit. In a 1999 national survey conducted by the Centers for Disease Control and Prevention (CDC), one in every eight middle-school students reported using some form of tobacco (*cigarettes*, *cigars*, *bidis*, or *kreteks*) in the past month (8). Bidis (or beedies) are brown, hand-rolled, flavored tobacco while kreteks (clove cigarettes) contain a mixture of tobacco and cloves; both are imported from Indonesia (17). Electronic cigarettes (E-cigarettes) are now available on the marketplace, which also can pose a threat to adolescents, though more research is needed to study the effects (29, 30). The role of nicotine as a gateway drug has been shown by research (31, 32). The DSM-5 lists a number of tobacco-related disorders: tobacco use disorder (mild, moderate, severe), tobacco withdrawal, other tobacco-induced disorders, and unspecified tobacco related disorders (18).

2019 YRBS

The 2019 YRBS reports that 24.1% of high school students had ever tried cigarette smoking with a prevalence of 25.3% in males and 22.9% in females (33). The prevalence was higher among white (25.6%) and Hispanic (26.1%) students than black (14.2%) students. The prevalence of ever smoked cigarettes changed from 70.1% in 1991 to 24.1% in 2019. This survey also revealed that 9.3% had smoked a whole cigarette for the first time before age 13 years and this dropped from 23.8% in 1991 to 7.9% in 2019. Also, 15.7% of students had smoked cigarettes on at least one day during the 30 days prior to the survey and this had dropped from 27.5% in 1991 to 6% in 2019. It was also noted that 1.3% of students had smoked cigarettes 20 or more days during the 30 days before the survey and this dropped from 12.7% in 1991 to 1.3% in 2019. Among the 6% who currently smoke cigarettes, 8.1% had smoked more than 10 cigarettes per day on the days they smoked during the 30 days before the survey; t his dropped from 18.0% in 1991 to 8.1% in 2019 (33).

Among the 6% who currently smoked cigarettes, 52.4% had tried to quit smoking cigarettes during the 12 months before the survey; this changed from 57.4% in 2001 to 52.4% in 2019. Also, 1.1% of students had ever smoked at least one cigarette daily for 30 days and this dropped from 20.0% in 2001 to 1.1% in 2019 (33). Also,6% had smoked cigarettes on at least one day during the 30 days before the survey.

The 2019 report also notes that 9.2% of students had smoked cigarettes or cigars on at least one day during the 30 days before the survey; this decreased from 22.0% in 1997 to 9.2% in 2019. It also noted that 10.5% of students had reported current cigarette use, current smokeless tobacco use, or current cigar use; this prevalence had decreased from 43.4% in 1997 to 10.5% in 2019 (33).

General issues

The smoke of cigars is more alkaline than that of cigarettes, dissolves more easily in saliva, and achieves the desired dose of nicotine without the need to inhale smoke into the lungs (8). Cigars are capable of providing high levels of nicotine at a rate fast enough to produce clear dependence, even if the smoke is not inhaled. The risk of lung cancer for cigar aficionados (well-known to cigarette smokers) is much higher than once thought. This rate increases more for cigar smokers if they were previous cigarette smokers. A class of carcinogenic compounds known as tobacco-specific, N-nitrosamines (TSNA) is present in cigar smoke at significantly higher levels than in cigarette smoke. Examination on a "per gram of tobacco smoke" basis reveals that tar, carbon monoxide, and ammonia are produced at greater quantities by cigars. When equal doses are applied, the tar produced by cigars exerts a greater tumor-producing activity in mice because of higher concentrations of carcinogenic polycyclic aromatic hydrocarbons.

Nicotine, an important component in tobacco, is highly addictive and a number of genes are involved such as the nicotinic receptor gene cluster on chromosome 15q25 (34). Current research shows that adolescents experience symptoms of nicotine dependence long before they become everyday smokers. Early and continued intervention, including the clinical use of such instruments as the HONC (*Hooked On Nicotine Checklist)*, is required because initiation of smoking during adolescence is related to drunkenness-oriented alcohol use and an increased risk for future substance abuse (8). The most powerful predictor of drunk driving in this research is regular smoking at age 14 (8).

Nicotine is absorbed over various sites: lungs, buccal mucosa, skin, and gastrointestinal tract. Approximately 10 mg of nicotine is found in one cigarette; when smoked, 1.0 to 3.0 mg of nicotine is absorbed by the user. Nicotine is rapidly taken up by the brain's nicotinic acetylcholine receptors that are found in numerous non-cholinergic presynaptic and postsynaptic areas. The tobacco addict has chronic exposure to many dangerous chemicals, including nicotine, tar, carbon monoxide, arsenous oxide, radioactive polonium, benzopyrene, and others. The addicted cigarette abuser becomes an adult with significant risks for the many well-known complications of this drug—lung cancer, emphysema, laryngeal carcinoma, other cancers, heart disease, and many other disorders. Lung cancer in female adult smokers is now more common than breast cancer.

A common condition noted in smokers and reverse smokers is keratosis of the mucosal palate posterior to the rugae. This was originally described in 1926 and is caused by the concentrated hot steam of smoke and chemicals producing a "smoker's patch." Reverse smoking has been associated with dysplastic and malignant changes over time. Recent research also notes negative effects, which occur from smoking during pregnancy, including lower birth weight and attention-deficit/hyperactivity disorder. Nicotine staining of the teeth, crow's feet from the occlusion of micro-arterioles near the eyes, bad breath, cough, and dyspnea are also well-recognized and widespread stigmata of smoking. Passive smoking is also known to be dangerous to those exposed to the smoking of others. Oral cancer is a serious consequence of using chewing tobacco.

Vaping devices such e-cigarettes, e-vaporizers, or electronic nicotine delivery systems are battery driven instruments that are used to inhale vapors that contain flavorings and other chemicals (8, 17). These are becoming increasingly popular among teens. The safety and use of these devices for quitting tobacco is doubtful and the US Food and Drug Administration (FDA) has even banned the sale of these devices to minors due to reports of safety concerns. The MTF (Monitoring the Future) study has reported a lifetime use prevalence of 24.3%, 41% and 45.6% among 8th,10th and 12th graders respectively (8, 17).

It is important for clinicians caring for adolescents to join the struggle to limit the use of tobacco by adolescents. For example, advertising to youth must be prevented, and efforts to reduce the acceptance of tobacco by society strengthened. The prevention and reduction of adolescent tobacco use and abuse must be encouraged on a national and statewide level. On a local level, a broad range program is recommended that targets the family, community, and schools.

Pharmacologic management

Table 7 reviews current pharmacologic management options for tobacco addicts who are motivated to quit using tobacco products (36). Clinicians should take every opportunity to remind tobacco-addicted teens that their habit is very dangerous and help is available when they are ready to stop. Psychosocial issues in the lives of teen smokers and underlying cues to smoking should be reviewed with the adolescent. Special situations may arise, such as the pregnant adolescent who also smokes. A variety of nicotine replacement (NT) products are produced, as reviewed in Tables 7 and 8; the rate of quitting smoking is doubled by use of these products for the motivated smoker (i.e., 30%), in contrast to those seeking to stop smoking without pharmacologic agents (i.e., 15%) (37). The choice of NT product is patient-driven; teens should not smoke while on NT products, though no overt negative sequelae have been reported in such cases.

Table 7. Pharmacologic products available in the USA to treat tobacco addiction*

Nicotine Medications	
Nicotine gum	• Nicorette OTC • Nicorette DS OTC
Nicotine patch	• Nicoderm CQ(SmithKline Beecham) OTC • Nicotrol Patch (McNeil) OTC • Habitrol (Novartis) • Prostep (Lederle)
Nicotine inhaler	• Nicotrol Inhaler (McNeil)
Nasal spray	• Nicotrol Nasal Spray (McNeil)
Non-Nicotine Medications Bupropion	Zyban SR (Glaxo Wellcome) sustained-release tablets

*Reprinted with permission from: Patel DR, Greydanus DE. Office interventions for adolescent smokers. Adolesc Med 2000;11(3):577-88 (37).

Table 8. Nicotine patch regimens*

Brand	Duration	Dosage
Nicoderm CQ and Habitrol	4 weeks then 2 weeks then 2 weeks	21 mg/24 hours 14 mg/24 hours 7 mg/24 hours
Prostep	4 weeks then 4 weeks	22 mg/24 hours 11 mg/24 hours
Nicotrol	8 weeks	15 mg/24 hours

*Reprinted with Permission from: Patel DR, Greydanus DE. Office interventions for adolescent smokers. Adolesc Med 2000;11(3):577-88 (37).

The *NT patch* is prescribed for two months (changed each morning), using a high strength patch for one month, and then the lower dose for one more month (see Table 8) (37). The patch is not placed over a site with hair. Up to half will develop local dermatitis, usually improved with local hydrocortisone application. The patch is applied only while awake if patch-induced secondary vivid dreams or insomnia develop. The NT gum (nicotine polacrilex) has a bitter taste that many teens do not like; some youth feel embarrassed while choosing the nicotine gum. If the tobacco addict smokes over 25 cigarettes a day, prescribe the 4 mg gum; eventually lower the patient to the two mg gum. Since acidic liquids reduce nicotine absorption, they should not be used for 15 minutes before gum use and while chewing. Instructions to give patients who chew this gum are provided in Table 9. Adverse effects of this gum, though temporary, include dyspepsia, mouth soreness, jaw ache and hiccups.

Table 9. Recommendations for use of nicotine gum

Chew a piece each hour for 6 weeks.
Then, chew a piece every 2 hours for 3 weeks.
Finally, chew a piece every 4 hours for 3 weeks.
Maximum limit is 30 pieces per day for the 2 mg gum and 20 pieces per day for the 4 mg gum.
Chewing instructions: • Chew slowly until a peppery taste appears (often after 15 chews) • Then put the gum between the cheek and buccal mucosa until the peppery taste has disappeared (often one minute) • Start chewing again and repeat the above cycle • Get rid of the gum when the peppery taste is gone (often 30 minutes).

The nicotine inhaler is designed to mimic the hand-to-mouth movement of the smoker; four mg of nicotine are delivered from the cartridge which contains about 10 mg overall (see Table 7). Low nicotine levels are produced and the user inhales 6-16 cartridges daily. Adequate nicotine absorption is accomplished with 80 inhalations over 20 minutes; absorption is through the oral mucosa. It is prescribed for 3 months and then slowly tapered off over three months. Adverse effects that often improve over time include coughing, dyspepsia, irritation of the mouth as well as throat, and nasal irritation.

The nicotine nasal spray is provided as one to two doses (1 to 2 mg of nicotine) per hour over three months; there is a rapid rise in nicotine serum levels (see Table 7). It is prescribed as a minimum of eight doses per day, not over 40 per day or over five inhalations per hour. Bronchospasm may occur and the nasal spray is not used for nicotine addicts with asthma. Other adverse effects include cough, rhinitis, nasal irritation, sneezing, and water eyes. The use of electronic cigarette for the cessation or reduction of smoking in adults remains under active research (38).

Non-nicotine therapy

The use of bupropion (see Table 7) in the nicotine addict who is motivated to quit smoking is helpful in up to 40% of cases; its relative success is attributed to the drug's ability to lower the classic nicotine craving while improving the nicotine-withdrawal problems of weight gain and depression (8). It was found to be twice as effective as placebo; however it is mostly indicated in age 18 years or older (8, 17). It is prescribed as Zyban in a sustained-release form that is provided as 150 mg a day for three days; if tolerated, it is increased to 150 mg twice daily. The dose should not exceed 300 mg a day. Additionally, the second dose should not be given less than 8 hours after the first to reduce the incidence of a seizure.

Though NT replacement therapies should not officially be started while the adolescent is still smoking, it is acceptable to start the teen smoker on bupropion while still using nicotine; a date of stopping the tobacco should still be negotiated while providing the bupropion. Bupropion is contraindicated in adolescents who have overt seizures and those with factors that increase the risk for seizures; the latter includes those with a history of epilepsy, an eating disorder, central nervous system tumor, and any medications that may lower the seizure threshold. Bupropion is contraindicated in those on monoamine oxidase (MAO) inhibitors. Bupropion adverse effects include insomnia, skin reactions, tremors, headaches, and dry mouth (8, 17).

Clonidine and nortriptyline may be useful to some late (older) adolescents and adult smokers to help them quit using tobacco (8, 17). Various other medications have been studied but not shown to help improve the craving for nicotine; these include buspirone, mecamylamine, naltrexone, doxepin, and oral dextrose. Another smoking cessation product is varenicline tartrate (Chantix®), an alpha-4 beta-2- nicotinic acetylcholine receptor partial agonist that binds to central nervous system receptors with a greater affinity than nicotine. It is FDA approved for adults with nicotine addiction and may be more effective than bupropion. Abstinence rates are 22% versus 16% for bupropion and 8% for placebo. In the short term, 44% of study patients quit smoking v. 30% using bupropion.

Starting dose is 0.5 mg per day for three days, twice a day for 4-7 days, then 1 mg twice daily. Chantix® decreases the pleasure of nicotine use and lessens the withdrawal craving. The major side effect is nausea, but weight gain is not a problem. There are reports of suicidality, agitation, hostility, and agitation (39). The use of cytisine,a partial agonist that binds the nicotinic acetylcholine receptor, is under study and has been found to be more effective in maintaining abstinence from nicotine when compared to NRT (40, 41). The use of a nicotine vaccine is also under active research (42, 43).

Marijuana (Cannabis)

Marijuana (cannabis) remains a popular euphoric and hallucinogenic drug for millions of youth as well as adults, and constitutes a major 'gateway drug' along with tobacco, alcohol, and others. It has many names, including "pot," "hash," "weed," "doobs," "BC Bud," "ganja," "grass," "smoke," and others. It is the most widely used illicit drug in the United States, accounting for up to 85% of the illicit drug trade. The 2014 YRBS reported that 35.6% of high school students had used pot one or more times during their life (2). Previous CDC surveys noted that the category of "ever used marijuana" had increased from 1991-1997 (31.3% to 47.1%); it did then decrease from 1997 to 2017 (47.1% to 35.6%) (2, 8, 17). The survey noted that 6.8% of students had tried pot for the first time before age 13 years and 19.8% of students had used pot one or more times during the 30 days prior to the survey. The prevalence of having ever used pot was higher among females (35.9%) versus males (35.2%) and higher among black and Hispanic youth versus white youth. In the 2013 National Survey on Drug Use and Health, marijuana was the most commonly consumed illicit drug with 35.8 million users 12 years of age and older over the past month of the survey (1, 17). From 2006 to 2019 the number of persons using daily cannabis increased multi-fold in this survey. The use of synthetic cannabinoids was also studied in the MTF study and found to be ranging from 2.6-3.3% in students from 8th to 12th grade.

This controversial drug is derived from *Cannabis sativa or C indica* (hemp plant) and the active euphoric chemical is delta-9-tetrahydrocannabinol or THC. It is present in the dried leaves, stems, seeds, flowers (sensimilla) and oil. This major lipophilic drug works on the cannabinoid receptors in the mesocortical and limbic systems. The marijuana of the 1960s and

1970s' hippie generation contained only 2% THC, while the Hawaiian sensimilla product was about 3% THC. Today's street pot can vary from 3 to 7%+ THC content, while cultivated sensimilla can contain 7 to 13%+. A popular brand of pot is BC Bud, a product imported by the ton from Canada at 3000-8,000 dollars per pound; it is grown in British Columbia and may contain up to 24% active ingredients. Many growers, commercial exporter consortiums, a significant fraction of the public and their elected officials, as well as active pot users are actively advocating for the legalization of marijuana that has occurred in various states in the United States (8).

Cannabis contains over 100 phytocannabinoids including cannabinol (or CBN – metabolite of THC), cannabidiol (or CBD--isomer of THC), cannabigerol (or CBG – alpha-2-adrenergic receptor agonist), tetrahydrocannabivarin (or THCV;THV – TCH homolog), and cannabichromene (or CBC) (8, 17, 44-46). Many other chemicals are found in this complex plant, including terpenoids, and endocannabinoids(such as 2-AG [2-arachidonoyl glycerol] and anandamide [arachidonoylethanolamide]).

Commercial preparations of synthetic cannabinoids include nabilone (schedule II drug), dronabinol (synthetic THC in sesame oil; schedule III drug), and nabiximols (phytocannabinoid marketed in Canada). Dronabinol capsules were approved on May 31, 1985 by the US Food and Drug Administration (FDA) for nausea and emesis management due to cancer chemotherapy; the US FDA also approved dronabinol on December 22, 1992 for persons with AIDS who have anorexia associated with weight loss. Oral nabilone was approved by the US FDA on December 26, 1985 for nausea and vomiting due to cancer chemotherapy. Though many other cannabis products are suggested for various other medical disorders, they are not approved by the FDA. Smoking marijuana is not approved by the FDA nor leading medical organizations because there is no research to support smoking pot and because of the many potential adverse side effects from cannabis smoking (44-46). In Canada the oromucosal spray, nabiximols, is indicated for management of cancer pain in addition to neuropathic pain and spasticity seen in persons with multiple sclerosis.

Though usually smoked, marijuana can also be eaten in such homemade concoctions as cookies, brownies, and spaghetti. The typical cannabis cigarette (joint) usually contains approximately 20 mg of THC obtained from about a gram of leaves and buds; however, much variation can be noted. The "blunt" is another popular way to smoke pot and consists of a cigarette with marijuana added to a hollowed cigarette. "Pot" is often combined with other drugs, such as phencyclidine, though glutethimide and methaqualone were also popular in the past as additives. PCP (phencyclidine) is frequently dissolved in an organic solvent, such as formaldehyde, in which a joint or hand-rolled cigarette is first dipped, dried, and then smoked. This preparation is variously referred to as "wet water," or "Sherms." This is a good reason for doing a urine drug test with informed consent and assent of a using teenager.

Marijuana use results in a potent sensation of euphoria ("buzz") that is noted within minutes of its use, and which can last for hours. Both THC and its metabolites are highly lipid soluble and are stored in fatty tissue; serum half-life is 19 hours. Marijuana can be found on urine drug screen and stool for as long as one month following regular use, and ten days after a single use. The behavioral effects are mediated by cannibinoid receptors and there is the release of dopamine in the nucleus accumbens. The effects of THC also include relaxation, time as well as perceptual distortions, and heightened sensory experiences such as listening to music, watching television, or eating ("getting the munchies"). Some drugs (alcohol or diazepam) may potentiate the sedative effects of marijuana, while other drugs (cocaine or amphetamines) worsen the stimulatory effects of cannabis.

A large number of potential adverse effects are seen with smoking cannabis, including cardiovascular, pulmonary, gastrointestinal (cannabis hyperemesis syndrome), dental, and central nervous system effects (8, 44-46). Cardiovascular adverse effects may include arteritis, cardiomyopathy, myocardial infarction, sudden cardiac death, transient ischemic accident (TIA), cardiovascular accident (CVA), and cardiac arrhythmias. Pulmonary side effects can include chronic cough, allergic hypersensitivity, bronchitis, bullous emphysema (COPD: chronic obstructive pulmonary disease), pneumothorax/pneumomediastinum, pulmonary dyplasia, pulmonary tuberculosis, other respiratory infections, and even dust disease (talcosis) in hemp workers.

Potential adverse dental effects can include dental caries, dental dysplasia, gingival enlargement, gingivitis, leukoedema, nicotinic stomatitis, oral infections, periodontal disease, poor dental health, uvulitis, and xerostomia. Potential adverse effects on the offspring of females smoking cannabis while pregnant include low birth weight, preterm labor, small for gestational age, treatment in a neonatal intensive care unit, and various childhood effects; the latter include inattention problems, problem-solving problems, aggression, executive function dysfunction, problems with memory as well as processing information, and depressive symptoms.

Cannabis poisoning can arise from consuming oral cannabis products and this is increasingly being seen in young children whose parents are pot smokers. Cannabis smoking (including spice drugs) increases risks for motor vehicle accidents (MVAs) and this can be worsened when combined with other drugs (i.e., alcohol, others). If one has smoked cannabis, 8 or more hours should pass before driving a motor vehicle. Pot smoking also increases road rage (8).

The central nervous system of young adolescents is very sensitive to cannabis and adverse effects may include decline in IQ, decreased coordination, distorted visuospatial perception, impaired executive function, impaired novel learning, impulsivity, inattention, memory loss, neuropsychiatric disorders (i.e., psychosis), and cannabis dependence (44-46). The DSM-5 has listed a number of cannabis-related disorders including cannabis use disorder (mild, moderate severe), cannabis intoxication (with or without perceptual disturbances), cannabis withdrawal, other cannabis-induced disorders, and unspecified cannabis-related disorders (DSM, 2013) (18).

Management of cannabis use disorder is mostly symptom-based as well as very difficult and there is no pharmaceutical agent approved for its management. Research continues to find medications that may be of help to those with cannabis use disorders and these include alpha 2 adrenergic agonists, antipsychotics (atypical), benzodiazepines, cannabidiol, dronabinol, gabapentin, lithium, lofexidine, nabilone, nabiximols, N-acetylcysteine (NAC), *N*-arachidonoylethanolamine (anandamide), nefazodone,2-arachidonoyl glycerol (2-AG), and others (8, 44-47).

The general principles of non-pharmacological management also apply to cannabis use disorders; these include use of modalities such as psycho-education, brief interventions, CBT (cognitive behaviour therapy)-based approaches, motivation enhancement treatment, and contingency management (CM) interventions (8). Therapy is typically prescribed and its efficacy may be low because of lack of motivation. Approximately 25% of the 19.8 million cannabis users in the United States meet the DSM-5 criteria for cannabis use disorders. Many fail to seek treatment and this tends to be due to failure to recognize the severity of their disorder and this denial may reflect their own brain dysfunction. Of the 7.6 million persons aged 12 or older who need treatment for an illicit drug use problem in 2013, only 1.5 million (19.5%) received management in a specialty program (44-46). Of the 6.1 million persons who needed but did not receive management, only 395,000 (6.4%) reported they were aware of a need for treatment.

Alcohol

Alcohol continues to be among the most used and abused "licit" substance (#1 choice of 29% youth) that enjoys a wide range of societal acceptance (17, 48). Alcohol is the leading cause of substance use morbidity and mortality contributing to over 88,000 deaths each year (8). Surveys have revealed that US high school seniors have a lifetime prevalence of over 80%, with over 50% noting alcohol use during the previous survey month, and 4% admitting to daily use (17). The average age that alcohol is first misused is age 12. The prevalence of alcohol use is higher among white and Hispanic youth than among black youth. It is important to ask youth if they drink and if so, describe their drinking pattern; repeated use of alcohol or other substances is not part of normal adolescent defiant behavior. The CRAFFT screening test and Alcohol Use Disorders Identification Test (AUDIT) for adolescent substance abuse are easy to use instrument for screening drug use (10).

About half of adolescents who are victims of a motor vehicle accidents or suicides were drinking before their death (8). The most common pattern of alcoholic consumption is binge drinking, as defined by 5 drinks in a row in males, and four in females. Blacking out spells is frequently a result of binge drinking behavior. Binge drinking is directly related to drunk driving, increased sexual activity (and teen pregnancy), smoking, dating violence, attempted suicide, and other substance abuse.

2019 YRBS

The 2019 YRBS revealed that 60.4% of high school students had had at least one drink of alcohol on at least one day during their life (1). This survey also revealed that 29.8% of students had at least one drink of alcohol on at least 1 day during the 30 days before the survey. Around 43.5% had usually obtained the alcohol they drank from someone who gave it to them during the 30 days before the survey. The prevalence of having ever drunk alcohol was higher in females versus males and higher in Hispanic youth than white or black youth.

The survey noted that 13.5% of students had had five or more drinks of alcohol in a row on at least 1 day during the 30 days prior to the survey (1). Also, 16.5% of high school students rode in a care at lease once with someone who had been consuming alcohol. Of the 64.3% of high school students who drove a car or other vehicle during the 30 days before the survey, 5.5% had driven after drinking alcohol during the 30 days prior to the survey.

Alcohol effects

Alcohol is a central nervous system depressant that also induces euphoria in the user; tolerance and psychological dependence may develop, in addition to physiologic dependence in alcoholics (8, 17). Alcohol drinks vary in their amount of this drug, ranging from 3% to 6% in beer, 12% in wine, and 50% in various liquors. Legal intoxication is usually 0.08 to 0.10 g/dl, though judgment may be impaired at a blood alcohol concentration (BAC) of 0.01 g/dl or lower. Central effects occur at 20-30 ng/dl. Acute intoxication may lead to respiratory depression, coma, and death. Adolescents should be educated about the dangers of alcohol consumption, including the deadly mixture of driving and drinking that kills "innocent" as well as alcohol-consuming victims.

Alcohol dependence is a serious psychiatric disorder in adults, and youth may be involved in this disorder as well. The genetics of alcohol dependence has been studied for decades and its molecular biologic basis is being revealed (49, 50). The abuse of alcohol depletes a number of so-called "comfort" hormones (opioid peptides, serotonin, gamma aminobutyric acid, dopamine) in addition to inducing stress hormone release (i.e., corticotropin releasing factor). Many adolescents do not stop at the social drinking or experimental stage and rapid progression can develop through the later stages of drug abuse. Youth who abuse alcohol tend to come from families where problem drinking occurs as well as families where problem drinking is absent. The DSM-5 lists a number of alcohol-related disorders: alcohol use disorder (mild, moderate, severe), alcohol intoxication, alcohol withdrawal, other alcohol-induced disorders, and unspecified alcohol related disorders (18).

Medical complications of problem drinking include intoxication, pancreatitis, gastritis, worsening of co-morbid medical disorders (i.e., diabetes mellitus, epilepsy, sleep dysfunction), and toxic psychosis (8, 17, 51). The alcohol withdrawal syndrome presents with such symptoms as tremors, seizures, hallucinations, and even overt delirium tremens. Youth who abuse alcohol may develop anemia, macrocytosis, and elevation in alkaline phosphatase, bilirubin, uric acid, glutamic-oxaloacetic, gamma glutamyl transpeptidase, or pyruvic transaminases. The diagnosis of alcohol abuse disorder is made mainly by a history of excessive alcohol use, and not on the basis of a positive serum or drug-screening test. The fetal alcohol syndrome and the effect of alcohol on neuronal migration and pruning (apoptosis) in the unborn fetus exposed to intrauterine alcohol are well-recognized consequences of alcohol consumption during pregnancy (8, 17). The mortality risk to the fetus is 5%, while the accidental risk of harm to family members of alcohol users is increased considerably.

Management of alcohol abuse

Acute alcohol ingestion is treated with gastric emptying, intravenous fluids, glucose, respiratory support, and sometimes, dialysis. The possibility of additional drug use is suggested by respiratory depression greater than that suggested by the available blood alcohol content (BAC); head injury may also have occurred in this situation.

The primary goal of alcohol use disorder management in adolescents is to achieve and maintain abstinence followed by a range of other measures for recovery. Management can be pharmacological and non-pharmacological (8, 17). Various medications used in the management of alcohol withdrawal syndrome include clorazepate, lorazepam, chlordiazepoxide, diazepam, and various antipsychotics. Medications approved for the management of adults with alcohol dependence for prophylaxis include acamprosate, naltrexone and disulfiram. Various medications have been used, but have not been approved for use in adults with alcohol dependence; these include calcium carbamide, tiapride, buspirone, carbamazepine, nalmefene, selective serotonin reuptake inhibitors, and tricyclic antidepressants (4, 8, 17).

Some of the non-pharmacological measures include psychoeducation of patient and family members; also useful are brief interventions, motivation enhancement therapy, CBT (cognitive behaviour therapy) based approaches, and contingency management (CM) interventions/motivational incentives (8). *Mothers Against Drunk Drivers* (*MADD*) and self-help groups (*Alcohol Anonymous* [*AA*] and *Alateen*) are important programs found in many communities that help with the wide-spread program of alcohol use and abuse in adolescents and adults (4, 8, 17). Attention to the sleep disruption seen in those abusing alcohol (and other drugs) is important in an overall management strategy as well (51).

Amphetamines

Amphetamines (Dexedrine, Benzedrine, Desoxyn, *chalk, meth, speed, Mollies, black beauties)* are classic central nervous system stimulants that lead to a variety of complications, as listed in Table 10 (8, 17). The DSM-5 lists a number of stimulant-related disorders with regard to amphetamine-type substance: stimulant use disorder-amphetamine-type substance (mild, moderate, severe), stimulant intoxication-amphetamine-type substance, stimulant withdrawal—amphetamine-type substance, other stimulant-induced disorders-amphetamine-type substance, and unspecified stimulant related disorder-amphetamine-type substance (18).

Amphetamines can be taken to develop euphoria, lessen fatigue, improve attention, loose weight, and/or allow continued sports performance. In the 2008 MTF, Johnson reported a decline in stimulant use with a prevalence of 4.5% in 8th graders and 6.8% in 12th graders. As per the MTF 2019 study the prevalence has been reported to be 6.8%,4.1% and 2.2% for use in lifetime, last year and month respectively for 8th graders. While for 12th graders it was 7.7,4.5 and 2% respectively (8, 17, 35). Data from India showed the general population prevalence to be 0.18% (52). The use of amphetamines has significantly decreased but is next in frequency of abuse to marijuana. Amphetamine can be abused in various forms—oral, subcutaneous, or intravenous. Amphetamine "look alikes" have become more available through mail order sites or from garage production using simple compounds such a phenylpropanolamine, pseudoephedrine, and ephedrine—including the herbal ma huang.

While the mechanism of action is not entirely known, amphetamines may act by inhibiting catecholamine re-uptake or facilitating the release of norepinephrine in the presynaptic cleft (8). Alternatively, they may act as monoxidase inhibitors. They are absorbed through the gastrointestinal tract within 30 minutes and within 5 minutes when used subcutaneously. An initial rush is followed by a prolonged euphoria, alertness, confidence, and excitation; also seen are flushing, sweating, temperature elevation, tachycardia, significant rise in blood pressure, and mydriasis. Tolerance is rapid and confusion, irritability, headache, insomnia, seizures, and weight loss may follow. Cerebral hemorrhage and cardiac arrhythmias have been reported. A drug-induced psychosis is well known in long time users, but has occurred following a single use. Acute overdose can be life-threatening and diagnosis as well as prompt treatment is necessary (see Table 11).

Table 10. Amphetamine adverse reactions

- Anorexia
- Anxiety
- Exhaustion
- Hyperactivity
- Hyperhidrosis
- Hypertension
- Insomnia
- Mydriasis
- Personality changes
- Tachycardia
- Tolerance
- Weight loss
- Withdrawal syndrome
- Restlessness, dysphoria, insomnia, irritability, hostility, and confusion.
- Generalized anxiety disorder and panic disorder,
- Psychotic symptoms like ideas of reference, paranoid delusions,
- and hallucinations.

Table 11. Management of amphetamine overdose

Activated charcoal /magnesium citrate for oral intoxication
Cooling blanket for hyperthermia
Medical control of hypertension and arrhythmias
Haloperidol or droperidol for agitation or delusions
Lorazepam (Ativan®) or diazepam (Valium®) for seizures
Urine acidification with ascorbic acid

An infected needle may lead to HIV/AIDS, endocarditis, hepatitis, and other infections (53). An abstinence or withdrawal syndrome is described in amphetamine abusers, with the development of severe apathy, depression, and hypersomnia. Amphetamine abusers develop tolerance and an overdose can lead to hyperthermia, hypertension, cardiac arrhythmias, seizures, and death. Table 11 outlines basic medical support for an amphetamine overdose; avoid the use of phenothiazines, since rapid decrease in blood pressure and increased seizures activity may result (8).

Clinicians using stimulant medications to manage adolescents with attention deficit hyperactivity disorder (ADHD) should appreciate the potential for abuse of short acting adderall (mixed amphetamine salts) and Ritalin (methylphenidate) (54). Ritalin is also called "the smart drug" and "vitamin R" by abusers, who crush the methylphenidate tablets and snort this chemical to obtain an intense euphoria; large doses can lead to seizure activity, stroke, and psychosis. Published guidelines should be followed carefully when providing stimulant medications to adolescents (8, 17). This should include the use of the long-acting preparations, such as Concerta®, which have formulations that reduce the risk for dispersion and the quick "buzz." Another stimulant addition with diminished abuse potential is lisdexamfetamine (Vyvanse®) a prodrug formulation. The long-acting preparations used for the treatment of ADHD do not produce tachyphylaxis, nor have they lead to addiction (8).

Apart from supportive symptomatic treatment, focus should be on establishing therapeutic alliance with patient and family. Management of dependence should preferably be in inpatient setting and various treatment modalities (i.e., individual, family, and group psychotherapy) are usually required to achieve long lasting abstinence. The specific amphetamine induced disorders (e.g., amphetamine-induced psychotic and anxiety disorder) with specific drugs such as antipsychotics and anxiolytics may sometimes be required for short term. Co-morbid disorders (i.e., depression, personality disorder, others) should also be dealt with using appropriate interventions.

Methamphetamine

This illicit drug (*meth, ice, crystal, fire, glass, chalk, crank*) is an N-methyl homolog of amphetamine and has become the stimulant favored by most adolescents, due to its potent stimulant effect on the central nervous system (55, 56). It is a highly addictive drug prepared by illicit drug laboratories using relatively inexpensive chemicals and sold on the streets as well as involving drug networks. The term "ice" or "crystal" comes from its production as clear, chunky *crystals* that look like *ice;* it can also be bought as an odorless, bitter-tasting, white powder that easily dissolves in liquids.

The 2013 YRBS noted that 3.2% of students had used this drug one or more times in their lifetime revealing a decreased prevalence of 9.1% in 1999 to 3.2% in 2013 (2). The prevalence has further reduced to 2.1% as per 2019 report. Methamphetamine is now responsible for one-quarter of illicit stimulant use.

This drug can be taken as a pill or its powder can be snorted, leading to a "high" or euphoria; when inhaled via smoking or taken intravenously, methamphetamine hydrochloride induces an immediate, potent euphoria that is described as a "flash" or "rush" lasting a few minutes. It is this intense feeling that abusers seek leading to rapid addiction with increased dosage and frequency of use. This is not the case with the long-acting mixed amphetamine salts preparation (Adderall XR) that is used to manage patients with ADHD.

Users of this drug note that there is increased wakefulness, less need for sleep, and increased physical activity; sometimes extreme anorexia may develop along with weight loss (8, 17). The temperature, respirations, pulse, and blood pressure are increased; there may be excited speech. Methamphetamine releases high levels of dopamine and thus can affect body movements and mood in these addicts. Central nervous system cells that contain dopamine and serotonin are damaged, eventually leading to low levels of dopamine, thought dysfunction, and a depressed mood ("blue Tuesdays"). Motor impairment or a Parkinsonian-like movement disorder can develop. Adverse reactions are many and some are listed in Table 12 (8). As with other illicit drugs that are taken intravenously, this drug can lead to various infectious diseases, including sexually transmitted diseases, such as hepatitis B and HIV/AIDS. Urine drug testing remains positive 48 hours and may reflect look alike designer drugs or prescription psychostimulants.

Management principles are similar to that of amphetamines (8, 17). The treatment of acute toxicity includes the support of cardiac and respiratory function. Orogastric lavage and activated charcoal may be indicated if oral ingestion of other substances is suspected. Droperidal or haloperidol are more effective than the benzodiazepines in blocking the behavioral effects of amphetamines and produce fairly rapid sedation. However, benzodiazepines are indicated for seizure management and thorazine is contraindicated. Blood pressure is best managed with labetelol or esmolol.

Management of this severe drug addiction is difficult and current research is seeking a medication to block the euphoric effects of methamphetamine to allow the addict to get off the drug, if there is motivation to stop. This antibody-type medication research is part of other addiction research studies seeking to neutralize the euphoric effects of drugs, such as cocaine, heroin, and others. Management of methamphetamine psychosis is difficult but important as is treatment of depression or anxiety related to the use of this drug in order to reduce risks for methamphetamine relapse (57). In addition to this, various psycho-therapeutic intervention as mentioned in amphetamines section are also useful.

Table 12. Adverse effects of methamphetamine

- Irritability
- Anxiety
- Confusion
- Memory loss
- Insomnia
- Tremors
- Convulsions
- Coma
- Hypertension
- Cardiac damage
- Rhabdomyolysis
- Paranoia and psychotic behavior
- Increased aggressiveness with violent behavior
- Cardiovascular collapse and death

Cocaine

This central nervous system stimulant is an alkaloid made from leaves of the South American plant, *erythroxylon coca* (8, 17). There are a number of ways to take this drug: intranasal, intravenous, inhalation, smoking, chewed (coca leaves), or swallowed. Previously, this drug was produced as a crystalline powder that is water soluble and developed from an alkaloidal paste of the plant's leaves. "Free base" and "crack" ("rock") are popular cocaine products used for smoking. Free-base cocaine is vaporized in a water piper (bong) or even a soda can with a hole in it. "Crack" is the street name for cocaine bicarbonate pellets that are pea-sized and produced using ammonia or sodium bicarbonate (baking soda); heating this concoction to remove its hydrochloride component produces a "crackling" sound. Crack may be crushed, tobacco added, and then this "cigarette" is smoked; other chemicals often added include mannitol, quinine, or marijuana. Over half of the cocaine used on the streets is now crack cocaine because cocaine powder is decomposed when ignited to smoke. Crack cocaine has become relatively inexpensive and very popular with adolescents.

The 2019 YRBS noted that 3.9% of students had used any form of cocaine one or more times during their life (1). The CDC surveys noted that the prevalence of ever used cocaine increased from 1991 to 1999 (5.9% to 9.5%) and decreased from 1999 to 2013 (9.5% to 5.5%) and further to 3.9% by 2019 (1, 2). The 2017 National Survey of Drug Use and Health indicated prevalence of 0.1% among 12 to 17 year old for current use (17). On the other hand, data from the Magnitude of Substance Use in India study conducted at All India Institute Of Medical Sciences (AIIMS, Delhi, India) found the prevalence to be 0.1% overall (52). The prevalence of ever-used cocaine was higher among male youth versus female youth. Approximately 23% of Americans report they have experience with cocaine before age 30 (8, 17). The DSM-5 lists a number of stimulant-related disorders with regard to cocaine: stimulant use disorder-cocaine (mild, moderate, severe), stimulant intoxication-cocaine, stimulant withdrawal—cocaine, other stimulant-induced disorders-cocaine, and unspecified stimulant related disorder-cocaine (18).

Table 13. Adverse effects of cocaine (8, 17)

1. Behavioural and Neuropsychological
• Anxiety
• Irritability and restlessness
• Confusion
• Agitation
• Irritability
• Dysphoria
• Paranoia
• Hypervigilance
• Grandiosity
• Psychotic symptoms like visual or tactile Hallucinations
• Executive dysfunction
• Impaired attention, and working memory
• Reduced social functioning and interactions; Seizures
• Frontal lobe infarctions
2. Physical
• Peripheral blood vessel constriction
• Pupillary dilation
• Hyperpyexia, tachycardia, and hypertension
• Cardiac complications
• Angina pectoris
• Myocardial infarction
• Ventricular arrhythmia
• Sudden death
• Nasal septum infection and perforation
• Intravenous needle complications (including hepatitis B, HIV/AIDS, endocarditis)
• Increased premature delivery
• Abruption (bleeding between placenta and uterine wall)
• Adverse neurodevelopmental sequelae in infants
• Vascular spasm-induced limb reduction anomalies and strokes

Cocaine is a topical anesthetic, a peripheral sympathomimetic, and a central nervous system stimulant; also, the drug interferes with neuronal catecholamine reuptake and dopamine reabsorption (8, 17). The popularity of cocaine is based on its ready availability and the potent euphoric feeling it produces; this high lasts 5 to 10 minutes if cocaine is smoked, in contrast to 10 to 30 minutes if taken intravenously. Because the high is short lived, the usual pattern of use is escalated and dependence is promoted. Urine and blood testing remains positive for 48-72 hours following its use. Once the euphoria is gone, irritability and fatigue set in. Users of this powerful drug develop severe psychological and physiological addiction along with tolerance. Serious physiological complications are infrequent and the death rate is low even in heavy long-term users; but, when they occur, they can be disastrous. A partial list of the serious side effects of cocaine is listed in Table 13 (8, 17).

As with other drugs, addicts look to mix various drugs together to intensify the pleasant or euphoric feeling of their drug of choice (8, 17). When alcohol is mixed with cocaine, *cocaethylene* is produced in the liver; this chemical heightens the cocaine euphoria (i.e., more potent and lasts longer), blunts some of the stimulant adverse cocaine effects, and increases the risk of sudden cardiac death 25 fold. The term, *speedballing*, refers to the mixture of cocaine and heroin (or morphine) and this combination also increases the risk for sudden death.

The method of using cocaine leads to various complications, as nasal perforation/infection with snorting and the infectious sequelae from intravenous use. The high abuse rate of cocaine is associated with increased risk of sexually transmitted diseases among adolescents and young adults; this includes HIV/AIDS, lymphogranuloma venereum (LGV), and chancroid (8). Smoking crack may lead to the development of a very aggressive paranoia. Sudden death occurs and is a constant risk, whether it is the first time or the user is very experienced with this drug; such death is probably due to a terminal ventricular arrhythmia. Use of cocaine during pregnancy can lead to a variety of adverse effects on the fetus including preterm-labor, placenta infarction, placental abruption, pre-eclampsia, impaired fetal growth, and neurodevelopmental defects (58).

Management of cocaine addiction

While acute intoxication is usually not severe, it may be complicated by the use of opioids, alcohol, marijuana, and other drugs. Initial management should focus on providing a safe, quiet and stimulation free environment. Emergency management includes the maintenance of an airway and naloxone if opiate use is suspected (8, 17). Treatment of arrhythmias may require lidocaine, phenytoin, or cardioversion. Lorazepam or diazepam can be used for severe agitation or seizures. Nitroprusside or labetalol can be used for hypertension. A cooling blanket and intravenous fluids may be used for hyperthermia; phenothiazines are contraindicated.

Cocaine addiction is a difficult central nervous system disorder to manage. If tachycardia and hypertension develop while on cocaine, short acting beta-blockers and short-acting direct vasodilators (as esmolol) may be helpful. Clinicians should avoid long-acting vasodilators, since cocaine intoxication is typically a short, self-limited phenomenon and use of these other drugs (as morphine, propranolol, thorazine) may lead to severe hypotension. Though naloxone is helpful for opioid addiction, it does not help with cocaine addiction.

Management of cocaine dependence includes assessment and treatment. Common screening instruments that can be used in children and adolescents include CRAFFT and the S2BI (screening to brief intervention); dependence can be confirmed by further detailed history and examination (8). Treatment can be both pharmacological and non-pharmacological. There are currently no FDA–approved pharmacologic agents for the treatment of cocaine use disorders; however, cocaine addicts with ADHD may observe that methylphenidate calms them down along with improving their concentration abilities. Indeed, reduction in cocaine use has been observed in some cocaine addicts who have ADHD and use methylphenidate.

Current addiction research seeks to find a way to stop the potent euphoric effects of cocaine and enable the motivated abuser to stop this drug. Dependence on cocaine involves various pathways (i.e., noradrenergic and dopaminergic) in the primitive midbrain reward center.

Multiple central nervous system (CNS) sites are involved with the addiction and thus any drug used to help the addict must work over many CNS areas. Table 14 lists proposed drug mechanisms that are being researched to potentially manage cocaine addiction by blocking this drug's many effects, including the use of vaccine technology (8, 17, 59).

Table 14. Potential mechanisms to manage cocaine addiction (8, 17)

• Bind to cocaine molecules and prevent movement into the CNS via the blood-brain barrier
• Change cocaine molecules into harmless (inactive) particles
• Remove the cocaine molecule as a vaccine using an antibody-type response
• "Catalytic" antibodies changing cocaine into inactive fragments

For example, research is looking at drugs called "peripheral blockers," such as dopamine D3receptor agonists (D3agonists), to prevent cocaine-induced CNS stimulation by neutralizing this drug in the blood; such drugs may help with addiction as well as with overdose and cocaine-induced seizures (8, 17). Oxytocin may be helpful via effects on the glutamate receptor systems (60). N-acetylcysteine is also under active research for the management of cocaine dependence.

If the addict uses other drugs, treatment of dependence on those other drugs may help. For example, naltrexone or disulfiram may help with alcohol abuse and be of benefit to the addict who uses both cocaine and alcohol.

Potentially beneficial non-pharmacological interventions/modalities include motivational interviewing, motivational enhancement therapy, cognitive behavioral therapy, contingency management and family focused interventions (8, 17).

Opioids

A number of opiate narcotics are abused by adolescents and adults, as reviewed in Table 15. The DSM-5 lists a number of opioid-related disorders: opioid use disorder (mild, moderate, severe), opioid intoxication, opioid withdrawal, other opioid-induced disorders, and unspecified opioid-related disorders (18).

Prescribed narcotics have been popular for many years, and are available in many ways, such as stealing them from home medicine supplies, obtained from emergency room or office clinicians by faking (exaggerating) injuries or illnesses (i.e., migraine headaches, dysmenorrhea), or simply buying the opiate of choice on the street. Most are obtained free from friends or bought from school mates. The 2008 MTF reports use by 10% of 12th graders with Vicodin being the choice of 9.7% (35). Oxycontin use was reported by 2.1 and 4.7% of 8th and 12th graders respectively. The most recent MTF (Monitoring the future) study is from 2018 and estimates that 3.4% of 12th graders report prescription opioid use in the past year. The magnitude was more or less stable from 2002 (9.4%) to 2009 (9.2%) in 12th graders; however, since then it has been declining steadily, decreasing to 7.9% in2012, 5.4% in 2015, and 3.4% in 2018. Trends have been similar in the NSDUH (National Survey on Drug Use and Health) and MTF (1, 17). Seven of the top 11 abused prescription medications are opiates (8, 17).

Table 15. Narcotic opiates

• Codeine
• Fentanyl
• Heroin
• Meperidine
• Methadone
• Morphine
• Oxycodone
• Pentazocine
• Propoxyphene
• Others

Clinicians may forget or not be aware of the addictive potential of such classic analgesics as Darvocet, Dilaudid, Percocet, Stadol, Vicodin, or Ultram. News media have covered the recent increased popularity of oxycodone (oxyContin), a narcotic that is abused by some in place of heroin; a variety of ways of abuse are noted, including chewing an oxycodone tablet, crushing the pill and either snorting the contents or intravenous use after boiling the powder (8). Its acceptance by addicts is reflected in the many street names it has acquired, including *OXY, OC, oxycotto, and killers*. Fentanyl is a prescribed narcotic that is ten times more potent than heroin and there are a number of reported overdoses from this drug.

Heroin

Inexpensive and potent heroin (diacetyl morphine hydrochloride) is available and comes from Mexico, Columbia, Afghanistan, and Pakistan. Heroin (*junk, smack, Mexican brown, China white*) can be abused in a snuff form, intravenously, or subcutaneously (skin-popping) (8, 17). China White is 2,000 times more potent than morphine and responsible for some 28 documented fatalities. Speedballing, as noted above, refers to the combination of heroin or morphine with cocaine in an effort to block the sedative effect of heroin. Use of both heroin and morphine is called "New Jack Swing." "Cheese" which blends black tar heroin and Tylenol PM has been associated with deaths in the United States.

Misuse of opioids includes two classes: the use of heroin and the misuse of prescription opioids. The mean age of heroin use dropped from 27 years of age in 1988 to 19 years of age in 1995. There was a doubling of high school seniors who used this drug from 1990 to 1996 at a time when the price of heroin was dropping along with a 40% increase in drug purity (8, 17). The 1999 YRBS noted that 2.4% of high school students had tried heroin on at least one occasion; this was broken down to 3.5% males and 1.3% females (8, 17). The 2003 Monitor the Future (MTF) Study recorded that 1.5% of high school seniors had a lifetime use of heroin, 0.8% over the past year and 0.4% over the past survey month. The lifetime heroin use for these seniors was 1.5% in the 2007 YRBS, and < 1% in the 2008 MTF Study (17).

The 2013 YRBS reported that 2.2% of students had used heroin one or more times during their life and this decreased from 2.9% in 2011 to 2.2% in 2013 (2). The 2019 report shows lifetime prevalence of opioid use of once or more to be 1.8% and that of prescription opiate use to be 7.2% (1). Data from India shows that the prevalence of current use of any opioid is 1.8%

among adolescents; heroin, pharmaceutical opioids and opium being most abused forms in that order (52).

Unfortunately, this use increases as these seniors leave school and also increases in those who drop out of school before graduation of their peers who stay in school.The typical situation is an adolescent who begins to snort this drug, then develops an intense craving for the resultant euphoria, and progresses to smoking or intravenous use (mainlining). An all-consuming addiction with tolerance develops, as noted by the saying: "*once is too much, 1000 times not enough*;" also classic, is the development of physical addiction, psychological dependence, and a narcotic withdrawal syndrome. This may follow initiation of abuse by as little as several weeks. Approximately 30% of adolescents who smoke heroin become mainlining adults. Those who smoke or snort this drug often mistakenly feel they are bypassing the dangerous effects of heroin by smoking. However, this is not true, and the younger the addiction starts, the greater is the risk for post-cessation relapse.

Opiate overdose presents with the triad of respiratory and CNS depression associated with miotic constriction of the pupils (8, 17). Mydriasis is seen with withdrawal which presents with flu-like symptoms, lacrimation, irritability, abdominal cramps and diarrhea. Cardiopulmonary failure with bradycardia, hypotension, and pulmonary edema can occur. A rapid response to the opiate antagonist naloxone is diagnostic of opiate overdose. Support of both respiratory and circulatory systems with airway maintenance is imperative. Correction of hypotension is necessary while monitoring for hypoglycemia, pulmonary edema, and arrhythmias. Thin-layer chromatography immunoassay will detect opiate metabolites for 2-3 days.

Table 16. Medical complications of heroin abuse

- Amenorrhea
- Endocarditis (from *Staphylococcus aureus*)
- False-positive VDRL
- Fat necrosis
- HIV/AIDS
- Hepatitis (B and C)
- Lipodystrophy
- Osteomyelitis
- Peptic ulcer disease
- Pulmonary edema and pneumonia
- Respiratory arrest
- Skin infections
- Tetanus
- Others

Table 16 lists some of the medical complications of heroin abuse, including an overdose that leads to death from respiratory depression and pulmonary edema. For example, an increase in heroin overdose deaths in 28 states was reported by the CDC for the period 2010 to 2012 (Rudd, 2014) (61). As per the CDC current data, the rates of drug overdose deaths involving heroin was lower in 2018 than in 2017 (from 4.9 in 2017 to 4.7 per 1,000,000 population in 2018) (1, 8, 17).

Clinicians should observe for the use of tattoos to obscure puncture wounds or needle-tract marks made by the heroin intravenous abuse; such mainlining and tattooing phenomena increase the infectious complications of needle use. A newborn withdrawal syndrome is described in newborns whose mothers abuse narcotics; heroin withdrawal in utero can lead to meconium aspiration, bile pneumonitis, and severe respiratory distress.

Management of opioid addiction

Addiction research of the last part of the 20th century led to the conclusion that opioid dependence is a neurobiological central nervous system disorder that involves brain receptors (8, 17). This science looks at *reward circuits* controlling such processes as hunger, thirst, reproduction, and even drug addiction. Drug-induced alterations in CNS opiate receptors lead to drug dependence and tolerance phenomena. Opiate addiction induces significant social dysfunction with complex biological and psychological components that are not corrected by incarceration. Unfortunately, the majority of such addicts are not in treatment designed to manage their brain disorder. These patients often need acute detoxification measures followed by residential and/or outpatient management of sufficient nature to blunt their often overwhelming need to find the narcotic euphoria. Community programs as the 12-Step groups (i.e., Narcotics Anonymous) can be very helpful to these individuals to stay off the drug (s).

Medication-assisted treatment (MAT) using medications such as buprenorphine, methadone, and naltrexone are effective when used along with other forms of treatment such as psychosocial interventions. Research on adolescents has shown decreased relapse rates, cost effectiveness, reduction in craving, and reduced withdrawal symptoms. Further the American Academy of Pediatrics (AAP) has advocated MAT for opioid-addicted adolescents. The opioid addict may benefit from the judicious use of various medications that are available as part of the overall management program (see Table 17) (8, 17). Naltrexone (*ReVia*, *Depade*) is an opiate antagonist that can help many with opiate addiction, including addicts with additional alcohol dependence. Methadone may block classic narcotic effects without giving the user the classic opiate euphoria; it can also remove withdrawal symptomatology and help with on-going desires for additional drugs. Clinicians have used this drug as a substitute agonist for opiate dependence since the 1960s. Pharmacokinetics allow once a day dosing and the patient officially must be at least 18 years of age or older. Daily doses may range from 40 mg to 400 mg and successful patients, while on methadone, are then able to maintain a more normal life, in contrast to the addict's chaotic life of only seeking money for another high (8, 17).

In search of longer-acting alternatives to methadone, addiction specialists have turned to levomethadyl acetate and buprenorphine, both of which are medications that are effective with narcotic addicts Clinicians can also use the sublingual combination of buprenorphine/naloxone (Suboxone) that provides benefit at least equal to that of methadone and seems more efficacious than detoxification/counseling (8, 17). The naloxone part of this dual treatment is used to stop diversion of the buprenorphine to intravenous administration. There have been some reports of ventricular tachycardia with prolonged QT intervals (*Torsade de pointes*) after taking LAAM and more research is needed to see if this drug is safe enough to be used. Longer acting preparations of buprenorphine and naltrexone (such as monthly injection and subdermal implants) have been recently approved for adults, however, they are yet to be tested in the adolescent population.

Table 17. Medications available for opioid addiction

• Naltrexone
• Methadone hydrochloride
• LAAM (levo-alpha-acetyl methadol or levomethadyl acetate)
• Buprenorphine
• Anti-depressant drugs (as selective serotonin reuptake inhibitors)
• Anti-stress medications (as buspirone)

Hallucinogenic drugs

Both the hallucinogens and dissociative drugs may alter a youth's state of mind and mood. Hallucinogens include psilocybin, psilocyn (*shrooms*, mushrooms), LSD, and mescaline (peyote); these drugs can cause auditory, visual, and tactile hallucinations. Dissociative drugs, such as ketamine or PCP, alter a persons' state of mind and mood, causing a "feeling of detachment" or "dissociate reaction," but do not cause hallucinations. The 2019 YRBS noted that 7% of surveyed students report having used a hallucinogenic drug one or more times during their lifetime YRBSS 2019) (1). As per the latest NSUDH data of 2018, approximately 376,000(1.5%) adolescents used hallucinogens at least once in the past year, which was lower than the percentages in 2015 and 2017 similar to trend that was found from 2001 to 2013 when the prevalence dropped from 13.3% to 7.1% respectively (1, 17). Of this group, nine percent reported use of LSD, 6 percent of ecstasy, and three percent of PCP. The Indian data from National Survey on Extent and Pattern of Substance Use in India shows only 0.12% of general population used any hallucinogen in the year before survey (52).

The DSM-5 lists a number of hallucinogen-related disorders: phencyclidine use disorder (mild, moderate, severe), other hallucinogen use disorder (mild, moderate, severe), phencyclidine intoxication, other hallucinogen intoxication, hallucinogen persisting perception disorder, other phencyclidine-induced disorders, other hallucinogen-induced disorders, unspecified phencyclidine-related disorder, and unspecified hallucinogen-related disorder (18).

PCP (*phencyclidine)* and LSD (*lysergic acid diethylamide*) are taken as pills to induce a potent reality distortion with synesthesia or alterations of sensory perception (involving sight and sound) and emotions (involving euphoria and intense fears), in addition to time and place. Tolerance is described in these individuals as are cases of psychosis and the well-known flashback that can be induced by antihistamines or marijuana. Overdosing can induce respiratory depression with coma and death. A recent addition to the "trip" scene is *Salvia divinorum* (Virgin Mary's Herb, Mary's leaf). This is a hallucinogenic ethnobiological plant grown in the southwest U.S. which may be smoked, squeezed into water, or steeped into a tea. It is absorbed through the mucus membranes and produces a "euphoric experience with God." It cannot be detected by current urinary drug screens (8).

Phencyclidine (PCP)

This drug has many street names, including *peace, pill, sternly, peace pill, angel dust, hog,* and *sheets*. PCP is an arylcyclohexalamine that can be made in illicit laboratories; it causes adrenergic potentiation by inhibition of neuronal catecholamines and exerts its unique effects by blocking *N*-methyl-D-aspartate (NMDA) receptors for the excitatory neurotransmitter glutamate (8, 17). PCP can be taken as tablets, liquid, or in a powder form, sometimes sprinkled on marijuana or cigarettes (*joints*) to augment pot's potency. It is a dissociative anesthetic with hallucinogenic, stimulant, and depressive properties. Since it is lipophilic it has a 72-hour half-life. PCP is the active ingredient and can be detected for up to eight days after ingestion. Clinical expression may include frank psychosis, mania, delirium, and late manifestations of depression. Agitation associated with vertical and horizontal nystagmus, miotic but reactive pupils, elevated blood pressure, gait ataxia, and delusions should suggest PCP intoxication.

Diagnosis can be confirmed with gas chromatography/mass spectrometry using blood levels with or without urine testing. Excretion is pH dependent (increased in acid pH). High doses of dextromethorphan, especially when mixed with benzodiazepines, have been associated with a similar toxicity to phencyclidine.

Management of a PCP-induced "trip" (bad reaction) involves keeping the patient in a dark, padded room with the provision of diazepam (10-20 mg orally, or 10 mg intramuscularly every four hours) (8, 17). Lorazepam (1-2 mg) may be used in intramuscular or intravenous methods of delivery for seizures. Haloperidol may be reserved for severe agitation. Death may be caused by PCP because of the development of hypothermia, seizures, trauma, severe hypertension or hypotension, and/or psychotic delirium/coma. However, most deaths are caused by accidental injury occurring during intoxication. Psychosis may be helped with D3 agonists and research seeks chemicals to act as "antibodies" to neutralize PCP molecules.

Lysergic acid diethylamine (LSD)

LSD is the most powerful hallucinogen and has earned many street names, including *acid, "L," sugar, dots, cubes, big "D,"* and *blotters*. LSD is found in morning glory seeds and rye fungus (*Ergot*). It is easy to produce by amateur chemists and easy to hide since it is odorless, tasteless, and colorless; because of this, it has become popular at marathon dances ("raves") where it can be given to unsuspecting victims. A dose as low as 20 mcg (placed on small objects as a sugar cube, paper blotter, or postage stamps) can lead to its classic euphoric or hallucinogen effects by increasing serotonin; sympathetic activity is potentiated with resultant tachycardia, fever, conjunctival injection, mydriasis, lacrimation, flushing, dry mouth, blurred vision, tremors, incoordination, and elevated blood pressure (8, 17). Onset of symptoms following an oral dose is 30-45 minutes. The half-life is three hours, but routine urine drug screens do not detect LSD. Most youth with a bad trip or unpleasant flashback respond to a reassurance and calm interaction with the clinician; if necessary, haloperidol has been given for major reactions, including prolonged seizure activity.

Tryptamines

Tryptamines include a number of naturally occurring Schedule I hallucinogenic substances obtained from "magic mushrooms" indigenous to South America, Mexico, and the United States. They can be synthetically produced and include psilocybin (0-phosphoryl-4-hydroxy-N, N-dimethyltryptamine) and psilocyn (4-hydroxy-n, n-dimethyltryptamine) (8, 17). These chemicals produce muscle relaxation, mydriasis, vivid auditory and visual distortions, as well as emotional liability. These drug effects are not well predictable and vary by the specific mushrooms used as well as the manner in which they are dried, brewed, and consumed. Users of tryptamines often experience a multitude of effects that include hallucinations, euphoria, dilated pupils, empathy, emotional distress, "feelings of love," and visual-auditory disturbances or distortions. Some experience gastrointestinal effects, as nausea, emesis, and diarrhea.

Dimethyltryptamine (DMT) occurs naturally in a variety of wild plants and seeds. It is usually smoked, sniffed, or injected. DMT is inactivated orally and rapidly metabolized. The drug experience is called a "businessman's trip" because its effects are for only one hour (8). Diethyltryptamine (DET) is an analogue of DMT and produces the same pharmacologic effects, but is less potent than DMT. Alpha-ethyltryptamine (AET) is another tryptamine class hallucinogen added to the list of Schedule I hallucinogens in 1994 (8, 17).

N,N-Diisopropyl-5-methoxytryptamine (referred as "Foxy-Methoxy") is an orally active tryptamine recently encountered in the United States (8, 17). Alpha-methyltryptamine (AMT), known as "spirals," was designated a Schedule I drug in 2003. Tryptamines, like "Foxy" and AMT, are very dose dependent, which means that the doubling of a moderate dose could result in effects similar to LSD. The duration of effects from 20 mg of AMT usually last between 12 and 24 hours, while the effects from 6 to 10 mg of Foxy reportedly last from 3-6 hours. 5-methoxy-alpha-methyltryptamine (*5-MeO-AMT*) is also a tryptamine. Other common names for 5-MeO-AMT are "alpha-O," "alpha" and "O-DMS."

Bufotenine (bufagin, bufotenin, 5-hydroxy-N-N-dimethyltryptamine) is a Schedule I substance found in certain mushrooms, seeds, and most notably, the skin glands of the green and red Cane Toad (*Bufomarinus*) (8, 17). In the 1960s-70s, the "toads milks" in northern Florida were obtained by daring to lick ("suck the toad") which lead to accidental handling of the toads. Historically, these toads were killed and their skin boiled to produce a bitter tasting broth. In Australia, the milk is dried into a powder and smoked. In South America, this substance is used as snuff. A mild, though frightening "trip" occurs as this 3-indoleamine works on serotonergic sites in the amygdale and ventral lateral geniculate. The toad can continuously replace the supply and, in general, most bufotenine preparations from natural sources can be extremely toxic (8).

MDMA (Ecstasy)

Phenethylamines are a family of over 100 chemicals that are hallucinogenic. MDMA (3,4 methylenedioxymethamphetamine) is a phenethylamine that resembles both a stimulant (methamphetamine) and a hallucinogen (mescaline) (8). The US Food and Drug Administration classified MDMA as a Schedule I drug in 1985 (8, 17). MDEA (3,4-methylenedioxy-N-ethyl-amphetamine) or *Eve* is a close congener of MDMA. There is also a designer version of the banned decongestant and "diet" drug, phenylpropanolamine; it is referred to as *U4ia* and is similar in action to MDMA with both stimulant and hallucinogenic effects.

MDMA was developed in 1912 by German scientists and synthesized as an appetite suppressant; it was utilized in the 1970s and 1980s in an attempt to improve psychotherapy. Concern over this drug developed as its severe side effects became evident. The 2013 YRBS reported that 6.6% of students had used ecstasy (MDMA) one or more times during their lifetime and this dropped from 11.1% in 2001 to 6.6% in 2013, which has further reduced to 3.6% as per the 2019 CDC report (1, 2).

MDMA produces an intense euphoria and energizing effect in users and thus is popular at dance or club halls (called "raves, trances, or dance parties that last all night); it is also popular with college students. It is a designer drug that abusers feel is safe at 1-2 mg/kg and produces prolonged effects; because of this, its availability and use is more common than cocaine at teenage raves (8, 17). Its effect is normally 3 to 6 hours, though it may be several days. Its purest form is as a white crystalline powder and if red or brown MDMA is found, this suggests impurities are present. MDMA has many street names, such as *ecstasy, XTC, X, hug drug, lover's speed, diamonds, clarity, dex, essence, roll, bean, M, E, and Adam.*

Table 18. Side effects of MDMA (8, 17)

• Hypertension and increased pulse
• Dehydration and possible heat stroke
• Fatigue
• Sleep dysfunction
• Muscle spasms
• Sweating
• Organ dysfunction: renal, liver, CNS, muscular
• Intracerebral hemorrhage
• Irreversible CNS damage with memory loss in chronic abuse
• Confusion and paranoia
• Psychosis
• Depression
• Anxiety, including panic attacks
• Euphoria
• Arousal
• Increased sociability/extroversion
• Enhanced self-awareness
• Sexual effects
• Mental confusion (MDMA current perspective)

MDMA has mescaline like effects, probably due to interaction with and destruction of serotoninergic neurons in the central nervous system that are involved with thought and memory (8, 17). This may result from the formation of quinones which can combine with glutathione and other thiols. MDMA produces an anxious state of "well-being," changes in perception, moderate derealization and depersonalization without producing psychomotor agitation. MDMA abuse may lead to cognitive dysfunction, memory impairment, and behavioral problems. If taken during pregnancy, the risk for congenital anomalies is increased. Users take MDMA to enhance sensual awareness and augmented psychic or emotional energy. A number of side effects are noted, as listed in Table 18 (8, 17).

MDMA can hide thirst and eventual death that may be due to dehydration (which is not uncommon and hence its association with water bottles at raves), hyperthermia, hyponatremia, or cerebral edema. High doses can lead to muscle breakdown, breakdown of muscles, malignant hyperthermia, renal failure, and cardiovascular failure at the raves. MDMA and some of the other "designer" drugs have been associated with intracerebral hemorrhage in adolescents and young adults who have undiagnosed vascular malformations. Also, anxiety (including paranoia and panic attacks) may last for weeks after drug cessation. MDMA is a popular date-rape drug (see below). Acute management requires diagnosis, rehydration, cardiovascular support, and the use of benzodiazapines for sympathomimetic effects (8, 17).

MDMA users may mix this drug with alcohol, marijuana, LSD, dextromethorphan, and other drugs. Preparations with camphor, menthol, and ephedrine are applied to the nasal mucosa or chest to enhance the desired MDMA effects. MDMA can also be taken in increasing doses in a "stacked" schedule similar to that used with anabolic steroids. The drug user may also take chemicals that are ecstasy-like in appearance, such as ketamine ("special K"), alpha-methyl fentanyl ("synthetic heroin," "china white") and ephedrine tablets ("herbal ecstasy," "Chinese ephedra," "Ma Huang"). Large amounts of these chemicals may lead to hypertension, cardiac arrhythmias, myocardial infarction, cerebrovascular accidents, and death. The ephedrine found in Herbal ecstasy products as found in "health" food stores has only recently been banned.

"Date rape" drugs

Novel and more creative uses for previously legitimate pharmaceuticals and "nutriceuticals" continue to emerge "on the street," including familiar drugs as marijuana (i.e., increased THC content), phencyclidine (PCP), crack cocaine (or opium) with Viagra, variations on MDMA described previously, short acting benzodiazepines ("benzos"), and those compounds readily made using recipes available on the internet and concocted by amateur chemists (8, 17). A variety of chemicals have been used to lower external and internal inhibitions and/or consciousness, helping to facilitate sexual assault. These so-called "date rape" drugs are named for their strong sedative and hypnotic effects that are enhanced with alcohol. They continue to be popular at all night dance parties or "raves," and thus, have also been called Club drugs or Party drugs. Some are sold in "nutrition" stores or via magazine ads as sleep aids, muscle builders, and even as "party drugs." A variety of drugs have been used, as partially listed in Table 19; this list includes MDMA-methylenedioxy-methamphetamine (*ecstasy*) previously discussed (8, 17).

Flunitrazepam (Rohypnol)

This is a potent benzodiazepine with sedative, anxiolytic, and anticonvulsant effects. It belongs to the same group as Halcion, Ambien, Xanax (*Z Bars*), klonopin, sonata, versed, and valium. Flunitrazepam is a central nervous system depressant produced commercially in Switzerland that reduces inhibition and results in memory loss (blackouts) with short term anterograde amnesia for activity that takes place while under the influence of the drug (8, 17).

Table 19. Club drugs (8, 17)

- Methylenedioxymethamphetamine (*Ecstasy*, MDMA)
- Rohypnol (Flunitrazepam; *Roofies, The Date Rape Drug, Roches, Rope*)
- Gamma-hydroxybutyrate (*GHB, Liquid Ecstasy*)
- Gamma-butryl lactone (*GBL, Blue nitro, Renewtrient*)
- Butanediol (*BD, soap, Revitalize plus*)
- Methamphetamine (*meth, ice, crystal, fire, glass, chalk, crank*)
- LSD (*acid, "L," sugar, dots, cubes, big "D,"* and *blotters*)
- Ketamine (Ketalar; *Special K, Cat Valiums*)

It can also lead to such adverse effects as urinary retention, drowsiness, confusion, dizziness, gastrointestinal dysfunction, visual disturbances, hypotension and others. It is available by prescription in Europe (not the United States) and used as a sedative for management of insomnia and also as a pre-surgery anesthetic.

Flunitrazepam is a tasteless, odorless, and colorless chemical that can be taken as a pill or dissolved in a beverage; anecdotal reports of snorting are noted as well (8, 17). One milligram can be secretly placed in a liquid to sedate a victim for 8 to 12 hours with unfortunate amnesia for the sexual assault that may follow the ingestion. The victim is seen voluntarily leaving with the rapist, recalls little if anything of the events, and is unable to testify in any later prosecution. It has become a popular and classic date rape drug used by gang members and even high school or college students operating at local parties. Its many street names include *forget-me pills, Rope, Roche, Mexican valium,* and *roofies.*

It is also an addictive drug used voluntarily by youth as an alternative or adjunctive drug to marijuana or LSD, as well as the self-treatment of anxiety. Its effects are enhanced with alcohol. If used on a regular basis, increasingly higher doses are needed for the desired euphoric effect. Its use has increased 50% over the past several years. In South Texas, along the United-States-Mexico border, it is frequently replaced by the more readily available Klonopin or Xanax, both of which are associated with blacking-out spells and "withdrawal seizures," especially when abused with alcohol and marijuana.

Gamma-hydroxybutyrate (GHB)

This is a CNS depressant that induces euphoria and lowered inhibition. It has many street names, including: Liquid X, Liquid E, Liquid XTC, Liquid Ecstasy, Natural Sleep-500, Organic Quaalude, G Caps, Gamma Hydrate, Georgia Home Boy, Growth Hormone Booster, Cherry Meth, Sodium oxybutyrate, Somatomax PM, Grievous Bodily Harm, G-Riffick, Oxy-Sleep, Scoop, Fantasy, Easy Lay, Soap, Salty Water, Vita G, Gamma OH, Somsanit, GHB; Liquid Ecstasy; G; Georgia home boy, caps, organic qualude, and goop (8, 17).

Like Rohypnol, GHB and its analogs are used as "date rape" drugs. It has a soapy or salty taste, and hence the name *salt* is used until it is mixed with any liquid, including water. Because it is colorless, tasteless, and odorless, it is easily and quietly slipped into an unattended party drink to induce sedation and amnesia. Effects develop in 10-20 minutes, peak in 1-2 hours, and last for four hours. GHB is rapidly cleared from the body and is undetected in subsequent rape investigations. The clinician providing care in an emergency situation must request that the laboratory specifically look for GHB. Adolescent females need to be warned about the danger of leaving drinks unattended.

It is used by bodybuilders and athletes because of beliefs that GHB will augment endogenous human growth hormone (HGH) release while sleeping. GHB is available in single doses that augment or mimic effects of alcohol; increasingly higher doses are needed for desired effects. The risk of seizures and death caused by GHB-induced respiratory depression is raised when mixing GHB with other drugs, such as alcohol, heroin, LSD, and psilocybin (8, 17). The CNS depression occurs because of increasing CNS dopamine and GABA (gamma-amino-butyric acid); the endogenous opioid system is also activated. It became a Schedule I substance in March of 2000 and in July 2002, GHB was approved by an FDA advisory committee for study in the treatment of cataplexy. Most of the GHB used in the United States is illegally manufactured in the United States. Law enforcement in every region of the United States reports that GHB has surpassed Rohypnol as the most common substance used in drug-facilitated sexual assaults.

Gamma-butyro-lactone (GBL)

Because the US Drug Enforcement Agency (DEA) is cracking down on GHB use, some are using GHB precursors, such as GBL as well as BD (1-4 butanediol), an industrial solvent; both are promoted to enhance sexual ability and pleasure (8, 7). Street names for GHL are many, including *Renewtrient, Revivarant, Reivivarant G, Blue Nitro, Blue Nitro Vitality, GH Revitalizer, Gamma G, Remforce, and Soap*; it is found in paint thinners and floor stripper products. BD leads to bradypnea and can induce emesis, aspiration, and coma. GBL and BD are both easily changed to GHB *in vivo*, and *in vitro* by adding water. Some producers are substituting BD for GHB, even though the FDA has identified BD as a potentially life-threatening drug. It is sold as a dietary supplement in a number of sleep aid and muscle enhancing products; names include *SomatoPro, NR63, Thunder Nectar, Enliven, GHRE, Weight Belt Cleaner, Revitalize Plus,* and *Serenity*. The FDA asked that products with GBL be recalled in January, 1999; some states, such as California, have told manufactures that it is illegal to sell these products or market them as a supplement or nutritional substance. GBL-related products have been associated with reports of at least 55 adverse health effects, including one death. In 19 of these cases, the consumers became unconscious or comatose, several requiring intubations for assisted breathing (8, 7).

Ketamine

This drug has been approved since 1970 in the role of an injectable airway-preserving veterinary anesthetic; it is taken orally to induce dissociative states, described as dream-like and hallucinatory (8, 17). Major action is by inhibition of NMDA receptors. Street names include *K, Cat Valium, Special K, and Vitamin K.* It can be obtained as a white powder that can be added to tobacco or marijuana or the powder can be snorted; intramuscular abuse is also described. The effects of ketamine last one half to two hours producing an "out of body" distortion of time and space. Ketamine in low doses can lead to dysfunction of learning ability, memory, and attention span; in high doses, it can lead to myalgia, paranoia, elevated blood pressure, delirium, motor function impairment, amnesia, long term flashbacks, and respiratory depression-induced death. There is no urine metabolite. There are also reports of methoxetamine abuse which is structural analogue of ketamine and has been linked to several deaths too (8, 7).

Inhalants

Inhalant drugs (see Table 20) are central nervous system depressants typically abused by young (ages 6-8, peaks at 14), often male, and homeless adolescents to induce temporary euphoria and excitement (62-64). These inhaled chemical vapors are viewed as easily available and as inexpensive substitutes or precursors to other drugs, such as alcohol or marijuana. Delivery is by "sniffing, huffing, or bagging."

Table 20. Types of inhalant drugs*

Solvents	Gases	Nitrites (Aliphatic nitrites)
Industrial or household solvents or solvent-containing products	Gases used in household or commercial products	Cyclohexyl nitrite (available to general public)
	Butane lighters	
	Propane tanks	
Paint thinners or solvents	Whipping cream aerosols or dispensers (whippets)	Amyl nitrite (available only with prescription)
Degreasers (dry-cleaning fluids)	Refrigerant gases	
Gasoline		
Glues	Household aerosol propellant and associated solvents	Butyl nitrite (Illegal substance)
Art or office supply solvents	Found in spray paints	
Correction fluids	Found in hair or deodorant sprays	
Felt-tip-maker fluid	Found in fabric protector sprays	
Electronic contact cleaners		
	Medical anesthetic gases	
	Ether	
	Chloroform	
	Halothane	
	Nitrous oxide	

* Greydanus DE, Patel DR. Substance abuse in adolescents: A complex conundrum for the clinician. Pediatric Clin North Am 2003;59(5):1179-223 (with permission) (64).

In 1995 the lifetime use was 21.6% for 8th graders versus 19.7% in 1999 and 17.3% in 2004. Approximately 5% of adolescent girls (age 12-17 years) used inhalants that included nitrous oxide vials (19.3%), glue sniffing (34.9%), correction fluid (23.4%), hair spray (23%), and inhalation of paints or sprays (6-16%) (8, 17). The 2019 YRBS reported that 6.4% had used any of the inhalants as compared to 8.9% of 2013 data; this included sniffing glue, breathing the contents of aerosol spray cans, or inhaling any paints or sprays to get high one or more times during their life (2). The prevalence dropped from 20.3% in 1995 to 86.4%% in 2019 (1). The Indian data from 2018 shows prevalence of 2.4% among adolescents of use during the year before the survey (52).

The main ingredient in airplane glue and some rubber cements is toluene (**8**). Another popular inhalant is gasoline, noted especially in rural areas of the United States and with Native American adolescents. Amyl nitrite, butyl nitrite, and other volatile nitrates are found in room deodorizers and are used by older adolescents to induce "aphrodisiac" effects.

Inhalant use is usually experimental and may occur as a group activity. Inhalation occurs after these substances are placed in a plastic bag ("bagging"), wrap, or inhaled from a soaked rag ("huffing") to induce the intoxicating (psychoactive) effects (8). Inhalants are considered CNS depressants in general similar to alcohol and barbiturates and have been thought to work through enhancing GABA activity and by altering fluidization of membranes. Absorption is rapid and the altered mental state lasts for 5-15 minutes. After a mild stimulatory effect, an inhibition reduction occurs, followed by unconsciousness. Death may occur from cardiac arrhythmias. Tolerance develops after long term use, though withdrawal is rare; dependence may develop (65).

Table 21. Effects of inhalants*

Hearing loss
• Toluene (paint sprays, glues, dewaxers)
• Trichloroethylene (cleaning fluids, correction fluids)
Peripheral neuropathies or Limb spasms
• Hexane (glues, gasoline)
• Nitrous oxide (whipping cream, gas cylinders)
CNS or Brain Damage: toluene
Bone Marrow Damage: benzene (gasoline)
Liver and Kidney Damage
• Toluene-containing substances
• Chlorinated hydrocarbons
• Correction fluids
• Dry-cleaning fluids
Blood Oxygen Depletion/ Methemoglobinemia
• Organic nitrites ("*poppers*," "amyl," "*bold*" and "*rush*")
• Methylene chloride
• Varnish removers
• Paint thinners
Loss of the sense of smell (nitrites)
Thermal burn injury with nebulized alcohol/Robitussin® ("RoboFires")
Death
Kaposi's sarcoma

* Adapted from Greydanus DE, Patel DR. Substance abuse in adolescents: A complex conundrum for the clinician. Pediatric Clin North Am 2003;59(5):1179-223 (with permission) (64).

Table 21 lists various complications known to occur with various inhalants (8, 17). The DSM-5 lists a number of inhalant-related disorders: inhalant use disorder (mild, moderate, severe), inhalant intoxication, other inhalant-induced disorders, and unspecified inhalant related disorders (18).

Most abusers of inhalants discontinue these drugs by stopping substance abuse in general or moving on to other drugs. Management of those who become chronic inhalant abusers is difficult, often being hindered by their many, varied behavioral and social problems. Inhalant intoxication usually does not require any medical attention; however, some frequent effects may require intervention and these include bronchospasm, arrhythmia, and physical trauma. There is no specific treatment for chronic effects of inhalant use such as cognitive and neurological effects. Inhalant induced psychosis or agitation are usually brief and treated supportively. Synopsis research on management is focusing on inhalant effects on dopaminergic, glutamatergic and GABAergic systems (65). Unfortunately death from volatile substance misuse may occur as seen, for example, with difluoroethane (66). Management of abuse is focused upon management of co-morbidities such as ADHD and conduct disorder.

Barbiturates

These are CNS depressants that are classified as sedative-hypnotic drugs. They act on the CNS by enhancing the neuroinhibitory action of gamma-aminobutyric acid (GABA) and producing relief from anxiety and sedation (8, 17). They are classified as ultra-short acting (thiopental), short acting (pentobarbital [*yellow jackets]*, secobarbital [*reds*]), and long acting (phenobarbital). The short acting barbiturates have a higher potential for abuse and are more lipid soluble than the long-acting formulations.

They can become addicting in 1 to 2 months and are deadly in high doses or when combined with opioids or alcohol. Abuse of these drugs leads to physical addiction, abstinence, and discontinuation syndrome, similar to that noted with alcohol abuse. The DSM-5 lists a number of "sedative, hypnotic, or anxiolytic"-related disorders: sedative, hypnotic, or anxiolytic use disorder (mild, moderate, severe); sedative, hypnotic, or anxiolytic intoxication; sedative, hypnotic, or anxiolytic withdrawal; other sedative, hypnotic, or anxiolytic -induced disorders; and unspecified sedative, hypnotic, or anxiolytic related disorders (18). Barbiturates were commonly abused before the introduction of benzodiazepines; however, due to higher abuse potential and fatal overdoses they are rarely abused at present. Certain other substances known as barbiturate-like substance include methaqualone (Mandrakes), meprobamate and chloral hydrate (8, 17). However, most of them have been banned in the United States.

Barbiturates are detoxified in the liver and/or excreted unchanged in the urine. Symptoms of acute use and overdose are similar to those of alcohol and include euphoria, slurred speech, lethargy, miosis, and ataxia. Overdosing leads to low blood pressure, bullous dermatological lesions, respiratory depression, coma, and death (8, 17). It is not commonly abused at current times and involves less than 3% of high school students. This reduced abuse probably reflects infrequent clinician prescription of these drugs, reduced availability on the streets, and the availability of many other illicit drugs. Barbiturates should usually not be prescribed to adolescents and then, only with extreme caution.

Conclusion

Substance abuse continues to be a widespread and very serious phenomenon for our adolescents and young adults in the United States and around the globe (4, 8, 17, 44-46, 67-72). Research continues to look at serious consequences of various drug use/abuse that includes tobacco, opioids, cocaine, hydrocarbons and others as reviewed in this discussion (73-81).

Many factors draw our youth into these deadly drugs, leading to many acute and chronic sequelae, ranging from addiction to death. The 21st century COVID-19 pandemic has complicated many facets for human mental health including substance use disorders (18, 82, 83). Testing for substance use is available and research is looking at various means of prevention including vaccination science (10, 43, 84, 85).

Youth must be clearly and carefully taught that drug use and abuse comes with considerable complications for their current and future life. They also must be taught that there is no scientific evidence that smoking cannabis is safe nor is medically beneficial (17, 46). They must also become aware of the dangers of the newer and designer drugs that are being produced in greater amounts that includes the dangers of vaping (86). Research continues in this critical condition of substance abuse in the 21st century (87-95).

Clinicians must join with other members of society to educate our patients to the many deadly and dangerous drugs of abuse that are available and work with society (including governments) to reduce the availability of drugs. The human instinct for pleasure at any cost must be tempered with education and direction from clinicians. Management of those addicted to drugs is a complex, often discouraging process. Like pharmacotherapy, psychosocial and behavioral therapies are equally important that involve a variety of health specialists. Group, family, and individual therapy all have a place in management and many need intensive treatment in drug abuse programs (8, 17).

Acknowledgment

This is an updated version of Greydanus DE, Reed WJ, Hawver EK. Substance use and abuse in adolescents. In: Greydanus DE, Patel DR, Pratt HD, Calles Jr JL, Nazeer A, Merrick J, eds. Behavioral pediatrics, 4th edition. New York: Nova Science, 2015:497-535 with permission.

References

[1] Substance Abuse and Mental Health Services Administration. Key substance use and mental health indicators in the United States: Results from the 2020 National Survey on Drug Use and Health. Rockville, MD: Center for Behavioral Health Statistics and Quality, Substance Abuse and Mental Health Services Administration, PEP21-07-01-003, NSDUH Series H-56, 2021. URL: https://www.samhsa.gov/data/.
[2] Kann L, Kinchen S, Shanklin SL, Flint KH, Hawkins J, Harris WA, et al. YRBS: Youth Risk Behavioral Surveillance-United States, 2013. MMWR 2014;63(4):1-169.
[3] Lui CK, Chung PJ, Ford CL, Grella DE, Mulia N. Drinking behaviors and life course socioeconomic status during the transition from adolescence to adulthood among whites and blacks. J Stud Alcohol Drugs 2015;76(1):68-79.
[4] Greydanus DE, Patel DR: Substance abuse in adolescents: Current concepts. Dis Mon 2005;51(7):392-431.
[5] Viteri OA, Soto EE, Bahado-Singh RO, Christensen CW, Chauhan SP, Sibai BM. Fetal anomalies and long-term effects associated with substance abuse in pregnancy: A literature review. Am J Perinatol 2015;32(5):405-16.
[6] Naim-Feil J, Zangen A. Addiction. HandbClinNeurol 2013;116:613-30.
[7] Müller CP, Homberg JR. The role of serotonin in drug use and addiction. Behav Brain Res 2015;277C:146-92.
[8] Greydanus DE, Reed WJ, Hawver EK. Substance use and abuse in adolescents. In: Greydanus DE, Patel DR, Pratt HD, Calles JL Jr., Nazeer A, Merrick J, eds. Behavioral pediatrics, 4thedition. New York: Nova Science, 2015:497-535.
[9] Lee D, Delcher C, Maldonado-Molina MM, Bazydlo LA, Thogmartin JR, Goldberger BA. Trends in licit and illicit drug-related deaths in Florida from 2001 to 2012. Forensic SciInt 2014;245C:178-86.
[10] Harris SK, Louis-Jacques J, Knight JR. Screening and brief intervention for alcohol and other abuse. Adolesc Med State Art Rev 2014;25(1):126-56.
[11] Patel DR, Greydanus DE: Substance abuse: a pediatric concern. Indian J Pediatrics 1999;66:557-67.
[12] Imtiaz S, Shield KD, Fisher B, Rehm J. Harms of prescription opioid use in the United States. Subst Abuse Treat Prev Policy 2014;9:43. doi: 10.1186/1747-597X-9-43.
[13] Levy S, Williams JF. Adolescent substance use: the role of the medical home. Adolesc Med State Art Rev 2014;25(1):1-14.
[14] Nielsen DA, Nielsen EM, Dasari T, Spellicy CJ. Pharmacogenetics of addiction therapy. Methods Mol Biol 2014;1175:589-624.
[15] Winters KC, Tanner-Smith EE, Bresani E, Meyers K. Current advances in the treatment of adolescent drug use. Adolesc Health Med Ther 2014;5:199-210.
[16] Urrila AS, Paunio T, Palomäki E, Marttunen M. Sleep in adolescent depression: physiological perspectives. ActaPhysiol (Oxf) 2015;213(4):758-77.
[17] Greydanus DE, Kaplan G, Patel DR, Merrick J. Substance abuse in adolescents and young adults: A manual for pediatric and primary care clinicians, Second edition. New York: Nova Science, 2019.

[18] American Psychiatric Association. Diagnostic and statistical manual of mental Disorders (DSM-5) Washington, DC: American Psychiatric Association, 2013.
[19] American Psychiatric Association. Diagnostic and statistical manual of mental disorders, Fourth edition, Text revision (DSM-IV-TR). Washington, DC: American Psychiatric Publications, 2000.
[20] Jones CM, Clayton HB, Deputy NP, Roehler DR, Ko JY, Esser MB, et al. Prescription opioid misuse and use of alcohol and other substances among high school students—Youth Risk Behavior Survey, United States, 2019.MMWR Suppl 2020;69(1):38-46.
[21] Ali F, Rehman H, Babayan Z, Stapleton D, Joshi DD. Energy drinks and their adverse health effects: A systematic review of the current evidence. Postgrad Med 2015; 127(3):308-22.
[22] Musselman ME, Hampton JP. "Not for human consumption": A review of emerging designer drugs. Pharmacotherapy 2014;34(7):745-57.
[23] Baumann MH, Solis E Jr, Watterson LR, Marusich JA, Fantegrossi WE, Wiley JL. Bath salts, spice, and related designer drugs: the science behind the headlines. J Neurosci 2014;34(46):15150-8.
[24] Nelson ME, Bryant SM, Aks SE. Emerging drugs of abuse. Emerg Med Clin North Am 2014;32(1):1-28.
[25] Urban DJ, Roth BL. DREADDs (Designer receptors exclusively activated by designer drugs): Chemogenetic tools with therapeutic utility. Annu Rev PharmacolToxicol 2015;55:399-417.
[26] Smith CD, Robert S. 'Designer drugs': update on the management of novel psychoactive substance misuse in the acute care setting. Clin Med 2014;14(4):409-15.
[27] Castaneto MS, Gorelick DA, Desrosiers NA, Hartman RL, Pirard S, Huestis MA. Synthetic cannabinoids: epidemiology, pharmacodynamics, and clinical implications. Drug Alcohol Depend 2014;144C:12-41.
[28] Banks ML, Worst TJ, Rusyniak DE, Sprague JE. Synthetic cathinones ("bath salts"). J Emerg Med 2014;46(5):632-42.
[29] Hajek P, Etter JF, Benowitz N, Eissenberg T, McRobbie H. Electronic cigarettes: review of use, content, safety, effects on smokers and potential for harm and benefit. Addiction 2014;109(11):1801-10.
[30] Knorst MM, Benedetto IG, Hoffmeister MC, Gazzana MB. The electronic cigarette; the new cigarette of the 21st century? J Bras Pneumol 2014;40(5):564-72.
[31] Rosenberg JM. A molecular basis fro nicotine as a gateway drug. N Engl J Med 2014;371(21):2038.
[32] Kandel D, Kandel E. The gateway hypothesis of substance abuse: developmental, biological and societal perspectives. ActaPaediatr 2015;104(2):130-7.
[33] Creamer MR, Everett Jones S, Gentzke AS, Jamal A, King BA. Tobacco product use among high school students - Youth Risk Behavior Survey, United States, 2019. MMWR Suppl 2020;69(1):56-63.
[34] Loukola A, Hällfors J, Korhonen T, Kaprio J. Genetics and smoking. Curr Addict Rep 2014;1(1):75-82.
[35] Johnston L, O'Malley PM, Bachman JG, Sckhlenberg JE. National survey results on druguse from the Monitoring the Future Study, 2003, 2006, 2007, 2008. Ann Arbor, MI:Institute for Social Research, University of Michigan, 2009.
[36] Collins GB, Jerry JM, Bales R. Quitting smoking: still a challenge, but new tools show promise. Cleve Clin J Med 2015;82(1):39-48.
[37] Patel DR, Greydanus DE: Office interventions for adolescent smokers. Adolesc. Med 2000;11(3):1-11.
[38] McRobbie H, Bullen C, Hartmann-Boyce J, Hajek P. Electronic cigarettes for smoking cessation and reduction. Cochrane Database Syst Rev 2014;12:CD010216.
[39] Greydanus DE, Calles JL, Jr., Patel DR: Pediatric and adolescent psychopharmacology: A practical manual for pediatricians. Cambridge, England: Cambridge University Press, 2008:241-77.
[40] Walker N, Howe C, Glover M, McRobbie H, Barnes J, Nosa V, et al. Cytisine versus nicotine for smoking cessation. N Engl J Med 2014;371(25):2353-62.
[41] Karnieg T, Wang X. Cysteine for smoking cessation. CMAJ 2018;190(19):E596.
[42] Jain R, Majumder P, Gupta T. Pharmacological intervention of nicotine dependence. Biomed Res Int. 2013;2013:278392.
[43] Le HT, Fraleigh NL, Lewicky JD, Boudreau J, Dolinar P, Bhardwaj N, et al. Enhancing the immune response of a nicotine vaccine with synthetic small "non-natural" peptides. Molecules 2020;25(6):1290.
[44] Greydanus DE, Hawver EK, Greydanus MM, Merrick J. Marijuana: Current concepts. Front Public Health 2013;1(42):1-17.

[45] Greydanus DE, Kaplan G, Patel DR, Merrick J. Special issue: The burden of substance abuse. Int Public Health J 2014;6(3):215-90.

[46] Greydanus DE, Kaplan G, Baxter LE, Sr., Patel DR, Feucht CL. Cannabis: The never-ending, nefarious nepenthe of the 21st century: What should the clinician know? Dis Mon 2015;61(5):1-80.

[47] Brezing C, Levin F. The current state of pharmacological treatments for cannabis use disorder and withdrawal. Neuropsychopharmacol 2018;43:173-94.

[48] Gutierrez A, Sher L. Alcohol and drug use among adolescents: an educational overview. Int J Adolesc Med Health 2015;27(2):207-12.

[49] Lopez-Leon S, González-Giraldo Y, Wegman-Ostrosky T, Forero DA. Molecular genetics of substance use disorders: An umbrella review. NeurosciBiobehav Rev 2021; 124:358-369.

[50] Ferraguti G, Pascale E, Lucarelli M. Alcohol addiction: A molecular biology perspective. Curr Med Chem 2015;22(6):670-84.

[51] Thakkar MM, Sharma R, Sahota P. Alcohol disrupts sleep homeostasis. Alcohol 2015; 49(4):299-310.

[52] Ambekar A, Agrawal A, Rao R, Mishra AK, Khandelwal SK, Chadda RK on behalf of the group of investigators for the National Survey on Extent and Pattern of Substance Use in India. Magnitude of Substance Use in India. New Delhi: Ministry of Social Justice and Empowerment, Government of India, 2019.

[53] Tung MK, Light M, Giri R, Lane S, Appelbe A, Harvey C, et al. Evolving epidemiology of injecting drug use-associated infective endocarditis: A regional centre experience. Drug Alcohol Rev 2015;34(4):412-7.

[54] Clemow DB, Walker DJ. The potential for misuse and abuse of medications in ADHD: a review. Postgrad Med 2014;126(5):64-81.

[55] Rawson RA. Current research on the epidemiology, medical and psychiatric effects, and treatment of methamphetamine use. J Food Drug Anal 2013;21(4):S77-81.

[56] London ED, Kohno M, Morales AM, Ballard ME. Chronic methamphetamine abuse and corticostriatal deficits revealed by neuroimaging. Brain Res 2015;1628(Pt A):174-85.

[57] Chiang M, Lombardi D, Du J, Makrum U, Sitthichai R, Harrington A, et al. Methamphetamine-associated psychosis: Clinical presentation, biological basis, and treatment options. Hum Psychopharmacol 2019;34(5):e2710.

[58] Smid MC, Metz TD, Gordon AJ. Stimulant use in pregnancy: An under-recognized epidemic among pregnant women. ClinObstetGynecol 2019;62(1):168-84.

[59] Alving CR, Matyas GR, Torres O, Jalah R, Beck Z. Adjuvants for vaccines to drugs of abuse and addiction. Vaccine 2014;32(42):5382-9.

[60] Sundar M, Patel D, Young Z, Leong KC. Oxytocin and addiction: Potential glutamatergic mechanisms. Int J Mol Sci 2021;22(5):2405.

[61] Rudd RA, Paulozzi LJ, Bauer MJ, Burleson RW, Carlson RE, Dao D, et al. Increase in heroin overdose deaths—28 states, 2010-2012. MMWR 2014;63(39):849-54.

[62] Curtis J, Metheny E, Sergent SR. Hydrocarbon toxicity. In: StatPearls. Treasure Island, FL: StatPearls Publishing, 2021 Jan–.

[63] Nakawaki B, Crano W. Patterns of substance use, delinquency, and risk factors among adolescent inhalant users. Subst Use Misuse 2015;50(1):114-22.

[64] Greydanus DE, Patel DR: Substance abuse in adolescents: A complex conundrum for the clinician. PediatrClin North Am 2003;59(5):1179-223.

[65] Duncan JR, Lawrence AJ. Conventional concepts and new perspectives for understanding the addictive properties of inhalants. J PharmacolSci 2013;122(4):237-43.

[66] Ossiander EM. Volatile substance misuse deaths in Washington State, 2003-2012. Am J Drug Alcohol Abuse 2015;41(1):30-4.

[67] Gaur N, Gautam M, Singh S, Raju VV, Sarkar S. Clinical practice guidelines on assessment and management of substance abuse disorder in children and adolescents. Indian J Psychiatry 2019;61(Suppl 2):333-49.

[68] Greydanus DE: Substance abuse in adolescents: Basic chemistry lessons gone awry. International Pediatrics 2002;17(1): 3-4.

[69] Greydanus DE, Kaplan G, Patel DR, Merrick J. Editorial: Substance abuse. Int Public Health J 2014;6(3):215-24.

[70] Comerci GB, Schwebel R: Substance abuse: Adolesc Med 2000;11(1): 79-101.

[71] Underwood JM, Brener N, Thornton J, Harris WA, Bryan LN, Shanklin SL, et al. Overview and Methods for the Youth Risk Behavior Surveillance System - United States, 2019. MMWR Suppl 2020;69(1):1-10.

[72] Hedegaard H, Miniño AM, Warner M. Drug overdose deaths in the United States, 1999-2018. NCHS Data Brief 2020:356:1-8.

[73] 2008 PHS Guideline Update Panel, Liaisons, and Staff. Treating tobacco use and dependence: 2008 update US Public Health Service clinical practice guideline executive summary. Respir Care 2008;53(9):1217-22.

[74] Ford JA. Prescription opioid misuse among adolescents. PediatrClin North Am2019; 66(6):1099-108.

[75] O'Connor PG: Treating opioid dependence—New data and new opportunities. N. Engl J Med 2000;343(18):193-5.

[76] Ryan SA. Cocaine use in adolescents and young adults. PediatrClin North Am 2019; 66(6):1135-47.

[77] Zhou L, Sun WL, Young AB, Lee K, McGinty JF, See RE. Oxytocin reduces cocaine seeking and reverses chronic cocaine-induced changes in glutamate receptor function. Int J Neuropsychopharmacol 2014;18(1):pyu009.

[78] Cressman AM, Natekar A, Kim E, Koren G, Bozzo P. Cocaine abuse during pregnancy. J ObstetGynaecol Can 2014;36(7):628-31.

[79] Deroche-Gamonet V, Piazza PV. Psychobiology of cocaine addiction: contribution of a multi-symptomatic animal model of loss of control. Neuropharmacology 2014;76 Pt B:437-49.

[80] Marasco CC, Goodwin CR, Winder DG, Schramm-Sapyta NL, McLean JA, Wikswo JP. Systems-level view of cocaine addiction: the interconnection of the immune and nervous systems. ExpBiol Med (Maywood) 2014;239(11):1433-42.

[81] Tormoehlen LM, Tekulve KJ, Nañagas KA. Hydrocarbon toxicity: a review. ClinToxicol (Phila) 2014;52(5):479-89.

[82] Hertz MF, Barrios LC. Adolescent mental health, COVID-19, and the value of school-community partnerships. InjPrev 2021 Feb;27(1):85-86.

[83] Taylor S, Paluszek MM, Rachor GS, McKay D, Asmundson GJG. Substance use and abuse, COVID-19-related distress, and disregard for social distancing: A network analysis. Addict Behav 2021;114:106754.

[84] Knight JR, Sherritt L, Shrier LA, Harris SK, Chang G. Validity of the CRAFFT substance abuse screening test among adolescent clinic patients. Arch PediatrAdolesc Med. 2002;156(6):607-14.

[85] Wolters A, de Wert G, van Schayck OC, Horstman K. Vaccination against smoking: an annotated agenda for debate. A review of scientific journals, 2001-2013.Addiction 2014;109(8):1268-73.

[86] Tai H, Swartz MD, Marsden D, Perry CL. The future of substance abuse now: relationships among adolescent use of vaping devices, marijuana, and synthetic cannabinoids. Subst Use Misuse 2021;56(2):192-204.

[87] Lovinger DM, Gremel CM. A circuit-based information approach to substance abuse research. Trends Neurosci 2021;44(2):122-35.

[88] Chun TH, Chernick LS, Ahmad FA, Ranney ML, Shenoi RP, Casper TC, et al.; Pediatric Emergency Care Applied Research Network. Adolescent substance abuse risk: A comparison of pediatric emergency care applied research network emergency department patients and 2 nationally representative samples. PediatrEmerg Care 2021; 37(9):e560-4.

[89] Taylor CB, Graham AK, Flatt RE, Waldherr K, Fitzsimmons-Craft EE. Current state of scientific evidence on Internet-based interventions for the treatment of depression, anxiety, eating disorders and substance abuse: an overview of systematic reviews and meta-analyses. Eur J Public Health 2021;31(31 Suppl 1):i3-10.

[90] Rizzal AF, Keliat BA, Wardani IY. Save the future: Enhancing substance abuse refusal skill in adolescent. Enferm Clin 2021;31(Suppl 2):S405-7. [English, Spanish].

[91] Compton WM, Han B. Substance Use Disorders Are Deadly. Am J Psychiatry 2022 Jan;179(1):11-13.

[92] Michienzi AE, Borek HA. Emerging agents of substance use/misuse. Emerg Med Clin North Am 2022;40(2):265-281.

[93] Nelson LF, Weitzman ER, Levy S. Prevention of substance use disorders. Med Clin North Am 2022 Jan;106(1):153-168.

[94] Matson PA, Ridenour T, Ialongo N, Spoth R, Prado G, Hammond CJ, et al. State of the art in substance use prevention and early intervention: Applications to pediatric primary care settings. Prev Sci 2022;23(2):204-211.

[95] Scott K, Becker SJ, Helseth SA, Saldanha IJ, Balk EM, Adam GP, et al. Pharmacotherapy interventions for adolescent co-occurring substance use and mental health disorders: a systematic review. Fam Pract 2022;39(2): 301-310.

Chapter 10

Cannabis: Current concepts and conundrums

Donald E. Greydanus*, MD, DrHC (Athens) and Maria Demma Cabral, MD

Department of Pediatric and Adolescent Medicine, Western Michigan University Homer Stryker MD School of Medicine, Kalamazoo, Michigan, United States of America

Abstract

Marijuana (cannabis) remains a controversial drug in the 21st century. This discussion considers current research on use of *cannabis sativa* and its constituents such as the phytocannabinoids. Topics reviewed include prevalence of cannabis use, other drugs consumed with pot, the endocannabinoid system, use of medicinal marijuana, medical adverse effects of cannabis, and psychiatric adverse effects of cannabis use. Treatment of cannabis use disorders and withdrawal is difficult and remains mainly based on psychological therapy; current research on pharmacologic management of problems related to cannabis consumption is also considered. The potential role of specific cannabinoids for medical benefit will be further clarified as the 21st century matures. However, potential dangerous adverse effects from smoking marijuana are well known and should be clearly taught to a public often confused by a media-driven false message and promise of benign pot consumption. *Caveat emptor!*

Introduction

A number of chemicals are inhaled for the development of euphoria, including cannabis (marijuana), methamphetamine, heroin, crack cocaine, phencyclidine, and nitrites (amyl and butyl) (1). Marijuana (cannabis, pot) has been known to *Homo sapiens* for thousands of years and concern has been raised over the past two centuries regarding its potential adverse effects – leading to various laws in the United States and other countries to control its production as well as consumption (2). The psychoactive chemical, *delta-9-tetrahydrocannabinol* (THC), was isolated in the mid-1960s while other aspects of the endocannabinoid system (cannabinoid

* ***Correspondence:*** Donald E Greydanus MD, DrHC(Athens), Professor and Founding Chair, Department of Pediatric and Adolescent Medicine, Western Michigan University Homer Stryker MD School of Medicine, 1000 Oakland Drive, Kalamazoo, MI, United States. Email: Donald.greydanus@med.wmich.edu.

In: Behavioral Pediatrics
Editors: Donald E. Greydanus, Dilip R. Patel, Ahsan Nazeer et al.
ISBN: 979-8-88697-060-9

receptors [CB1 and CB2] and key endogenous cannabinoids [2-arachidonoyl glycerol and anandamide]) were identified over 20 years later. Though use of qualified phytocannabinoids is being increasingly linked to improvement of some health conditions, frequent users of cannabis are at increased risk for adverse effects which can lead to additional health problems (3). Research is identifying components of cannabis which are not psychoactive and may become established parts of the pharmacopoeia as the 21st century continues.

Cannabis sativa plant

The products of cannabis are made from the easily grown hemp plant, *Cannabis sativa*, and the psychoactive ingredient, *delta-9-tetrahydrocannabinol* (THC), is at the heart of the complex cannabis controversy in this and the past century. There are three important subsets of the cannabis plant which are *cannabis sativa*, *cannabis indica* and *cannabis ruderalis*. In contrast to cannabis indica and cannabis ruderalis, *cannabis sativa* is a taller and slimmer plant that gives a "head high" and is more stimulating, euphoric as well as uplifting. *Cannabis indica* is a shorter plant, rich in THC, and induces more relaxation with aiding in sleep. *Cannabis ruderalis* produces low THC content with high CBD (cannabidiol; *vida infra*) content, and is thought of as a more traditional "hemp" plant.

THC-induced euphoria can last minutes to hours. The enzyme, Δ1-tetrahydrocannabinolic acid synthase, catalyzes the oxidative cyclization of cannabigerolic acid (CBGA) into Δ1-tetrahydrocannabinolic acid that is the precursor of THC (4). This enzyme controls the psychoactivity of *cannabis sativa* due to THC which is present in the *cannabis sativa's* dried leaves, seeds, stems, flowers (sensimilla), and oil (4, 5). The pot of the 1960s-1970s contained 1-2% THC while the Hawaiian sensimilla product was 3%; this is in contrast to current versions with much higher THC percentage as measured by the Potency Monitoring Project and other research (5, 6). A survey in Japan revealed an average potency of 11.2% with a maximum potency of 22.6% (7). The cannabis industry has genetically modified the sativa plants to produce higher THC content and, in so doing, decreased CBD content. High-potency cannabis is referred to as "skunk."

Cannabis remains a popular global drug that is easily obtained around the world. Movements are increasing to legalize this drug because of the research noting positive medical benefits as well as the intense euphoria it produces along with a popular though false impression that this is a "safe" drug (8, 9). Cannabis remains a controversial drug though it has been legalized in many states in the US; however, it remains federally illegal. The illegal history of cannabis places it in conflict with the popular notion that pot is a harmless chemical—a notion made fashionable or trendy by many media and Hollywood personalities who may promote its use to enhance their *joie de vivre*.

Such promotions seem to be effective as noted by the popularity of this illicit drug. However, marijuana (cannabis) has been prohibited in the United States since the 1937 Marijuana Tax Act and is classified by the US Drug Enforcement Agency (DEA) as an illegal Schedule I drug. Cannabis has been decriminalized in many countries and states. It has been legalized in many states as "medical "cannabis while recreational legalization has happened in some states and also in Canada. Each state that has legalized cannabis is responsible for writing the rules and regulations with regard to growing, resting, and dispensing both the medical and recreational cannabis.

Prevalence

Prevalence data for cannabis can be determined in various ways such as self-report data, wastewater (sewage) analysis, and sales of cigarette paper (10, 11). Research notes that marijuana is the most commonly used illicit drug on earth (12, 13). The most frequently used substances among American adolescents are tobacco, alcohol, and marijuana. Marijuana ("*weed, pot, hash, BC Bud, Ganja, grass, smoke, doobs*," others) is an illicit schedule I drug that constitutes about three-fourths of the illegal drug utilization in the United States (14-16).

Many studies have been done to confirm the high use of cannabis among adolescents and young adults of the world (1, 17). The United States Centers for Disease and Prevention (CDC) YRBSS (Youth Risk Behavioral Surveillance System) reported a lifetime use (once or more times) among US high school students of 31.3% in 1991 that increased to 47.2% in 1999, was 36.8% in 2009, and then 35.2% in the 2017 survey (1, 18). Use of marijuana by US high school students that occurred 30 days before the survey ranged from 14.7% in 1991 to 26.7% in 1999, 20.8% in 2009, and 19.8% in 2017 (18). Other studies note marijuana use by adolescents that range from 28% in New York City versus 38% across the United States (19). Prevalence of cannabis use disorders (CUDs) have increased in veterans in the United States and these CUDs are higher in states that allowed cannabis for medical purposes (1).

Consumption of cannabis (marijuana)

Marijuana is typically smoked as a *joint* but can be taken orally in various foods, teas or capsules which may be used as "medicinal" marijuana. It can be prepared in food for oral consumptions, as in brownies, cookies, or spaghetti. Various oral consumptions are found in different countries. For example, in eastern Iran, there is a special solid "pie" called *majoon birjandi*, which is consumed by adolescents to reach a cannabis-induced euphoria (20).

Currently, there are many preparations of both THC and CBD (cannabidiol) products on the market. THC has been extracted from the cannabis plant and the THC content of these products is up to 90%. The term, dab, is a name provided to pot products that need a dab or oil rig to smoke (vape) this drug and dabs can include resin, shatter, wax, and other hash oil products. There are a variety of other products including creams, topical patches, suppositories, cannabis-soaked tampons, inhalers and food products.

The marijuana (bhang) cigarette is rolled from the *cannabis sativa* plant (upper leaves, tops, and stems) that is cut and dried. *Hashish* refers to dried exudate that comes from the top and underside of the plant leaves while concentrated hashish distillate is called *hashish oil*. *Sensimilla* is another potent marijuana product that is made from the seedless female flower of the cannabis plant. The "typical" marijuana cigarette includes about 20 mg of THC that is produced from a gram of *cannabis sativa* leaves and buds; however, much variation in potency can be found (*vida supra*). THC can be found in the body for up to two weeks after use of a single pot cigarette. A *blunt* is a cigarette or cigar form made from tobacco and filled with marijuana in a process called *boosting*; this can be used to boost the effects of other drugs such as alcohol (1). Vaping has become popular with various cannabis users as well (21, 22).

Cannabis and other drug use

Pot is often combined with consumption of alcohol or diazepam which increases cannabis sedative effects. Addition of various other drugs enhances the euphoric effects. For example, marijuana is often mixed with various drugs such as nicotine, cocaine, opioids, or hallucinogens (as LSD [lysergic acid diethylamide]). It is also mixed with drugs such as phencyclidine (PCP) in which the joint is dipped (hand-rolled) into PCP dissolved in an organic solvent (as formaldehyde); after drying it is smoked – called "*water, wet, or sherms.*" Such additions add to the complications of pot use. Other additives include glutethimide and methaqualone which have been popularized in the past. Persons abusing marijuana who also take disulfiram due to alcohol abuse can develop increased psychoactive effects of cannabis due to THC blockage by the disulfiram (23). Methamphetamines and cocaine are frequently being used as additives, as well.

Cannabis users also smoke tobacco and research notes this occurs for a variety of reasons, including shared genetic factors, the similar cue of smoking for both, and withdrawal symptoms that are seen to some extent in both (24). One study of 467 adults who regularly smoked both cannabis and tobacco noted that one-third started with cannabis first; also, nearly half initiated tobacco before cannabis, and most cannabis smokers who stopped tobacco did so after taking up regular cannabis consumption (25).

Table 1. Types of cannabinoids

Endogenous cannabinoid agonists
1, 2-AG (2-arachidonoyl glycerol)
2. Anandamide (arachidonoyl ethanolamide)
Phytocannabinoids
1. Cannabidiol (CBD) (isomer of THC)
2. Cannabinol (CBN) (metabolite of THC)
3. Cannabigerol (CBG) (alpha-2-adrenergic receptor agonist)
4. Tetrahydrocannabinolic acid (THC biosynthetic precursor)
5. Cannabichromene (CBC) (agonist of TRPA1 [transient receptor potential ankyrin 1])
6. Others (>100)
Other cannabinoids
1. Dronabinol (synthetic THC in sesame oil) (Schedule III drug); FDA-approved for AIDS-associated anorexia and anti-emetic)
2. Nabilone (THC-like; Schedule II drug) (FDA-approved for nausea and emesis due to cancer chemotherapy)
3. Nabiximols (phytocannabinoid marketed in Canada; THC + CBD in oral mucosal spray) (used in Canada for cancer pain, neuropathic pain and spasticity with multiple sclerosis; others)
Synthetic cannabinoids (cannabinoid designer drugs; cannabimimetics) (SEE TEXT)

As noted, those who consume marijuana also tend to use other drugs and it may serve as a gateway drug from early experimentation in adolescence to other drug use (26, 27). For example, two different studies report that 45% of college students who illegally used prescription drugs also abused marijuana, while 24% to 57% also abused alcohol (28). Cannabis initiation usually follows alcohol use though cannabis use can start before alcohol use, and African Americans (versus European-Americans) have an increased risk for this cannabis-first trend (29). Other research notes increased risk for cannabis-related problems in African American females versus European-Americans (29). Some research identifies declining socioeconomic position from childhood to adulthood as a risk factor for cannabis as well as tobacco consumption (30).

Some researchers report that patients seen in a pain clinic are at increased risk for use of marijuana. For example, one study of these patients with 21,746 urine specimens found 13.0% incidence of urine with cannabis (tetrahydrocannabinol); also, 4.6% were positive for cocaine and 1.07% were positive for methamphetamine (31). A case-crossover research design study noted that cannabis was a trigger for onset of cocaine use even when genetic influences and various environmental conditions were held constant (32). There are indications that concurrent use of opioids and cannabis products by patients with a history of chronic pain may lead to a higher risk of opioid misuse (33). A follow-up study with more than 33,000 people seems to suggest that there is an increase in non-medical opioid use, as well as an increase in opioid use disorder (34).

Cannabinoids

Cannabis sativa contains over 100 cannabinoids as well as over 400 other chemicals including benzopyrene, a known carcinogen. Table 1 lists some of the known cannabinoids (1). The cannabinoids of the *cannabis sativa* plant include *cannabidiol* (CBD), *cannabigerol* (CBG), and *cannabinol* (CBN) which, in contrast to THC, are not psychoactive. Cannabidiol (CBD) may activate central nervous system (CNS) limbic and paralimbic regions that can reduce autonomic arousal and feelings of anxiety; this is in contrast to THC that can be anxiogenic (1). Cannabigerol is found in higher concentrations in hemp and has been used to lower intraocular pressure. Plants grown outdoors have a higher concentration of THC, CBN, and CBD (35).

Other research also notes that THC and cannabidiol influence different central nervous system (CNS) regions and thus, have different effects on cannabis users (1, 36). In addition to anxiolytic effects, cannabidiol has been shown to have anti-emetic, anti-inflammatory, and antipsychotic effects (1). There is no effect on vital signs (i.e., blood pressure, pulse, body temperature), gastrointestinal transit, or psychological functioning. Doses up to 1,500 mg per day as well as chronic use of CBD have been reported as being well tolerated by humans (1).

There can be hepatic drug metabolism inhibition, reduced activities of some drug transporters (i.e., p-glycoprotein), and lowered capacity of fertilization (1, 36). CBD is a potent inhibitor of CYP3A4 and CYP2D6 and this can lead to changes in serum concentrations of many drugs; these include cyclosporine, warfarin, benzodiazepines, sildenafil, haloperidol, other anti-psychotics, anti-retrovirals, selective serotonin reuptake inhibitors (SSRIs), other antidepressants, opioids, and beta-blockers (1, 36).

Euphoria is produced from effects of this lipophilic drug on cannabinoid receptors (endocannabinoid system [ECS]: CB 1 and CB 2) in mesocortical and limbic systems; THC also effects the striatum and lateral prefrontal cortex as well as the inferior frontal gyrus (1, 37). Cannabinoid receptors are also found in the liver, gastrointestinal tract, skeletal tissue, and adipose tissue. There are endogenous ligands for cannabinoid receptors (i.e., N-palmitoethanolamide and anandamide) that act like neurotransmitters (26). Part of the complexity of the cannabis issue is the presence of the endogenous endocannabinoid system (ECS) and this system is now reviewed.

Table 2. Potential benefits of cannabis based on research studies

Remedy for inflammation
Remedy for pain (including chronic pain & neuropathic pain)
Remedy for diarrhea (as in Crohn's disease)
Treatment for dystonia
Treatment for multiple sclerosis
Treatment for rheumatoid arthritis
Treatment for glaucoma
Treatment for emesis due to chemotherapy
Treatment for epilepsy
Improvement of anorexia in AIDS patients
Treatment for Huntington's Disease
Management of inflammatory bowel disease
Beneficial effect on atherosclerosis
Reduce brain infarct size
Block negative memories in posttraumatic stress disorder
Reduce cardiac reperfusion injury
Adjuvant treatment for prostate carcinoma
Others

Endocannabinoid system

The endocannabinoid system consists of CNS cannabinoid receptors and their endogenous ligands; ligands (Latin: binding) refers to triggering molecules that bind to a target protein site (1). This system is a major signaling system in the brain and peripheral tissues affecting multiple physiologic as well as behavioral processes (38).

Endocannabinoids (endogenous cannabinoid receptor agonists) include arachidonic acid derivatives: 2-AG (2-arachidonoyl glycerol) and anandamide (arachidonoyl ethanolamide [AEA]) (Table 2) (39-41). AEA and 2-AG are the two most researched endocannabinoids. The complex effects of this system on emotional and cognitive behavior may be strongly influenced by various environmental factors (42).

The endocannabinoid system is identified both as a cause of psychiatric disorders but also research suggests that proper manipulation of this system may be pharmacologically useful in management of some psychiatric disorders — such as depression, anxiety, anorexia nervosa, and others utilizing cannabidiol, for example (43).

The endocannabinoid system is involved in processes of brain reward that are related to drug abuse — as noted in animal and human research; this includes cue-induced relapse of drug abuse (43). This CNS system is involved in various functions involving memory, emotions, movement, cell proliferation, and other important cell functions (1). Key neuron classes that express high levels of CB1 receptors are GABAergic interneurons in such CNS areas as the cerebral cortex, amygdala, and hippocampus; these areas also contain cholecystokinin, an important neuropeptide (1). The endocannabinoid system is involved with stress and the HPA axis (44).

The cannabinoid CB (1) receptor (CB1R) is mainly found in the central nervous system and the CB (2) receptor is expressed in immune system cells; both receptors are G-protein coupled receptors and are involved in adenylate cyclase inhibition (45, 46). The CB1R is a G-protein coupled receptor that is associated with most of the CNS endocannabinoid signaling (47). It is widely found in the cerebellum, basal ganglia, and limbic system; the hippocampus has the highest concentration of cannabinoid receptors. Chronic drug use, including cannabis, leads to decreased neurogenesis in the hippocampus that leads to impairment in the ability to learn new information (48).

Cannabinoid receptors are found in other tissues including the heart, lungs, endocrine glands, arteries, immune system, sympathetic ganglia, gastrointestinal tract, and reproductive tract (1, 39). The activation of CB1 receptors can inhibit amino acid and monoamine neurotransmitter release. Certain lipid derivatives (i.e., 2-arachidonoylglycerol [2-AG] and anandamide [AEA]) can function as endogenous ligands for CB 1 receptors and lead to excitation in such areas as the cerebellum and hippocampus by inhibition suppression (44).

Most drugs of abuse alter brain levels of endocannabinoids. Since blockade of this system can change the reward behavior associated with some drugs of abuse, the CNS endocannabinoid system is under active research to develop medications that may be helpful in treatment of drug abuse—including drug relapse (43). Cannabis as potential medication ("medicinal marijuana") is now considered.

Medicinal cannabis

Conclusions regarding the "benign" or "malignant" effects of cannabis use influence different countries' policies regarding legalization or criminalization of cannabis use (49). This is also complicated by use of cannabis products in a "medicinal" manner and thus, effects to find the most "appropriate" variety (varieties) of cannabis that are available (50). A plethora of medicinal benefits have been identified with marijuana use over past centuries (51-53) (see Table 2). The concern over the addictive and psychotomimetic qualities of THC placed active research on potential medical benefits of this plant on the backburner until recently (53). However, increased understanding of the cannabinoid signaling system has led to renewed research on potential medicinal uses of cannabis (1, 54).

Studies are looking at potential benefits of cannabinoids (phytocannabinoids) in management of neuropsychiatric diseases, neuropathic pain, hypertension, post-stroke neuroprotection, multiple sclerosis, epilepsy, cancer, and other disorders; this is based on potential anti-inflammatory, immunomodulatory and neuroprotective effects of these chemicals (1, 43, 54-65). Cancer research, for example, has identified that cannabinoids can inhibit cancer growth, angiogenesis, and metastasis (62). Cannabinoid-like anti-inflammatory products may be useful as material for wound dressing due to anti-inflammatory effects (63). Cannabidiol is under research as a new class of anti-inflammatory bowel disease drug (64).

A number of cannabis products are being manufactured by pharmaceutical companies, including sativex (THC + cannabidiol), marinol (dronabinal; THC; Schedule III drug), and cesamet (THC, Schedule II) (see Table 1) (53). The latter two have been approved for use in the anorexia-cachexia syndrome as well as for nausea and vomiting (53). Dronabinol is a synthesized gelatin capsule that has been used to treat glaucoma by lowering intraocular pressure or relieve chemotherapy-induced emesis (1). Marijuana has been used to treat the wasting syndrome associated with HIV/AIDS (9). One tablet formulation of THC is namisol (>98% THC) which has been studied to ameliorate pain and spasms in adults with multiple sclerosis as well as relieve nausea, and emesis in HIV or cancer patients (1).

Cannabis has been used since ancient times for treatment of epilepsy and research has been looking at the anti-epileptic features of the phytocannabinoid—cannabidiol (CBD) (66). The legal and regulatory status of CBD in the United States has been in flux as various states legalize cannabis and societal pressure mounts regarding legalizing cannabis (67, 68). In 2018 the US FDA approved of cannabidiol (CBD; epidiolex®) in an oral solution for management of two types of rare but severe epilepsy seen in the Dravet syndrome and the Lennox-Gastaut syndrome (69). Also in 2018, the US Drug Enforcement Administration placed FDA-approved drugs that contain cannabidiol (and no more than 0.1% tetrahydrocannabinols) in schedule V of the Controlled Substances Act (CSA) (70).

Though cannabis users noted lowering of anxiety and feelings of anxiety, much research remains to be accomplished to identify which if any cannabinoid products may be therapeutically and safely used as pharmacologic management of individuals with anxiety disorders (1). Current research is looking at such anxiety disorders as social anxiety disorder, post-traumatic stress disorder (PTSD), panic disorder, and obsessive-compulsive disorder (1). For example, there is increasing clinical evidence that low doses of CB1 receptor agonists have anxiolytic effects while high doses have the opposite effects (71). Research suggests that the phytocannabinoid chemical, cannabidiol (CBD), may be useful in blocking negative or fear memory associated with posttraumatic stress disorder in a process called *reconsolidation blockage* (70).

Some research identifies a lower mortality rate among adults with schizophrenia and related psychotic disorders in those who smoked cannabis versus those who did not smoke cannabis (1). Research on smoked, vaporized, and oral cannabis products for potential improvement of health are continuing; this includes the use of the phytocannabinoid, CBD (cannabidiol) (1, 72, 73).

Synthetic cannabinoids (cannabinoid designer drugs; cannabimimetics)

A number of designer drugs have become available in the 21st century and cannabis has become involved in this trend as well. These synthetic cannabinoids (called "legal highs," "spice drugs," "K2" drugs) are similar to THC found in the *cannabis sativa* plant and produce similar effects to smoking cannabis since they bind to the same cannabinoid brain and peripheral organ receptors as THC (74-79). These herbal blends have been noted since 2008 in various "herbal" smoking products; they are sold via the internet and in retail outlets (called "head shops") that focus on drug paraphernalia sold for cannabis and other drug use. Brand names include such exotic names as *aroma*, *yucatan fire*, *spice gold*, and others (1, 80).

Though available in some countries, advertised as "safe," (since they do not resemble the chemical structure of THC) and considered legal in various locations, they are potentially dangerous drugs – having up to 10 times the strength of delta-9-THC (1, 81, 82). In a moving as well as dangerous cat and mouse game, sellers change the synthetic cannabinoids in attempts to avoid putting up for sale a specific product identified as illegal in a specific country or area. As one synthetic cannabinoid is banned, others are produced to take their place as there are over 140 different spice drugs that are produced (73). They may be marked as some type of "incense" or "herbal" product and even "air fresheners" but potential adverse reactions remain (76). Toxicology screens looking at THC may miss the presence of these cannabinoid designer drugs (76, 78).

They are typically tobacco and cannabis free but produce similar cannabis effects that can include withdrawal symptoms, anxiety, intoxication, psychosis, death, and others (*vida infra*)

(1, 75, 77, 83). Some reports suggest that increased hallucinations and paranoia are noted with these "spice" synthetic cannabinoids and new onset as well as worsening of known psychosis have been reported (1, 78). Part of the potential danger is that they can contain various added but often unknown chemicals that are part of the manufacturing process. However, some of the products found on the internet do not have significant amounts of impurities and adverse effects are due to the synthetic cannabinoids themselves and the potential additives (84).

Cannabis lab testing

Those smoking 3.55% pot develop a peak plasma level near 160 mg/ml 10 minutes after beginning to ingest this product; the THC is removed from the plasma to body tissues leading to its euphoric effects and then to body fat as long-term storage (6). THC is then eliminated over several weeks in the urine and feces. Urine tests can be used to establish the presence of cannabinoid metabolites and can be positive in casual users for up to 10 days versus 14 to 30 days for chronic pot users (26). Current drug testing (using high-performance liquid chromatography with diode-array detection) can identify low THC content in cannabis seedlings right after germination; however, chemotype determination of THC can occur as the plant ages – at three weeks and beyond (85).

Cannabis testing can be used to verify past pot use but not the presence of cannabis intoxication, dependence, or abuse. Testing may also note suppression of testosterone and luteinizing hormone (LH), though it is unclear what such tests actual mean from a clinical viewpoint. Passive inhalation of cannabis does not result in a positive urine test for THC. Urine testing for THC does not identify the presence of synthetic cannabinoids (1).

THC-COOH (11-nor-9-carboxy-THC) is the main secondary THC metabolite developed after cannabis is taken; it is not psychoactive but has a long-half life and can be detected for days and in heavy cannabis users, for weeks after consumption. It is an important metabolite used in blood or urine testing for identification of cannabis; urine THC-COOH testing has been used to identify cannabis abstinence and a positive test can be confirmed with gas chromatography-mass spectrometry THC blood testing that indicates recent cannabis exposure (6). Whole blood and plasma testing can also reveal 11-hydroxy-THC after smoking cannabis. Polymerase chain reaction (PCR) testing is available to police authorities to identify where specific *C sativa* samples came from in order to assist with forensic studies and investigations (86). In addition to urine as well as blood testing, saliva and hair testing for cannabis are possible—the latter for evaluation of chronic cannabis exposure (1, 87, 88).

Cannabis can also be detected in maternal hair and her offspring's meconium in a pregnant person who has been consuming cannabis; cannabis can also be detected in breast milk of a lactating mother who consumes cannabis (88). Such drug use is important as research notes potential negative consequences in the offspring of cannabis smoking mothers that includes increased risk for low birth weight, small for gestational age, and admission to a neonatal intensive care unit (NICU); childhood effects that may occur include inattention problems, memory and processing difficulties, problem-solving dysfunction, and executive function dysfunction (1, 89-91).

Medical adverse effects

Though some have questioned the data on negative effects of cannabis use, most authors conclude that use of cannabis has significant risks for the user in both dose-dependent and/or idiosyncratic fashions (1, 92). Identifying adverse effects of cannabis is challenging because studying an illicit drug can be problematic as can separating out cannabis effects from other drugs that are often taken simultaneously (such as tobacco or alcohol); also, there is variation in techniques of cannabis consumption (1, 92).

A case of an infant with altered consciousness after exposure to cannabis smoke (passive inhalation) has been reported (1, 93). Another 10-month-old infant consumed oral cannabis and presented with cannabis poisoning – drowsiness, generalized hypotonia, and restlessness; this infant had high blood as well as urine levels of cannabis products and recovered with symptomatic management that included clinical monitoring for the first 24 hours after the ingestion (94). Twelve toddlers, all less than six years of age and hospitalized for accidental cannabis poisoning, presented similarly with drowsiness and hypotonia; they all had favorable medical outcomes, but the majority were referred to social services due to concerns for neglect (95).

Table 3. Potential adverse effects of marijuana*

Addiction (Physiologic)
Withdrawal syndrome
Dependence (Psychological) and with heavy use, tolerance
Variety of negative psychological reactions:
(anxiety, hallucinations, violent behavior, depression, fear)
Overt precipitation of psychosis or depression
Insomnia (can be chronic and improved with trazodone)
Memory spans that are impaired
Blunted reflexes
Flu-like reaction (after stopping this drug after 24 to 60 hours, lasting up to 2 weeks)
Confusion and cognition impairment
Alteration of time perception
Amotivational syndrome (lose interest in school or work success)
Physiologic responses can include cough, bronchospasm, bronchitis
Cannabinoid induced hyperemesis
Cardiovascular: pericarditis, myocarditis, others (see text)
Others (see text)

* Used with permission from Greydanus DE, Feucht CL, Hawver EK. Substance abuse disorders. In: Greydanus DE, Patel DR, Omar HA, Feucht C, Merrick J, eds. Adolescent medicine: Pharmacotherapeutics in general, mental, and sexual health. Berlin: De Gruyter, 2012:180.

A number of side effects are possible for the cannabis consumer including increased mortality rates (see Table 3). Chronic use can lead to weight gain from overeating and reduced physical activity. Acute cannabis use can lead to suppression of rapid eye movement (REM) and diffuse slowing of background EEG activity (26). The smoke of cannabis can be irritating to conjunctival, nasopharyngeal, and bronchial tissue leading to injected conjunctiva, chronic cough, sinusitis, pharyngitis, and (chronic) bronchitis (96). Adolescents or young adults who present with acute or chronic cough should be screened for cannabis use in addition to more classic causes; these include asthma, gastroesophageal reflux, respiratory tract infections, and cannabis allergy (97, 98). Cannabis allergy can present in various ways and suspicion for such a diagnosis in cannabis users is important for those with allergic components to plants (such as *cannabis sativa*) that can include contact dermatitis (98, 99).

Chronic use of cannabis has not been shown to effect thyroid function while potential reduction in sperm concentration has been noted in some studies (1, 100). Acute pancreatitis linked to cannabis use has been reported with presentations of epigastric pain, nausea, and emesis (1, 101). Abdominal pain due to colonic perforation and subsequent peritonitis has been reported as a complication of cannabis body packing in attempts to illegally smuggle illicit drugs from one country to another (1).

Cannabis hyperemesis syndrome

Cannabinoid hyperemesis is noted in some cannabis users who present with usually sudden, severe, and cyclic (intractable) emesis that resolves with intravenous fluids, anti-emetics, and cannabis cessation. As the cannabis strength and use frequency increases, the syndrome of cannabinoid hyperemesis has increased (1). There can be cyclic nausea and abdominal pain as well and after a careful evaluation, the cause is linked to cannabis use (102). It was first described in Australia in 2004 and may be missed in patients presenting with hyperemesis and abnormal patterns of bathing (103). Though cannabinoids have been used to treat chronic nausea and emesis, a paradoxical effect on the gastrointestinal tract in noted in this cannabis hyperemesis syndrome and three parts (phases) are described: prodromal, hyper-emetic, and recovery phases (104).

The hyperemesis phase is usually resolved in 48 hours. Patients may report temporary symptomatic improvement with prolonged hot showers or bath exposure and thus, compulsive hot water bathing has become part of the cannabis (cannabinoid) hyperemesis complex (102, 105-108). Diagnostic confusion with the cyclic vomiting syndrome may occur and fatal cases are reported (104, 105).

Management includes antiemetic agents, benzodiazepines, antipsychotics and topical capsaicin (107, 108). If cannabis use resumes, the hyperemesis complex may reoccur (1, 104). It not known why some cannabis using patients develop this syndrome and others do not. Traditional anti-emetics are less effective in management and the only known permanent treatment is cannabis abstinence. Once developed, it may take months for resolution of symptoms (106).

Dental effects of cannabis

Pot users tend to have increased risks for dental caries, oral infections, and periodontal disease (109-111). Gingival hypertrophy, similar to phenytoin-related enlargement, has been described in asymptomatic chronic male users (111). Dysplastic changes and premalignant lesions can be identified in oral mucosa of cannabis users (109). Use of local anesthetics in patients intoxicated with cannabis intensifies and prolongs pot-induced tachycardia (109).

Exposure to smoking (cannabis or tobacco) leads to contact with many carcinogens (pro-carcinogens) such as polycyclic aromatic hydrocarbons (112). Cannabis users often smoke tobacco and drink alcohol that increases carcinogen exposure and risk of oral squamous cell carcinoma representing 95% of malignant lesions in the mouth (112).

Pulmonary effects

Some research identifies an anti-inflammatory effect from consumption of the *C sativa* plant. For example, one study of 5,115 adult males that took place over 20 years noted that occasional and low cumulative cannabis use was not associated with adverse effects on pulmonary function (113). Murine studies suggest that cannabidiol has an immunosuppressive and anti-inflammatory effect on acute lung injury because of an increase in extracellular adenosine (114).

However, it is known that marijuana, as well as tobacco, contains a toxic combination of gases and other substances that can be injurious to the pulmonary system (1, 5, 14, 22, 23, 115). Marijuana smokers usually smoke fewer "joints" than tobacco smokers consume cigarettes; however, methods of cannabis smoking may place more cannabis particulate matter into the lungs than noted with typical cigarette smoking (115). Those with cannabis dependence will continue to use it despite chronic cough, excessive sedation, or other marijuana-related problems.

Combining marijuana with tobacco leads to known tobacco-effects via exposure to the smoke. As the use and production of cannabis products have increased in various states that have legalized cannabis, there has been an increase in the number of contaminations; such contaminants include molds, heavy metals, insecticides and various other chemicals with unknown long-term complications for human health (116).

Pot use can induce some bronchodilation but regular or heavy cannabis consumption can result in generalized airway inflammation with evidence of respiratory epithelial cell injury and damage to alveolar macrophages leading to pulmonary infection (115). Sharing of cannabis water pipes has led to the development of pulmonary tuberculosis (TB) (1). Smoking cannabis that contains fungal spores can result in pulmonary aspergillosis in those with immune-compromised conditions (1, 117).

Dose-related large airway dysfunction with hyperinflation and obstruction of airflow has been described; one cannabis joint has been noted to be equivalent to 2.5 to 5 cigarettes in terms of this pulmonary dysfunction (1). Macrophage injury can result in cytokine and nitric oxide impairment. Smokers of cannabis are typically exposed to more carbon monoxide and tar than cigarette smokers; this effect is not related to the THC content (1). Also, Δ-THC can interfere with airway clearance due to negative effects on a key airway component—the ion channel CFTE (cystic fibrosis transmembrane conductance regulator) (119).

Heavy and/or chronic users of cannabis may have persistent cough, bronchitis, (bullous) emphysema (chronic obstructive lung disease [COPD]), pulmonary dysplasia, pneumothorax, tuberculosis (TB), and other respiratory infections (26, 115, 119-121). Cannabis smoking can lead to increased airway resistance and large airway inflammation – though causal links to COPD or macroscopic emphysema remain controversial and unproven (1, 92, 93, 118). Smoking both tobacco and marijuana increases risks for abnormal tracheobronchial histopathology and COPD (1).

Cannabis and cancer

Marijuana smoke contains toxic chemicals in amounts similar to or higher than that found in tobacco and is identified as having potential respiratory tract carcinogens (1, 26, 93, 96, 122). Research reports chronic inflammatory and precancerous airway changes in a dose-dependent relationship as well as increase in airway cancer in cannabis users (90). Anecdotal reports of upper and lower respiratory airway cancer have been published (116, 122). For example, a case of small-cell lung cancer was reported in a 22-year old male who smoked one marijuana joint three times a week for three years (123).

However, specific link of cannabis to lung cancer remains unproven (1, 92, 93, 124). Current literature suggests that cannabis-only smokers are at lower risk of lung cancer than tobacco-only smokers (125). On the other hand, some epidemiologic data does place an independent role of cannabis smoking in the development of lung cancer (1, 126, 127). The search in this area continues and clarification awaits further research data (127).

Cardiovascular effects

Cannabinoids have complex and varying effects on blood pressure depending on which cannabinoid is being studied (33). Acute effects of cannabis include increase in heart rate along with an increase (usually mild) in blood pressure and then decreased vascular resistance-induced orthostatic hypotension (1, 55). Individuals with coronary heart disease may have increased cardiovascular adverse effects from cannabis use (89). Cannabis-induced ST segment elevation mimicking the Brugada syndrome has been reported (128). Other drugs, both licit and illicit (i.e., cocaine), have been linked with the Brugada syndrome as well (1).

Reported cardiovascular effects linked to cannabis include anecdotal cases of acute coronary syndrome, myocardial infarction, congestive heart failure, arrhythmias, and myopericarditis (55, 96, 129-135). Patients with angina may have decreased time with chest pain onset due to the acute effects of cannabis use; as noted, myocardial infarction may be triggered by the acute effects of cannabis use (1, 55). Patients at high risk for coronary heart disease should be advised to avoid using cannabis (55). Further research is indicated to explore the cardiovascular effects of cannabis (134, 135).

Studies on cannabis also provide evidence of positive or "neutral" effects from cannabis consumption. For example, though inhalation of marijuana may induce acute coronary symptoms, ingestion of cannabinoids may have a positive effect on atherosclerotic heart disease via effects on the endocannabinoid system (ECS) (1). Also, cannabis use has not been specifically linked to increased hospitalization due to cardiovascular disease or increased mortality from cardiovascular etiology (55). If a patient has a cardiac death and has a positive urine test for cannabinoid, a plasma THC level should also be done before seeking to link the cannabis history with the cardiac death.

Motor vehicle accidents

Those driving under the influence of cannabis (combined with alcohol consumption as well) are at increased risk (two-times or more) of motor vehicle accidents leading to potential death and injury (89, 90, 96, 136-142). Those who consume cannabis without other drugs also place themselves at increased risk for motor vehicle crashes (1). Individuals driving under marijuana influence may experience distortion of on-coming vehicle headlights resulting in motor vehicle crashes. Driving impairment worsens with increasing amounts of cannabis consumed (1). Research notes that chronic daily cannabis smokers have observable impairment up to 3 weeks after stopping the cannabis (140).

Each state that legalizes marijuana has developed a state-specific DUI (driving under the influence) criteria. In the state of Colorado, this is set at 5 ng/ml of delta-9 THC; recreational use of this drug was legalized in Colorado in 2012 (141). A 2017 survey by the Colorado Department of Transportation indicated that 69% of self-identified marijuana users admitted to driving after marihuana consumption (141). DUI testing for marijuana is complicated because delta-9 THC is rapidly metabolized and getting blood samples are typically delayed. The maximum blood level of THC drops an average of 73.5% within the first 25 minutes after starting to smoke a pot joint; within an hour, THC levels drop below 5 ng/ml for occasional users and within two hours it drops below 5 ng/ml for chronic users (142). Thus, actual calculations of marijuana-impaired drives can be very difficult to obtain.

Sports doping

Athletes can and do use cannabis as part of recreational or anticipated sports doping effects (1, 143, 144). Those involved in sports should understand that cannabis is a drug banned by the World Anti-Doping Agency (WADA) despite history of pot use in the Olympics. It has been on the list of prohibited drugs of the International Olympic Committee since 1999 in certain sports (1, 75). In 2004, cannabinoids were prohibited in all competitive sports. Research has shown potential performance enhancement by improving tissue oxygenation and decreasing sports-related fear or anxiety as well as potential benefit with pain management and concussion-induced symptomatology (1, 143).

Cannabis smoking results in reduced exercise test duration during maximal exercising and increased heart rate at less than maximal exercise levels (55). Cannabis-induced increase in blood pressure and reduced psychomotor activity can also decrease overall athletic performance. Management of urine samples from athletes can be problematic because of the intricacies of interpreting urine samples due to the complexities of prolonged cannabis excretion (1).

Adverse effects: Psychiatric

Adverse neuropsychological effects of cannabis use must be separated out from the acute effects of cannabinoids, effects of heavy cannabis consumption, and psychiatric disorders worsened or even caused by cannabinoids (1). Specific effects in individual cannabis users are difficult to predict because of the heterogeneity or non-uniformity of different studies that have been done to seek neuroimaging effects in cannabis use; some authors have concluded it is difficult to prove major effects of cannabis on brain structure (145, 146). Some research suggests that identified cannabis-related neurocognitive performance defects disappear after 25 days of cannabis abstinence and/or is of minimal significance in many persons (1, 147). Evaluation of cannabis effects in chronic users must also consider the presence of tolerance that develops in these persons as well (148).

However, other recent research studies are noting that cannabis users demonstrate important deficits in prospective memory and executive functioning that exist beyond acute cannabis intoxication (1). The presence of cannabis and nicotine use disorders in parents appears to increase the risk for major depressive disorder in their late adolescent offspring (149). Studies in animals and humans suggest a subtle (versus gross) effect on cognitive functioning with later development of hyperactivity, reduced attention span, impulsivity, depression, and substance use disorders (150). Most frequently reported adverse effects of cannabis use include mental slowness, reduced reaction times, and increased anxiety (89). Dysfunction occurs to dopamine and opioid neurotransmitter systems (151).

Animal and human research concludes that the developing brain, with its high neuronal plasticity, is vulnerable to exposure to exogenous cannabinoids – particularly in the perinatal/prenatal period and during young adolescence (43, 151-158). Animal and human studies suggest that *early* onset of cannabis use (i.e., early adolescence) can increase risks for cognition dysfunction, CNS changes (i.e., low striatal dopamine release), neuropsychiatric disorders, cannabis dependence, and consumption as well as addiction to additional illicit drugs (152, 155). Persistent or problematic marijuana use can lead to major interference with daily life activities whether at work, in school, or in one's home.

Cannabis consumption often develops in adolescence and early adulthood which, as noted, is a vulnerable time for subsequent adverse brain effects (1, 47, 156-158). For example, cannabinoid receptors are abundant in the CNS white matter in adolescence as well as young adulthood; long-term cannabis use during this time-period can lead to impaired axonal fiber connectivity with negative effects on the white matter of the brain (1). Cannabis use in early adolescence may alter CB1R signaling with potentially increased risk for development of psychiatric disorders (47). Early adolescent cannabis use has been linked with adolescent drop out behavior in school as well as increased depression and decreased educational accomplishment in young adulthood; reduced motivation is reported with cannabis consumption (1, 156, 158).

Some research links other CNS problems with heavy cannabis use. For example, one study identified regional brain abnormalities (in the hippocampus and amygdale) in long-term, heavy pot smokers—data found in both human and animal studies (158). Animal studies noted hippocampal-dependent short-term memory deficits that occurred in some but not all rats given chronic cannabinoid administration (1).

Cannabis and ADHD

Comorbidity between cannabis use and attention-deficit/hyperactivity disorder (ADHD) are classically noted in the literature and research reports that cannabis use can impair attention span (159). One report of 162 adolescents studied during inpatient management of problems related to drug dependence (i.e., marijuana, heroin, alcohol, or cocaine abuse) revealed attention deficit hyperactivity disorder (ADHD) in 34% of them (160). A study from different medical centers that focused on 600 adolescents (ages 13 to 16 years of age) who were undergoing management for marijuana-related problems reported that 38% also had ADHD (161). Such studies support the theory that ADHD and adolescent substance abuse disorder (including cannabis dependence) can be seen as a developmental disorder with similar underlying physiologic mechanisms (1, 5, 14, 19, 23).

Table 4. 2013 DSM-5 cannabis related disorders (26)

Cannabis Use Disorders (mild, moderate and severe)
Cannabis intoxication (with and without perceptual disturbances)
Cannabis withdrawal
Other cannabis-induced disorders
Unspecified cannabis-related disorders

Cannabis-related psychiatric disorders

The 2013 American Psychiatric Association's DSM-5 (Diagnostic and statistical manual of mental disorders, 5th edition) identified cannabis-related disorders as listed in table 4: cannabis use disorder, cannabis intoxication, cannabis withdrawal and others (26, 162). In the DSM-5 category of SUD or substance use disorder (as cannabis or other drugs) the separation of the terms "abuse" and "dependency") was placed into the single entity of substance use disorder (SUD) with separations of mild (meeting 2-3 of specific criteria), moderate (4-5 of criteria) and severe (6 or more of DSM-5 criteria)—as discussed elsewhere (1, 26). Cannabis use disorders are more common in males versus females and are most prevalent in the 18 to 30 years old group (1, 26).

Research has suggested that the earlier term, dependency or dependency rate, was seen in at 7-10% of regular users and that a susceptibility gene, NRG1, has been associated with cannabis dependence in African Americans (1, 90). Some data reveal that 9% who try cannabis will become dependent (addicted) and 17% of cannabis smokers who initiate this drug as adolescents will become addicted; cannabis higher in THC is associated with increased dependence (142, 163). Those with cannabis dependence can consume cannabis in potent forms for years and spend several hours a day in finding as well as taking it; there can be physiologic dependence and also psychologic dependence (26).

Cannabis intoxication may last longer with oral cannabis versus smoking it. Intoxication may even last up to 24 hours due to effects of enterohepatic circulation and/or slow release of fat soluble THC and other cannabinoids from fatty tissue (1, 5). The timing of intoxication onset with cannabis edibles is unpredictable due to many factors. Many people consume an excessive amount of cannabis due to the delayed onset and then are highly intoxicated once they metabolize all that has been ingested. After the cannabis is consumed, side effects will persist and may last longer versus smoking it.

Depersonalization and de-realization episodes are described in cannabis users (1, 26). Anecdotal cases of cannabis-induced depersonalization in adolescents have been reported (1). A history of conduct disorder in childhood or adolescence and antisocial personality disorder are risk factors for substance use disorder including cannabis-related disorders (1, 26).

Differentiation of cannabis-induced disorders from primary mental health disorders can be difficult. Ataxia and aggression are more likely to be seen with phencyclidine (PCP) intoxication versus cannabis intoxication; aggression with nystagmus or ataxia is more likely to be from alcohol intoxication (1, 26).

Demonstrating a direct link between cannabis use and the development of overt depression has been problematic and not clearly proven (164). Regular cannabis consumption (particularly daily use) in adolescence has been linked with increased risks for anxiety disorders in adolescents and young adults, even after the cannabis was stopped (154). World Health Organization (WHO) surveys from 2008 demonstrated that the highest rates of anxiety occurred in the two countries with the highest cannabis abuse rates – the United States and New Zealand (165). Anxiety is linked to regular or heavy use of cannabis and further research is needed to unravel this connection in more detail (1). For example, anxiety can arise due to fear of being discovered by law enforcement officials; there can be episodes resembling panic attacks.

Cannabis withdrawal syndrome

Chronic cannabis users can develop psychological addiction and a withdrawal syndrome comparable to heroin addiction (8). A heavy marijuana user (whether an adolescent or adult) who suddenly stops this drug, can develop a recognizable withdrawal syndrome as reported by various research studies (166-172). Withdrawal symptoms can develop within 48 hours of cessation and include irritability, restlessness, anxiety, aggression, and sleep difficulties (89). Withdrawal symptoms tend to subside in 2 to 12 weeks after cannabis abstention (89). As noted, a CNR1 (cannabinoid receptor 1) gene has been linked with abstinence-induced withdrawal symptoms (173). Heavy cannabis use has been linked with a smaller amygdala and hippocampus while those with the CNR1 gene may be predisposed to smaller hippocampal volume following heavy cannabis use (173). Some smoke pot to control problems with anger (169-172).

Withdrawal symptoms are due to the cessation of THC and are relieved with taking delta-9-THC or simply smoking marijuana (166, 174). Adolescents undergoing treatment for cannabis dependence experience withdrawal symptoms most acutely during the first week of cannabis absence and this tends to ease over the next month of abstinence (166, 175). Research notes that the majority of heavy pot users report several symptoms after stopping cannabis and this can complicate effective management – especially since cannabis dependent users may resort to consuming various others drugs to relieve the symptoms of cannabis withdrawal (166, 176, 177).

Addiction

The identification and isolation of THC in 1964 enhanced specific research into effects of cannabis on humans and animals (43). Endogenous cannabinoids (particularly CB1 receptor activation) stimulate neural mechanisms in the central nervous system (CNS) similar to how other reward-enhancing drugs induce drug addiction (1, 178-180). This core reward system is part of the addiction mechanism that use of cannabis develops in the unwary pot smoker as well as in consumers of other illicit drugs of addiction (181, 182). This mechanism involves the meso-accumbens reward circuitry of the central nervous system (CNS) as well as neural firing of the neurotransmitter, dopamine. Some research notes that THC can induce striatal effects on dopamine as noted with other drugs of abuse (183). Though some studies suggest dependence develops faster in cocaine versus cannabis users, recent research concludes there is no such difference (184).

Addiction also involves prefrontal cortex (PFC) dysfunction with frontostriatal dysfunction and the erosion of the ability to stop the addiction; more research is needed to identify potential impact of cannabinoids in the PFC and its potential role in cannabis dependence (185-187). A nucleotide polymorphism has been identified in a cannabis receptor-1 gene (CNR1) – rs2023239, that is associated with cannabis dependence, cannabis craving, and withdrawal symptoms due to cannabis abstinence (173). Some neuropeptides called orexins (hypocretins) originate in the lateral hypothalamus and are linked to features of drug addiction (i.e., cannabis, nicotine) that include drug craving, relapse, and withdrawal (188).

Cannabis and psychosis

Chronic use of cannabis, particularly with the newer synthetic cannabis products, as well as the newer high potency cannabis, is associated with increased rates of psychosis (1, 154, 189-191). Frequent cannabis use increases the risk by two times (or more) for schizophrenia and psychotic symptoms; this is perhaps by cannabis-induced disruption of the endocannabinoid system in which the normal signaling and functioning of this endogenous system is disturbed (192). Cannabis (marijuana) is commonly used by those with schizophrenia and can cause paranoia in approximately 40% of these persons experimenting with this drug (193). Patients with schizophrenia who consume cannabis are hospitalized at rates higher than those who do not use cannabis (194).

Cannabis-induced schizophrenia is currently theorized as being due to dysfunction of late postnatal brain maturation in which glutamatergic transmission dysfunction leads to abnormal prefrontal neuro-circuitry (195). Exposure of adolescents to cannabis at certain times in adolescence and at certain doses may lead to prefrontal cortical circuitry abnormalities with the result of inducing schizophrenia in susceptible adolescents (195).

One research group reports a mean time of 7.0 +/- 4.3 years between onset of cannabis use and onset of psychosis (190). Those at risk for psychosis may be vulnerable to brain volume loss (i.e., cerebellum, prefrontal cortex, and cingulate) due to use of cannabis (196). Self-mutilation can also occur with cannabis-induced psychosis (197). Those with psychosis who use cannabis may not notice improved psychotic symptoms with cessation of their cannabis (198).

Most cannabis users do not develop psychosis and this cannabis-psychosis link appears to be via a complex environmental-genetic-molecular interaction possibly involving anandamide dysfunction and other biological factors (191, 199, 200). Most research suggests a link between cannabis use and risk for suicide in patients with psychosis and also those without psychosis (201). The development of schizophrenia and use of cannabis share a variety of similarities, including neuropsychological deficits, reduced motivation, hallucinations, and initiation in late adolescence (202).

Cannabis is also a very common illicit drug for individuals with psychosis and disruptive disorders to consume (13, 203). Those with psychosis have a higher rate of cannabis use than the general population, probably in attempts to utilize the cannabis-induced euphoria to deal with negative aspects of schizophrenia, such as boredom and depression (12). Cannabis can also prompt the onset of psychotic symptoms in otherwise healthy people as well; this includes paranoia and/or delusional thinking due to effects of THC on striatal and prefrontal function.

Thus, use of marijuana can have opposite effects on different users. Some research fails to find a clear association between use of cannabis and symptoms of psychosis, especially with low or moderate cannabis use (204). A major component of cannabis, *cannabidiol* (*CBD*), has been shown by some research to have *anti-psychotic* effects (205). The presence of CBD may explain the lack of psychosis development in many cannabis users. Studies with cannabidiol (versus THC) suggest a modulating effect based on functional MRI brain imaging (1). Schizophrenic patients using cannabis may be particularly sensitive to brain damage from cannabis consumption – though cannabidiol (CBD) may provide a protective effect from brain volume loss (202). Further study is needed, although some researchers speculate that CBD may have therapeutic potential for the treatment of psychosis and schizophrenia (206). There is increasing concern with the newer commercially available retail THC products that have virtually no CBD.

Management

The "hedonic" CNS dysregulation seen in drug addiction studies in animals and human subjects underscores the concept of drug addiction as a brain disease and the necessity of *prevention* before this complex brain dysfunction arises (12, 182, 207). Indeed, it is difficult to convince an addicted cannabis user to stop smoking this plant and thus, *prevention* via intensive and comprehensive education is the best option currently available. Unfortunately, cannabis dependence is difficult to treat successfully and few who seek to stop their cannabis addiction succeed in long-term cessation (180). One of the ironic reasons for this reality is that chronic cannabis consumers classically have cognitive impairments leading to defects in their decision-making skills (208).

However, there are steps therapists can take in helping this phenomenon of a nation and a world obsessed with smoking pot. Continued education of the dangers of cannabis should take place on a persistent and relentless basis. It should be understood that some literature and some people conclude that the negative impact of smoking cannabis is limited (209). Cannabis consumers may be cognizant of such literature which may encourage them to continue to use this so-called" safe illicit drug. Thus, teaching about the potential problems of cannabis should always be provided by healthcare providers to help offset this destructive message of "benign" pot consumption including unproven messages of some about "cures" or "treatments" for various illnesses.

Treatment specifically for cannabis use is needed as management of other or co-existing drug dependence (such as heroin, tobacco, or alcohol, for example) does not necessarily reduce levels of cannabis consumption (210). Comprehensive school-based prevention programs teaching about drug use, including cannabis, can be beneficial in lowering youth drug experimentation and addiction (211, 212). Increased education about high-risk adolescent behaviors for adolescents and their parents can be useful in prevention efforts (213). Intense education is needed for groups at high risk for drug abuse, such as males, young adults, and individuals with increased psychological stress (214).

Behavioral principles for management in adolescence can be directed by factors shown to suggest higher risk for cannabis use including genetic factors, family history, minimal parental supervision, drug availability, high-risk peer group, and those with a need for higher thrill-seeking activities (215, 216). Groups at high risk of mental health problems are those with combined drug use, such as comorbid cannabis and methamphetamine; thus, this group should receive intense management (217). Comprehensive behavioral management can also be of help in reducing cannabis use in those arrested for cannabis possession (218). Screening of these persons for suicide risk is recommended and lower cannabis use can reduce risks for suicide in those with and without psychosis (201). Patients with psychosis and cannabis smoking should undergo behavioral therapies to improve both problems and not just one (219).

If life-time abstinence from cannabis is not possible, delaying its use (especially heavy use) as long as possible after adolescence and young adulthood is recommended; this may result in less white matter damage from cannabis consumption than noted during cannabis smoking in the second and third decade of life (156). Management can also focus on reducing cannabis use if abstinence is not possible, since adverse effects tend to be increased with heavy use of cannabis (91). Therapy should seek underlying factors in use of cannabis or other drugs. For example, research notes that socially anxious males are at increased risk for cannabis consumption as part of a mechanism to deal with or avoid social situations (220). Thus, therapy can be directed at reasons for this avoidance behavior and the acquisition of successful strategies to improve their social anxiety that may reduce the need for ongoing cannabis consumption.

Often recommended behavioral management strategies (such as cognitive behavioral therapy and contingency management) have their limitations and combination of these techniques does not increase success in helping those with cannabis dependence (221). However, research notes that youth with cannabis use disorder benefit more from CBT (versus family therapy) if they are older teenagers (i.e., 17-18 years of age) and do not have pre-existing psychiatric disorders; in the same study, multidimensional family therapy was more helpful (versus CBT) for those who were younger (i.e., under age 17) and/or had a past year history of disruptive disorders (i.e., opposition defiant or conduct disorder) (222).

However, one should continue to provide the cannabis consumer with hope and encouragement that overcoming this drug addiction is possible despite its widespread acceptance in society. Research does show that such benefit is more likely with intensive or prolonged behavioral therapy, especially cognitive-behavioral therapy and motivational interviewing (1, 223). Also, it should be understood that even brief (i.e., four) sessions of motivational interviewing with cognitive behavioral therapy delivered via telephone can be beneficial, at least in the short run, for *motivated* cannabis users who called in seeking help with treatment (224).

The primary care clinician (PCC) can be helpful by utilizing an approach called SBIRT that was developed by the US Substance Abuse and Mental Health Services Administration and the US Institute of Medicine (1). This program consists of appropriate screening, brief intervention and referral to treatment by persons/programs with extensive skills in the management of substance abuse disorders (1, 225, 226). Impactful implementation of such a recommended program allows the primary care clinician to identify as well as improve the substance use and abuse situations of many of the adolescent as well as adult patients in the PCC practice.

Behavioral therapies can be useful in the motivated cannabis addict and such counseling seeks to help the cannabis consumer gain control over his/her addiction at the CNS level by enhancing neuroanatomical progression from ventral striatal (nucleus accumbens) to dorsal striatal control (182). Even brief interventions may have positive benefit in less cannabis use at 3-month follow-up (3) and another study at 12-month follow-up (17).

Also, therapy seeks to help the addict deal with cannabis craving and relapse triggers, such as becoming re-exposed to various drugs of addiction; it is also important to help this person deal with stress and with finding as well as avoiding old clues (cues) in his/her milieu, such as key persons, places, or objects (182, 207). In addition, genetic factors have a role in why some develop addiction and are recalcitrant to management strategies (207). Involvement of families, schools, communities, and peer groups are critical in seeking to reduce and prevent cannabis smoking in adolescents. It is unclear what the interactions are between abuse of illicit drugs and use of prescription drugs, but the potential drug interactions should be considered in overall prevention and treatment plans (1).

Pharmacologic therapies

There are no FDA-approved pharmacologic agents for management of cannabis dependence (227). Traditionally, pharmacologic agents have not been specifically beneficial in treating marijuana addiction whether dependence or withdrawal symptoms (228). However, a careful assessment of each patient is necessary and a reduction in cannabis use can be noted in some patients with standard pharmacotherapy (1). There is no evidence that one anti-depressant, anxiolytic, or antipsychotic is more effective than another. Cannabis use disorders are common in those with schizophrenic spectrum disorders; however, there is no current literature that guides clinicians in the best treatment approaches for this dual diagnosis (229). Knowledge, however, is slowly emerging to guide pharmacologic therapies for cannabis-induced problems in the 21st century (1).

Individuals with co-occurrence of cannabis and tobacco use tend to have higher abstinence rates if treatment includes measures aimed at dual abstinence (24). Thus, pharmacotherapy for nicotine addiction may help the individual stop marijuana use as well by removing use of and thus, influence of tobacco. Pot-associated persistent insomnia may be improved with use of trazodone. Research is looking at new methods of treatment that will emerge from the study of the genetics of addiction including gene-milieu interplay and role of genetic variation (1, 230).

Cannabis intoxication

Pharmacologic management typically centers on use of benzodiazepines or atypical antipsychotics. Propranolol and rimonabant (*vida infra*) have been reported to be beneficial in management of acute, physiologic effects of cannabis *intoxication*; use of flumazenil and cannabidiol (CBD) is under current study in this regard (231).

Cannabis withdrawal

Pharmacologic management for cannabis withdrawal continues to be under active research (1, 162, 232). Dronabinol (synthetic THC in sesame oil) may relieve cannabis *withdrawal* symptoms but not relapse (1). Adding dronabinol and lofexidine (alpha-adrenergic receptor agonist) can lower the severity of withdrawal and lower relapse rates in those with cannabis dependence (1). The anti-depressant, mirtazapine, can also help those undergoing cannabis withdrawal and part of the management in cannabis withdrawal involves dealing with the concomitant insomnia—including utilizing mirtazapine (1, 232, 233). The centrally acting alpha agonist, guanfacine, may be helpful with cannabis withdrawal as well (234).

Cannabis-associated psychosis

Cannabidiol has been shown in animal and human studies to have anti-psychotic effects and it may become a useful pharmacotherapeutic agent for schizophrenia management (1, 205). Research has therapeutically targeted the cannabinoid (CB1) receptor since delta-9-THC is a partial CB1 receptor agonist. Treatment of patients with psychotic disorders and cannabis use should include seeking to reduce or stop the cannabis use, perhaps using cannabinoid agonist medication (219). Those with psychosis can be provided with appropriate anti-psychotic medications.

Cannabis use disorder

Pharmacologic management of cannabis use disorder includes use of various drugs (162, 235). Nabilone is a synthetic THC analogue with improved bioavailability over dronabinol and is under current research as a potential medication for *marijuana use disorder* as it may lead to a positive mood and limited adverse cognitive effects in marijuana smokers (1). Olanzapine can reduce psychomimetic effects of THC in some individuals and its potential benefit is under study (236).

Rimonabant and the anxiolytic buspirone have provided some efficacy in cannabis addicts on maintenance therapy. Rimonabant is a CB1-selective cannabinoid receptor antagonist/inverse agonist that has been under research for obesity treatment as well as treatment of nicotine and marijuana addiction (237). It is not available in the United States and was pulled from the European market in October of 2008 due to a high risk to benefit ratio; concerns have been identified regarding major psychiatric adverse effects (i.e., depression and suicide) as well as overall efficacy (166). Research looking at the endocannabinoid system (ECS) as a target for management of addiction disorders including cannabis use disorder will continue as this early part of the 21st century continues (237).

Cannabis use disorder is higher in those who smoke cigarettes as well as cannabis and thus, management of CUD includes cessation of both cannabis and tobacco (238). The links between cigarette smoking and cannabis smoking are complex and dangerous including links between electronic nicotine delivery systems (ENDS) and cannabis vaping (238-240). Parents should know that cannabis use disorder in the father increases risks for the offspring to use cannabis (241).

Oxytocin

Animal research notes that various drugs, including cannabis, can induce chronic changes in markers of oxytocin function with resultant social behavior dysfunction. Oxytocin is a neurohypophyseal hormone that has been under research in the regulation of drug abuse (1). This neuropeptide may serve as a neuromodulator on neurotransmission of dopamine in the nucleus accumbens as well as effects on the hippocampus (1). Central nervous system oxytocin pathways may offer a way of improving mood and social deficits found in some individuals with drug addiction (242). Research suggests that use of intranasal oxytocin may be useful in correcting the negative cannabis (and other illicit drug) effect on social behavior and perhaps protect the individual from addictive disorders. (243).

NAC

N-acetylcysteine (NAC) has been shown to be useful in management of cannabis-dependent adolescents and young adults due to modulation of glutamate in the nucleus accumbens; it is suggested as an adjuvant treatment (1,200 mg per day) along with psychological management (244).

Others

Research has failed to validate the use of *naltrexone* for the treatment of cannabis dependence. *Entacapone* is a member of the drug class called nitrocatechols that is used in the management of Parkinson's disease. It is an inhibitor of COMT (catechol-O-methyltransferase) and is under research as a possible drug for cannabis dependence.

Other drugs under research include lithium, dronabinol, URB597 (fatty acid amide hydrolase [FAAH] inhibitor), methyllycaconitine or MLA (nicotinic alpha-7-receptor antagonist), and endocannabinoid metabolizing enzymes (245). The use of cannabinoid replacement therapy with nabiximols is also under study as well as reduction of cannabis consumption if abstinence is not feasible or attainable (246, 247).

Conclusion

Polydrug use and addictions, including cannabis use, continues to be major phenomena in the 21st century world (17, 18, 248-253). Cannabis consumption continues to be high that included a 24% prevalence among United States 8th to 12th graders in 2017 (189). Research over the past decades has revealed a number of potential adverse effects in acute and chronic use of cannabis that can harm the human being throughout life from the womb to the tomb (1, 5, 8, 14-16, 23,

26). Generalized consumption of the unprocessed *cannabis sativa* plant can lead to considerable public health risks including increased schizophrenia, other psychoses, dependence, cognitive dependence and other risks as noted in this review (1, 254-259).

Many questions remain in the research on cannabis including the epigenetic effects of drug abuse including cannabis in a cause and consequence reverberation (260). Increase use of cannabis is found in adolescents who had emotional abuse as children; this is especially noted in females (261). Increasing cannabis potency (including synthetic varieties) leads to worsening health effects in all ages including adolescents and young adults (1, 262, 263).

The negative effects of contaminants found in the cannabis plant sometimes linked to the cultivation process are under study (264, 265). Clinicians are currently seeing heavy metal toxicity, chemical/insecticide exposure, and atypical fungal infections that are acquired from the use of contaminated marijuana products (both legal and illegal) (266-268). Women should be encouraged not to use cannabis and other illicit drugs during pregnancy since it can lead to negative problems in the baby that continue through childhood and beyond (1, 269-272). The tragic role of cannabis and fatal car crashes must also be considered (273).

The unproven role of *medical* cannabis continues to be explored as some wish to smoke or vape cannabis for health issues while pharmaceutical companies produce various phytocannabinoids (CBD, CBN, others) for oral or mist consumption (50-72, 274-278). The issue of drug-to-drug interactions must be further explored (i.e., *cytochrome P450, UDP-glucuronosyltransferases*, others) (279). The impact of medical and recreational cannabis in various states of the United States is under study as it leads to more cannabis consumption with tragic trajectories of car accidents and other effects found in patients of all ages in the emergency rooms, acute care clinics and primary care clinics across the United States (1, 136-141, 189, 280-285).

With the wave of cannabis legalization, the cannabis industry has created new, even novel ways to consume and use cannabis products. Some of these means include inhalers, vape pens, creams as well as topicals, oral/edibles and less traditional methods such as THC-infused tampons and rectal suppositories.

Such a milieu in the second and third decade of the 21st century poses risks for our children and youth. Indeed, there is growing public opinion regarding the so-called benign and even positive impact of cannabis consumption with increasing legalization for medicinal as well as recreational use. This raises the clear need for improved methods of prevention and management of cannabis use disorder as well as other complex complications of cannabis consumption (1, 189, 286-292).

The neuropsychological profile of cannabis with its potential negative impact on the adolescent brain must be considered and further studied as society develops a more tolerant view of cannabis with many adolescents having a chronic exposure to this product from adolescence through adulthood (293-295). Indeed, continued clinician guidance is needed for current cannabis consumption as *cannabis sativa (cannabis ruderalis, cannabis indica)*, a controversial plant known for thousands of years, remains disputatious and contentious in the 21st century (1, 5, 8, 14-16, 23, 296-305).

References

[1] Greydanus DE, Kaplan G, Baxter LE Sr., Patel DR, Feucht CL. Cannabis: The never-ending, nefarious nepenthe of the 21st century: What should clinician know? Dis Mon 2015;61(4):118-75.

[2] Anthony JC. Steppingstone and gateway ideals: a discussion of origins, research challenges, and promising lines of research for the future. Drug Alcohol Depend 2012;123(Suppl 1):S99-104.

[3] Fischer B, Jones W, Shuper P, Rehm J. 12-month follow-up of an exploratory "brief intervention" for high-frequency cannabis use among Canadian university students. Subst Abuse Treat Prev Policy 2012;7(1):15.

[4] Shoyama Y, Tamada T, Kurihara K, Takeuchi A, Taura F, Arai S, et al. Structure and function of Δ1-tetrahydrocannabinolic acid (THCA) synthase, the enzyme controlling the psychoactivity of Cannabis sativa. J Mol Biol 2012;423(1):96-105.

[5] Greydanus DE, Reed WJ, Hawver EK. Substance use and abuse in adolescents. In: Greydanus DE, Patel DR, Pratt HD, Calles Jr JL, Nazeer A, Merrick J, eds. Behavioral pediatrics, fourth edition. New York: Nova Science, 2015:497-535.

[6] Goullé JP, Saussereau E, Lacroix C. Delta-9-tetrahydrocannabinol pharmacokinetics. Ann Pharm Fr 2008;66(4):232-44.

[7] Tsumura Y, Aoki R, Tokieda Y, Akutsu M, Kawase Y, Kataoka T, et al. A survey of the potency of Japanese illicit cannabis in fiscal year 2010. Forensic Sci Int 2012;221(1-3):77-83.

[8] Greydanus DE, Patel DR. Substance abuse in the adolescent. In: Greydanus DE, Patel DR, Pratt HD, eds. Essential adolescent medicine. New York: McGraw-Hill, 2006:704-5.

[9] Clark PA, Capuzzi K, Fick C. Medical marijuana: Medical necessity versus political agenda. Med Sci Mont 2011;17(12):RA249-61.

[10] Steppan M, Kraus L, Piontek D, Siciliano V. Are cannabis prevalence estimates comparable across countries and regions? A cross-cultural validation using search engine query data. Int J Drug Policy 2013;24(1):23-9.

[11] Baz-Lomba JA, Salvatore S, Gracia-Lor E, Bade R, Castiglioni S, Castrignanò E. Comparison of pharmaceutical, illicit drug, alcohol, nicotine and caffeine levels in wastewater with sale, seizure and consumption data for 8 European cities. BMC Public Health 2016;16(1):1035.

[12] Kolliakou A, Fusar-Poli P, Atakan Z. Cannabis abuse and vulnerability to psychosis: targeting preventive services. Curr Pharm Des 2012;18(4):542-9.

[13] Teesson M, Slade T, Swift W, Mills K, Memedovic S, Mewton L, et al. Prevalence, correlates and comorbidity of DSM-IV cannabis use and cannabis use disorders in Australia. Aust NZ J Psychiatry 2012;46(12):1182-92.

[14] Greydanus DE, Feucht CL, Hawver EK. Substance abuse disorders. In: Greydanus DE, Patel DR, Omar HA, Feucht C, Merrick J, eds. Adolescent medicine: Pharmacotherapeutics in general, mental, and sexual health. Berlin: De Gruyter, 2012:157-99.

[15] Greydanus DE, Patel DR. Substance abuse in adolescents: a complex conundrum for the clinician. Pediatr Clin North Am 2003;59(5):1179-223.

[16] Greydanus DE, Patel DR. Substance abuse in adolescents: Current concepts. Dis Mon 2005; 51(7):392-431.

[17] European Monitoring Centre for Drugs and Drug Addiction. European Drug Report 2017: Trends and developments. Luxembourg: Publications Office of the European Union, 2017. URL: www.emcdda.europa.eu.

[18] Kann L, McManus T, Harris WA, Shanklin SL, Flint KH, Queen B, et al. Youth risk behavior surveillance--United States, 2017. MMWR Surveill Summ 2018;67(8):1-114.

[19] Ivanov I, Pearson A, Kaplan K, Newcorn J. Attention deficit hyperactivity disorder and comorbid substance abuse. In: Greydanus DE, Calles Jr JL, Patel DR, Nazeer A, Merrick J. eds. Clinical aspects of psychopharmacology in childhood and adolescence, Second edition, New York: Nova Science, 2017:61-80.

[20] Mehrpour O, Karrari P, Afshari R. Recreational use and overdose of ingested processed cannabis (Majoon Birjandi) in the eastern Iran. Hum Exp Toxicol 2012;31(11):1188-9.

[21] Tashkin DP. Vaping cannabis and chronic obstructive pulmonary disease. Ann Am Thorac Soc 2018;15(10):1137-8.

[22] Knapp AA, Lee DC, Borodovsky JT, Auty SG, Gabrielli J, Budney AJ. Emerging trends in cannabis administration among adolescent cannabis users. J Adolesc Health 2019;64(4):487-493.

[23] Greydanus DE, Feucht C, Hawver EK. Substance abuse and adolescence. Int J Child Health Hum Dev 2012;5(2):149-79.

[24] Agrawal A, Budney AJ, Lynskey MT. The co-occurring use and misuse of cannabis and tobacco: a review. Addiction 2012;107(7):1221-33.

[25] Simmons MS, Tashkin DP. The relationship of tobacco and marijuana smoking characteristics. Life Sci 1995;56(23-24):2185-91.

[26] American Psychiatric Association. Diagnostic and statistical manual of mental disorders, DSM-5, 5th ed. Arlington, VA: American Psychiatric Association, 2013.

[27] Olthuis JV, Darredeau C, Barrett SP. Substance use initiation: the role of simultaneous polysubstance use. Drug Alcohol Rev 2013;32(1):67-71.

[28] Barrett SP, Darredeau C, Pihl RO. Patterns of simultaneous polysubstance use in drug using university students. Hum Psychopharmacol 2006;21(4);255-63.

[29] Sartor CE, Agrawal A, Lynskey MT, Duncan AE, Grant JD, Nelson EC, et al. Cannabis or alcohol first? Differences by ethnicity and in risk for rapid progression to cannabis-related problems in women. Psychol Med 2013;43(4):813-23.

[30] Bowes L, Chollet A, Fombonne E, Galéra C, Melchior M. Lifetime SEP and tobacco and cannabis use. Eur J Public Health 2013;23(2):322-7.

[31] Pesce A, West C, Rosenthal M, West R, Crews B, Mikel C, et al. Marijuana correlates with use of other illicit drugs in a pain patient population. Pain Physician 2010;13(3):283-7.

[32] O'Brien MS, Comment LA, Liang KY, Anthony JC. Does cannabis onset trigger cocaine onset? A case crossover approach. Int J Methods Psychiatr Res 2012;21(1):66-75.

[33] DiBenedetto DJ, Weed VF, Wawrzyniak KM, Finkelman M, Paolini J, Schatman ME, et al. The association between cannabis use and aberrant behaviors during chronic opioid therapy for chronic pain. Pain Med 2018;19(10):1997-2008.

[34] Olfson M, Wall MM, Liu SM, Blanco C. Cannabis use and risk of prescription opioid use disorder in the United States. Am J Psychiatry 2018;175(1):47-53.

[35] Aizpurua-Olaizola O, Omar J, Navarro P, Olivares M, Etxebarria N, Usobiaga A. Identification and quantification of cannabinoids in Cannabis sativa L. plants by high performance liquid chromatography-mass spectrometry. Anal Bioanal Chem 2014;406(29):7549-60.

[36] Turner SE, Williams CM, Iversen L, Whalley BJ. Molecular pharmacology of phytocannabinoids. Prog Chem Org Nat Prod 2017;103:61-101.

[37] Oomen PP, van Hell HH, Bossong MG. The acute effects of cannabis on human executive function. Behav Pharmacol 2018;29(7):605-16.

[38] Ronan PJ, Wongngamnit N, Beresford TP. Molecular mechanisms of cannabis signaling in the brain. Prog Mol Biol Transl Sci 2016:137:123-47.

[39] Murillo-Rodriquez E, Pastrana-Trejo JC, Salas-Crisóstomo M, de-la-Cruz M. The endocannabinoid system modulating levels of consciousness, emotions and likely dream contents. CNS Neurol Disord Drug Targets 2017;16(4):370-9.

[40] Mechoulam R, Parker LA. The endocannabinoid system and the brain. Annu Rev Psychol 2013; 64:21-47.

[41] Tsuboi K, Uyama T, Okamoto Y, Ueda N. Endocannabinoids and related N-acylethanolamines: biological activities and metabolism. Inflamm Regen 2018;38:28. doi: 10.1186/s41232-018-0086-5.

[42] Marco EM, Garcia-Gutiérrez MS, Bermúdez-Silva FJ, Moreira FA, Guimarães F, Manzanares J, et al. Endocannabinoid system and psychiatry: in search of a neurobiological basis for detrimental and potential therapeutic effects. Front Behav Neurosci 2011;55:63-70.

[43] Fattore L, Spano MS, Deiana S, Melis V, Cossu G, Fadda P, et al. An endocannabinoid mechanism in relapse to drug seeking: a review of animal studies and clinical perspectives. Brain Res Rev 2007;53(1):1-16.

[44] Micale V, Drago F. Endocannabinoid system, stress and HPA axis. Eur J Pharmacol 2018; 834:230-9.

[45] Marriott KS, Huffman JW. Recent advances in the development of selective ligands for the cannabinoid CB (2) receptor. Curr Top Med Chem 2008;8(3):187-204.

[46] Guindon J, Hohmann AG. The endocannabinoid system and cancer: therapeutic implication. Br J Pharmacol 2011;163(7):1447-63.

[47] Caballero A, Tseng KY. Association of cannabis use during adolescence, prefrontal CB1 receptor signaling, and schizophrenia. Front Pharmacol 2012;3:101-4.

[48] Chambers RA. Adult hippocampal neurogenesis in the pathogenesis of addiction and dual diagnosis disorders. Drug Alcohol Depend 2013;130:1-12.

[49] Hall W. The adverse health effects of cannabis use: what are they, and what are their implications for policy? Int J Drug Policy 2009;20(6):458-66.

[50] Hazelkamp A, Fischedick JT. Cannabis-from cultivar to chemovar. Drug Test Anal 2012;4(7-8):660-7.

[51] Naftali T, Lev LB, Yablecovitch D, Half E, Konikoff FM. Treatment of Crohn's disease with cannabis: an observational study. Isr Med Assoc J 2011;13(8):455-8.

[52] Collen M. Prescribing cannabis for harm reduction. Harm Reduct J 2012;9(1):1.

[53] Fernandez-Ruiz J. Cannabinoid drugs for neurological diseases: what is behind? Rev Neurol 2012;54(10):613-28.

[54] Mücke M, Phillips T, Radbruch L, Petzke F, Häuser W. Cannabis-based medicines for chronic neuropathic pain in adults. Cochrane Database Syst Rev 2018;3:CD012182.

[55] Bonomo Y, Souza JDS, Jackson A, Crippa JAS, Solowij N. Clinical issues in cannabis use. Br J Clin Pharmacol 2018;84(11):2495-8.

[56] Maroon J, Bosts J. Review of the neurological benefits of phytocannabinoids. Surg Neurol Int 2018; 9:91. doi: 10.4103/sni.sni_45_18.

[57] Hofmann ME, Frazier CJ. Marijuana, endocannabinoids, and epilepsy: Potential and challenges for improved therapeutic intervention. Exp Neurol 2011;233:112-25.

[58] Calvaruso G, Pellerito O, Notaro A, Giuliano M. Cannabinoid-associated cell death mechanisms in tumor models. Int J Oncol 2012;41(2):407-13.

[59] Rice J, Cameron M. Cannabinoids for treatment of MS symptoms: State of the evidence. Curr Neurol Neurosci Rep 2018;18(8):50.

[60] Wade D. Evaluation of the safety and tolerability profile of Sativex: is it reassuring enough? Expert Rev Neurother 2012;12(4 Suppl):9-14.

[61] Śledziński P, Zeyland J, Słomski R, Nowak A. The current state and future perspectives of cannabinoids in cancer biology. Cancer Med 2018;7(3):765-75.

[62] Treister-Goltzman Y, Freud T, Press Y, Peleg R. Trends in publications on medical cannabis from the year 2000. Popul Health Manag 2019;22(4):362-8.

[63] Styrczewska M, Kulma A, Ratajczak K, Amarowicz R, Szope J. Cannabinoid-like anti-inflammatory compounds from flax fiber. Cell Mol Biol Lett 2012;17(3):479-99.

[64] Mouhammad ZA, Kolko M. Should ophthalmologists recommend medical cannabis to patients with glaucoma? Ugeskr Laeger 2018;180(29):V11170861. [Danish].

[65] Bonini SA, Premoli M, Tambaro S, Kumar A, Maccarinelli G, Memo M, et al. Cannabis sativa: A comprehensive ethnopharmacological review of a medicinal plant with a long history. J Ethnopharmacol 2018;227:300-15.

[66] Russo EB. Cannabis and epilepsy: An ancient treatment returns to the fore. Epilepsy Behav 2017; 70(Pt B):292-7.

[67] Mead A. The legal status of cannabis (marijuana) and cannabidiol (CBD) under US law. Epilepsy Behav 2017;70(Pt B):288-91.

[68] Corroon J, Kight R. Regulatory status of cannabidiol in the United States: A perspective. Cannabis Cannabinoid Res 2018;3(1):190-4.

[69] FDA approves first drug comprised of an active ingredient derived from marijuana to treat rare, severe forms of epilepsy. Silver Spring, MD: US Food and Drug Administration, 2018.

[70] Drug Enforcement Administration, Department of Justice. Schedules of controlled substances: Placement in Schedule V of certain FDA-approved drugs containing cannabidiol; Corresponding change to permit requirements. Final order. Fed Regist 2018;83(189):48950-3.

[71] Tambaro S, Bortolato M. Cannabinoid-related agents in the treatment of anxiety disorders: current knowledge and future perspectives. Recent Pat CNS Drug Discov 2012;7(1):25-40.
[72] Grof CPL. Cannabis, from plant to pill. Br J Clin Pharmacol 2018;84(11):2463-7.
[73] Noreen N, Muhammad F, Akhtar B, Azam F, Anwar MI. Is cannabidiol a promising substance for new drug development? A review of its potential therapeutic applications. Crit Rev Eukaryot Gene Expr 2018;28(1):73-86.
[74] Papaseit E, Pérez-Mañá C, Pérez-Acevedo AP, Hladun O, Torres-Moreeno MC, Muga R, et al. Cannabinoids: from pot to lab. Int J Med Sci 2018;15(12):1286-95.
[75] Cooper ZD. Adverse effects of synthetic cannabinoids: Management of acute toxicity and withdrawal. Curr Psychiatry Rep 2016;18(5):52.
[76] Castellanos D, Thornton G. Synthetic cannabinoid use: recognition and management. J Psychiatr Pract 2012;18(2):86-93.
[77] Tait RJ, Caldicott D, Mountain D, Hill SL, Lenton S. A systematic review of adverse events arising from the use of synthetic cannabinoids and their associated treatment. Clin Toxicol (Phila) 2016; 54(1):1-13.
[78] Deng H, Verrico CD, Kosten TR, Neilsen DA. Psychosis and synthetic cannabinoids. Psychiatry Res 2018;268:400-12.
[79] Karila Petit A, Cottencin O, Coscas S, Reynaud M. Synthetic drugs: The new low-cost landscape of drugs. Rev Prat 2012;62(5):664-6.
[80] Rosenbaum CD, Carreiro SP, Babu KM. Here today, gone tomorrow....back again? A review of herbal marijuana alternatives (K2, Spice), synthetic cathinones (bath salts), Kratom, Salvia divinorum, methoxetamie, and piperazines. J Med Toxicol 2012;8(1):15-32.
[81] Funada M. Pharmacological properties and dependence liabilities of synthetic cannabinoids. Nihon Arukoru Yakubutsu Igakkai Zasshi 2010;45(3):167-74.
[82] Johnson LA, Johnson RL, Alfonzo C. Spice: A legal marijuana equivalent. Mil Med 2011;176 (6):718-20.
[83] Schneir AB, Cullen J, Ly BT. "Spice" girls: synthetic cannabinoid intoxication. J Emerg Med 2011;40(3):296-9.
[84] Ginsburg BC, McMahon LR, Sanchez JJ, Javors MA. Purity of synthetic cannabinoids sold online for recreational use. J Anal Toxicol 2012;36(1):66-8.
[85] De Backer B, Maebe Verstraete AG, Charlier C. Evolution of the content of THC and other major cannabinoids in drug-type cannabis cuttings and seedlings during growth of plants. J Forensic Sci 2012;57(4):918-22.
[86] Köhnemann S, Nedele J, Schwotzer D, Morzfeld J, Pfeiffer H. The validation of a 15 STR multiplex PCR for Cannabis species. Int J Legal Med 2012;126(4):601-6.
[87] Salomone A, Gerace E, E'Urso F, Di Corcia D, Vincenti M. Simultaneous analysis of several synthetic cannabinoids, THC, CBD, and CBN, in hair by ultra-high performance liquid chromatography tandem mass spectrometry. Method validation and application to real samples. J Mass Spectrom 2012;47(5):604-12.
[88] Cortes L, Almeida L, Sabra S, Muniesa M, Busardo FP, Garcia-Algar O, et al. Maternal hair and neonatal meconium to assess gestational and prenatal exposure to drugs of abuse and psychoactive drugs. Curr Pharm Biotechnol 2018;19(2):136-43.
[89] Crume TL, Juhl AL, Brooks-Russell A, Hall KE, Wymore E, Borgelt LM. Cannabis use during the perinatal period in a state with legalized recreational and medical marijuana: The association between maternal characteristics, breastfeeding patterns, and neonatal outcomes. J Pediatr 2018; 197:90-6.
[90] Baker T, Datta P, Rewers-Felkins K, Thompson H, Kallem RR, Hale TW. Transfer of inhaled cannabis into human breast milk. Obstet Gynecol 2018;131(5):783-8.
[91] Brown RA, Dakkak H, Seabrook JA. Is breast best? Examining the effects of alcohol and cannabis use during lactation. J Neonatal Perinatal Med 2018;11(4):345-356.
[92] Adverse effects of cannabis. Prescrire Int 2011;20(112):18-23.
[93] Howden ML, Naughton MT. Pulmonary effects of marijuana inhalation. Expert Rev Respir Med 2011;5(1):87-92.

[94] Molly C, Mory O, Basset T, Patural H. Acute cannabis poisoning in a 10-month-old infant. Arch Pediatr 2012;19(7):729-32.

[95] Pélissier F, Claudet I, Pélissier-Alicot AL, Franchitto N. Parental cannabis abuse and accidental intoxications in children: prevention by detecting neglectful situations and at-risk families. Pediatr Emerg Care 2014;30(12):862-9.

[96] Mallaret M, Dal'Bo-Rohrer D, Demattéis M. Adverse effects of marijuana. Rev Prat 2005;55(1): 41-9.

[97] Davis GP, Gunderson EW. Evaluation of chronic cough should consider cannabis use. Am Fam Physician 2012;85(7):680-2.

[98] DeCuyper II, Faber MA, Lapeere H, Mertens C, Rihs HP, Van Gasse AL, et al. Cannabis allergy: A diagnostic challenge. Allergy 2018;73(9):1911-4.

[99] Foster E, Nguyen C, Norris P. Contact buzz: Allergic contact dermatitis to cannabis. Dermatitis 2018;29(4):223-4.

[100] Hsiao P, Clavijo RI. Adverse effects of cannabis on male reproduction. Eur Urol Focus 2018;4(3):324-8

[101] Haffar S, Murad MH, Bazerbachi F. Canna is-induced acute pancreatitis: Evaluation of causation in a systemic review. Pancreas 2018;47(6):e31.

[102] Simonetto DA, Oxentenko AS, Herman ML, Szostek JH. Cannabinoid hyperemesis: a case series of 98 patients. Mayo Clin Proc 2012;87(2):114-9.

[103] Fleig S, Brunkhorst R. Hyperemesis and a high water bill. Z Gastroenterol 2011; 49(11): 1479-81.

[104] Galli JA, Sawaya RA, Friedenberg FK. Cannabinoid hyperemesis syndrome. Curr Drug Abuse Rev 2011;4(4):241-9.

[105] Nourbakhsh M, Miller A, Gofton J, Jones G, Adeagbo B. Cannabinoid hyperemesis syndrome: Reports of fatal cases. J Forensic Sci 2019;64(1):270-4.

[106] Sorensen CJ, DeSanto K, Borgelt L, Phillips KT, Monte AA. Cannabinoid hyperemesis syndrome: diagnosis, pathophysiology, and treatment. J Med Toxicol 2017;13(10:71-87.

[107] Richards JR. Cannabinoid hyperemesis syndrome: Pathophysiology and treatment in the emergency department. J Emerg Med 2018;54(3):354-63.

[108] Graham J, Barberio M, Wang GS. Capsaicin cream for treatment of cannabinoid hyperemesis syndrome in adolescents: A case series. Pediatrics 2017;140(6):e20163795

[109] Cho CM, Hirsch R, Johnstone S. General and oral health implications of cannabis use. Aust Dent J 2005;50(2):70-4.

[110] Maloney WJ. Significance of cannabis use to dental practice. J Mich Dent Assoc 2011;93(11):44-8.

[111] Rawal SY, Tatakis DN, Tipton DA. Periodontal and oral manifestations of marijuana use. J Tenn Dent Assoc 2012;92(2):26-32.

[112] Lopes CF, de Angelis BB, Prudente HM, de Souza BV, Cardoso SV, de Azambuja Ribeiro RI. Concomitant consumption of marijuana, alcohol, and tobacco in oral squamous cell carcinoma development and progression: Recent advances and challenges. Arch Oral Biol 2012;57(8):1026-33.

[113] Pletcher MJ, Vittinghoff E, Kalhan R, Richman J, Safford M, Sidney S, et al. Association between marijuana exposure and pulmonary function over 20 years. JAMA 2012;307(2):173-81.

[114] Ribeiro A, Ferraz-de-Paula V, Pinheiro ML, Vitoretti LB, Mariano-Souza DP, Quinteiro-Filho WM, et al. Cannabidiol, a non-psychotropic plant-derived cannabinoid, decreases inflammation in a murine model of acute lung injury: role for the adenosine A (2A) receptor. Eur J Pharmacol 2012; 678(1-3):78-85.

[115] Tashkin DP. Airway effects of marijuana, cocaine, and other inhaled illicit agents. Curr Opin Pulm Med 2001;7(2):43-61.

[116] Colorado State Web Portal. URL: https://www.colorado.gov/pacific/marijuana/marijuana-basics.

[117] Szyper-Kravitz M, Lang R, Manor Y, Lahav M. Early invasive pulmonary aspergillosis in a leukemia patient linked to aspergillus contaminated marijuana smoking. Leuk Lymphoma 2001; 42(6):1433-7.

[118] Greydanus DE, Alsukhon J, Leonov A. Cannabis smoking and the lung. BAOJ Aller Immunol 2017;3:012.

[119] Chang SW, Wellmerling J, Zhang X, Rayner RE, Osman W, Mertz S, et al. The psychoactive substance of cannabis Δ9-tetrahydrocannabinol (THC) negatives regulates CFTR in airway cells. Biochim Biophys Acta Gen Subj 2018;1862(9):1988-94.

[120] Tashkin DP. Marijuana and lung disease. Chest 2018;154(3):653-63.

[121] Ribeiro L, Ind PW. Marijuana and the lung: hysteria or cause for concern? Breathe (Sheff) 2018;14(3):196-205.

[122] Van Hoozen BE, Cross CE. Marijuana. Respiratory tract effects. Clin Rev Allergy Immunol 1997; 15(3):243-69.

[123] Kothadia JP, Chhabra S, Marcus A, May M, Saraiya B, Jabbour SK. Anterior mediastinal mass in a young marijuana smoker: a rare case of small-cell lung cancer. Case Report Med 2012; 2012:754231. doi: 10.1155/2012/754231.

[124] Yu-Hui JH, Zuo-Feng Z. An epidemiologic review of marijuana and cancer; an update. Cancer Epidemiol Biomarkers Prev 2015;24(1):15-31.

[125] Chen AL, Chen TJ, Braverman ER, Acuri V, Kemer M, Varshavskiy M, et al. Hypothesizing that marijuana smokers are at significantly lower risk of carcinogenicity relative to tobacco-non-marijuana smokers: evidence based on statistical reevaluation of current literature. J Psychoactive Drugs 2008;40(3):263-72.

[126] Quoix E. What is new in the epidemiology of lung cancer: non-smokers, women, and the role of cannabis. Rev Pratt 2009;59(7):920-4.

[127] Bigay-Gamé L, Bota S, Greillier L, Monnet I, Madroszyk A, Corre R, et al.; GFPC Investigators. Characteristics of lung cancer in patients younger than 40 years: A prospective multicenter analysis in France. Oncology 2018;95(6):337-43.

[128] Kariyanna PT, Jayarangaiah A, Hegde S, Marmur JD, Wengrofsky P, Yacoub M, et al. Marijuana induced Type I Brugada pattern: A case report. Am J Med Case Rep 2018;6(7):134-6.

[129] Lee J, Sharma N, Kazi F, Youssef I, Myers A, Marmur JD, et al. Cannabis and myocardial infarction: Risk factors and pathogenic insights. Scifed J Cardiol 2017;1(1). pii: 1000004.

[130] Singh A, Saluja S, Kumar A, Agrawal S, Thind M, Nanda S, et al. Cardiovascular complications of marijuana and related substances: A review. Cardiol Ther 2018;7(1):45-59.

[131] Rodríguez-Castro CE, Alkhateeb H, Elfar A, Saifuddin F, Abbas A, Siddiqui T. Recurrent myopericarditis as a complication of marijuana use. Am J Case Rep 2014;15:60-2.

[132] Nappe T, Hoyte C. Pediatric death due to myocarditis after exposure to cannabis. Clin Pract Cases Emerg Med 2017;1(3):166-70.

[133] Pacher P, Steffens S, Haskó G, Schindler TH, Kunos G. Cardiovascular effects of marijuana and synthetic cannabinoids: the good, the bad, and the ugly. Nat Rev Cardiol 2018;15(3):151-66.

[134] Piano MR. Cannabis smoking and cardiovascular health: It's complicated. Clin Pharmacol Ther 2017;102(20:191-3.

[135] Rezkalla S, Kloner RA. Cardiovascular effects of marijuana. Trends Cardiovasc Med 2019; 29(7):403-7.

[136] Ramaekers JG. Driving under the influence of cannabis: An increasing public health concern. JAMA 2018;319(14):1433-4.

[137] Steinemann S, Galanis D, Nguyen T, Biffl W Motor vehicle crash fatalities and undercompensated care associated with legalization of marijuana. J Trauma Acute Care Surg 2018; 85(3):566-71.

[138] Aydelotte JD, Brown LH, Luftman KM, Mardock AL, Teixeira PGR, Coopwood B, et al. Crash fatality rates after recreational marijuana legalization in Washington and Colorado. Am J Public Health 2017;107(8):1329-31.

[139] Martin JL, Gadegbeku B, Wu D, Viallon V, Laumon B. Cannabis, alcohol and fatal road accidents. PLoS One 2017;12(11):e0187320.

[140] Bosker WM, Karschner EL, Lee D, Goodwin RS, Hirvonen J, Innis RB, et al. Psychomotor function in chronic daily cannabis smokers during sustained abstinence. PLoS One 2013; 8(1):e53127.

[141] Colorado Department of Public Safety. Driving under the influence of drugs and alcohol. Denver, CO: Division of Criminal Justice, 2018. URL: https://cdpsdocs.state.co.us/ors/docs/reports/2018-DUI_HB17-1315.pdf.

[142] Volkow ND, Baler RD, Compton WM, Weiss SR. Adverse health effects of marijuana use. N Engl J Med 2014;370(23):2219-27.

[143] Ware MA, Jensen D, Barrette A, Vernec A, Derman W. Cannabis and the health and performance of the elite athlete. Clin J Sport Med 2018;28(5):480-4.

[144] Brisola-Santos MB, Gallinaro JG, Gil F, Sampaio-Junior B, Marin MC, de Andrade AG, et al. Prevalence and correlates of cannabis use among athletes--A systematic review. Am J Addict 2016; 25(7):518-28.

[145] Martin-Santos F, Fagundo AB, Crippa JA, Atakan Z, Bhattacharyya S, Allen P, et al. Neuroimaging in cannabis use: a systemic review of the literature. Psychol Med 2010;40(3):383-98.

[146] Crippa JA, Lacerda AL, Amaro E, Busatto Filho G, Zuardi AW, Bressan RA. Brain effects of cannabis—neuroimaging findings. Rev Bras Psiquiatr 2005;27(1):70-8.

[147] Scott JC, Slomiak ST, Jones JD, Rosen AFG, Moore TM, Gur RC. Association of cannabis with cognitive functioning in adolescents and young adults: A systematic review and meta-analysis. JAMA Psychiatry 2018;75(6):585-95.

[148] Colizzi M, Bhattacharyya S. Cannabis use and the development of tolerance: A systematic review. Neurosci Biobehav Rev 2018;93:1-25.

[149] Marmorstein NR, Iacono WG, McGue M. Associations between substance use disorders and major depression in parents and late adolescent-emerging adult offspring: An adoption study. Addiction 2012;107(11):1965-73.

[150] Harvey MA, Sellman JD, Porter RJ, Frampton CM. The relationship between non-acute adolescent cannabis use and cognition. Drug Alcohol Res 2007;26(3):309-19.

[151] Sundram S. Cannabis and neurodevelopment: implications for psychiatric disorders. Hum Psychopharmacol 2006;21(4):245-54.

[152] Schneider M. Puberty as a highly vulnerable developmental period for the consequences of cannabis exposure. Addict Biol 2008;13(2):253-63.

[153] Dinieri JA, Hurd YL. Rat models of prenatal and adolescent cannabis exposure. Methods Mol Biol 2012;829:231-42.

[154] De Aquino JP, Sherif M, Radhakrishnan R, Cahill JD, Ranganathan M, D'Souza DC. The psychiatric consequences of cannabinoids. Clin Ther 2018;40(9):1448-56.

[155] Abush H, Ghose S, Van Enkevort EA, Clementz BA, Pearlson GD, Sweeney JA, et al. Associations between adolescent cannabis use and brain structure in psychosis. Psychiatry Res Neuroimaging 2018;276:53-64.

[156] Pacheco-Colón I, Limia JM, Gonzalez R. Nonacute effects of cannabis use on motivation and reward sensitivity in humans: A systemic review. Psychol Addict Behav 2018;32(5):497-507.

[157] Lichenstein SD, Musselman S, Shaw DS, Sitnick S, Forbes EE. Nucleus accumbens functional connectivity at age 20 is associated with trajectory of adolescent cannabis use and predicts psychosocial functioning in young adulthood. Addiction 2017;112(11):1961-70.

[158] Yücel M, Solowij N, Respondek C, Whittle S, Fornito A, Pantelis C, et al. Regional brain abnormalities associated with long-term heavy cannabis use. Arch Gen Psychiatry 2008;65(6):694-701.

[159] Wallace AL, Wade NE, Hatcher KF, Lisdahl KM. Effects of cannabis use and subclinical ADHD symptomology on attention based tasks in adolescents and young adults. Arch Clin Neuropsychol. 2019;34(5):700-5.

[160] Gordon SM, Tulak F, Troncale J. Prevalence and characteristics of adolescent patients with co-occurring ADHD and substance dependence. J Addict Dis 2004;23:31-40.

[161] Dennis M, Godley SH, Diamond G, Tims FM, Babor T, Donaldson J, et al. The Cannabis Youth Treatment (CYT) Study: main findings from two randomized trials. J Subst Abuse Treat 2004; 27(3):197-213.

[162] Brezing CA, Levin FR. The current state of pharmacological treatments for cannabis use disorder and withdrawal. Neuropsychopharmacology 2018;43(1):173-94.

[163] Freeman TP, Winstock AR. Examining the profile of high-potency cannabis and its association with severity of cannabis dependence. Psychol Med 2015;45(15):3181-9.

[164] Horwood LJ, Fergusson DM, Coffey C, Patton GC, Tait R, Smart D, et al. Cannabis and depression: an integrative data analysis of four Australasian cohorts. Drug Alcohol Depend 2012; 126(3):369-78.

[165] Degenhardt L, Chiu WT, Sampson N, Kessler RC, Anthony JC, Angermeyer M, et al. Toward a global view of alcohol, tobacco, cannabis, ad cocaine use. Findings from the WHO World Mental Health Surveys. PLoS Med 2008;5(7):e141.
[166] Schlienz NJ, Budney AJ, Lee DC, Vandrey R. Cannabis withdrawal: A review of neurobiological mechanisms and sex differences. Curr Addict Rep 2017;4(2):75-81.
[167] Budney AJ, Hughes JR, Moore BA, Vandrey R. Review of the validity and significance of cannabis withdrawal syndrome. Am J Psychiatry 2004;161(11):1967-77.
[168] Budney AJ, Hughes JR. The cannabis withdrawal syndrome. Curr Opin Psychiatry 2006;19(3): 233-8.
[169] Crowley TJ, MacDonald MJ, Whitmore EA. Cannabis dependence, withdrawal, and reinforcing effects among adolescents with conduct symptoms and substance use disorders. Drug Alcohol Depend 1998;50(1):27-37.
[170] Vandrey RG, Budney AJ, Hughes JR, Liguoria A. A within-subject comparison of withdrawal symptoms during abstinence from cannabis, tobacco, and both substances. Drug Alcohol Depend 2008;92(1-3):48-54.
[171] Arendt M, Rosenberg R, Fjordback L, Brandholdt J, Foldager L, Sher L, et al. Testing the self-medication hypothesis of depression and aggression in cannabis-dependent subjects. Psychol Med 2007;37(7):935-45.
[172] Calles JL Jr, Nazeer A. Aggressive and violent behavior. In: Greydanus DE, Calles JL Jr, Patel DR, Nazeer A, Merrick J, eds. Clinical aspects of psychopharmacology in childhood and adolescence. New York: Nova Science, 2011:103-13.
[173] Schacht JP, Hutchinson KE, Filbey FM. Associations between cannabinoid-receptor-1 (CNR1) variation and hippocampus and amygdale volumes in heavy cannabis users. Neuropsychopharmacology 2012;37(11):2368-76.
[174] Haney M, Hart CL, Vosburg KD. Marijuana withdrawal in humans: effects of oral THC or divalproex. Neuropsychopharmacology 2004;29(1):158-70.
[175] Milin R, Manion I, Dare G, Walker S. Prospective assessment of cannabis withdrawal in adolescents with cannabis dependence: A pilot study. J Am Acad Child Adolesc Psychiatry 2008; 47(2):174-8.
[176] Cornelius JR, Chung T, Martin C, Wood DS, Clark DB. Cannabis withdrawal is common among treatment seeking adolescents with cannabis dependence and major depression, and is associated with rapid relapse to dependence. Addict Behav 2008;33(11):1500-5.
[177] Hood L. Social factors and animal models of cannabis use. Int Rev Neurobiol 2018;140:171-200.
[178] Gardner EL. Addictive potential of cannabinoids: the underlying neurobiology. Chem Phys Lipids 2005;121(1-2):267-90.
[179] Cooper ZD, Haney M. Cannabis reinforcement and dependence: role of cannabinoid CB1 receptor. Addict Biol 2008;13(2):188-95.
[180] Cooper ZD, Haney M. Actions of delta-9-tetrahydrocannabinol in cannabis: relation to use, abuse, dependence. Int Rev Psychiatry 2009;21(2):104-12.
[181] Zehra A, Burns J, Liu CK, Manza P, Wiers CE, Volkow ND, et al. Cannabis addiction and the brain: a review. J Neuroimmune Pharmacol 2018;13(4):438-52.
[182] Gardner EL. Addiction and brain reward and antireward pathways. Adv Psychosom Med 2011;30: 22-60.
[183] Bossong MG, van Berckel BN, Boellaard R, Zuurman L, Schuit RC, Windhorst AD, et al. Delta 9-tetrahydrocannabinol induces dopamine release in the human striatum. Neuropsychopharmacology 2009;34(3):759-66.
[184] Horey JT, Mariani JJ, Cheng WY, Bisaqa A, Sullivan M, Nunes E, et al. Comparison of substance use milestones in cannabis-and cocaine-dependent patients. J Addict Dis 2012; 31(1):60-6.
[185] Goldstein RZ, Volkow ND. Dysfunction of the prefrontal cortex in addiction: neuroimaging findings and clinical implications. Nat Rev Neurosci 2011;12(11):652-69.
[186] Goldstein RZ, Volkow ND. Drug addiction and its underlying neurobiological basis: neuroimaging evidence for the involvement of the frontal cortex. Am J Psychiatry 2002;159(10):1642-52.
[187] Feil J, Sheppard D, Fitzgerald PB, Yücel M, Lubman DI, Bradshaw JL. Addiction, compulsive drug seeking, and the role of frontostriatal mechanisms in regulating inhibitory control. Neurosci Biobehav Rev 2010;35(2):248-75.

[188] Rotter A, Bayerlein K, Hansbauer M, Weiland J, Sperling W, Kornhuber, et al. Orexin A expression and promoter methylation in patients with cannabis dependence in comparison to nicotine-dependent cigarette smokers and nonsmokers. Neuropsychobiology 2012;66(2):126-33.
[189] Bagot KS, Chang A: Marijuana and psychosis: Policy implications for treatment providers. J Am Acad Child Adolesc Psychiatry 2018;57(8):613-4.
[190] Galvez-Buccollini JA, Proal AC, Tomaselli V, Trachtenberg M, Coconcea C, Chun J, et al. Association between age at onset of psychosis and age at onset of cannabis use in non-affective psychosis. Schizophr Res 2012;139(1-3):157-60.
[191] Giovanni M, Giuseppe DI, Gianna S, Domenico DB, Luisa DR, Massimo DG. Cannabis use and psychosis: theme introduction. Curr Pharm Des 2012;18(32):4991–8.
[192] Leweke FM, Koethe D. Cannabis and psychiatric disorders: it is not only addiction. Addict Biol 2008;13(2):264-75.
[193] Nazeer A, Calles Jr JL. Schizophrenia in children and adolescents. In: Greydanus DE, Calles Jr JL, Patel DR, Nazeer A, Merrick J, eds. Clinical aspects of psychopharmacology in childhood and adolescence, second edition. New York: Nova Science, 2017:191-204.
[194] Van Dijk D, Koeter MW, Hijman R, Kahn RS, van den Bring W. Effect of cannabis use on the course of schizophrenia in male patients: a prospective cohort study. Scizophr Res 2012;137(1-3):50-7.
[195] Bossong MG, Niesink RJ. Adolescent brain maturation, the endogenous cannabinoid system, and the neurobiology of cannabis-induced schizophrenia. Prog Neurobiol 2010;92(3):370-85.
[196] Rapp C, Bugra H, Riecher-Rössler A, Borgwardt S. Effects of cannabis use on human brain structure in psychosis: a systematic review combining in vivo structural neuroimaging and post-mortem studies. Curr Pharm Des 2012;18(32):5070-80.
[197] Khan MK, Usmani MA, Hanif SA. A case of self amputation of penis by cannabis induced psychosis. J Forensic Leg Med 2012;19(6):355-7.
[198] Barrowclough C, Emsley R, Eisner E, Beardmore R, Wykes T. Does change in cannabis use in established psychosis affect clinical outcome? Schizophr Bull 2013;39(2):339-48.
[199] Leweke FM. Anandamide dysfunction in prodromal and established psychosis. Curr Pharm Des 2012;18(32):5188-93.
[200] Decoster J, van Os J, Myin-Germeys I, De Hert M, van Winkel R. Genetic variation underlying psychosis-inducing effects of cannabis: critical review and future directions. Curr Pharm Des 2012; 18(32):5015-23.
[201] Serafini G, Pompili M, Innamorati M, Rihmer Z, Sher L, Girardi P. Can cannabis increase the suicide risk in psychosis? A critical review. Curr Pharm Des 2012;18(32):5165-87.
[202] Hermann D, Schneider M. Potential protective effects of cannabidol on neuroanatomical alterations in cannabis users and psychosis: a critical review. Curr Pharm Des 2012;18(32):4897-905.
[203] Lev-Ran S, Aviram A, Braw Y, Nitzan U, Ratzoni G, Fennig S. Clinical correlates of cannabis use among adolescent psychiatric inpatients. Eur Psychiatr 2012;27(6):470-5.
[204] Auther AM, McLaughlin D, Carrión RE, Naqachandran P, Correll CU, Cornblatt BA. Prospective study of cannabis use in adolescents at clinical high risk for psychosis: Impact of conversion to psychosis and functional outcome. Psychol Med 2012;42(12):2485-97.
[205] Zuardi AW, Crippa JA, Bhattacharyya S, Atakan Z, Martin-Santos R, et al. A critical review of the antipsychotic effects of Cannabidiol: 30 years of translational investigation. Curr Phar Des 2012;18(32):5131–40.
[206] Manseau MW, Goff CG. Cannabinoids and schizophrenia: Risks and therapeutic potential. Neurotherapeutics 2015;12(4):816-24.
[207] Blum K, Gardner E, Oscar-Berman M, Gold M. "Liking" and "Wanting" linked to reward deficiency syndrome (RDS): hypothesizing differential responsivity in brain reward circuitry. Curr Pharm Des 2012;18(1):113-8.
[208] Bailén AJR, Quesada PS, Valladares MA. Decision making in cannabis users. Adicciones 2012;24(2):161-72.
[209] Van Ours JC, Williams J. The effects of cannabis use on physical and mental health. J Health Econ 2012;31(4):564-77.

[210] Schifano F, Martinotti G, Cunniff A, Reissner V, Scherbaum N, Ghodse H. Impact of an 18- month, NHS-based, treatment exposure for heroin dependence: Results from the London Area Treat 2000 Study. Am J Addict 2012;21(3):268-73.

[211] Porath-Waller AJ, Beasley E, Beirness DJ. A meta-analytic review of school-based prevention for cannabis use. Health Educ Behav 2010;37(5):709-23.

[212] Teesson M, Newton NC, Barrett EL. Australian school-based prevention programs for alcohol and other drugs: A systemic review. Drug Alcohol Rev 2012;31(6):731-6.

[213] De Looze M, Harakeh Z, van Dorsselaer SA, Raaijmakers QA, Vollebergh WH, Bogt TF. Explaining educational differences in adolescent substance use and early sexual debut: The role of parents and peers. J Adolesc 2012;35(4):1035-44.

[214] Yap MB, Reavley NJ, Jorm AF. Young people's beliefs about the harmfulness of alcohol, cannabis, and tobacco for mental disorders: findings from two Australian national youth surveys. Addiction 2012;107(4):838-47.

[215] Gillespie NA, Lubke GH, Gardner CO, Neale MC, Keanler KS. Two-part random effects growth modeling to identify risks associated with alcohol and cannabis initiation, initial average use, and changes in drug consumption in s sample of adult, male twins. Drug Alcohol Depend 2012; 123(1-3):220-8.

[216] Abdoul H, Le Faou AL, Bouchez J, Touzeau D, Lagrue G. Cannabis cessation interventions offered to young French users: Predictors of follow-up. Encaphale 2012;38(2):141-8.

[217] Scott LA, Roxburgh A, Bruno R, Matthews A. Burns L. The impact of comorbid cannabis and methamphetamine use on mental health among regular ecstasy users. Addict Behav 2012;37(9): 1058-62.

[218] Friedmann PD, Green TC, Taxman FS, Harrington M, Rhodes AG, Katz E, et al. Collaborative behavioral management among parolees: drug use, crime & re-arrest in the Step'n Out randomized trial. Addiction 2012;107(6):1099-108.

[219] Baker AL, Thornton LK, Hides L, Dunlop A. Treatment of cannabis use among people with psychotic disorders: a critical review of randomised control trials. Curr Pharm Des 2012;71(3): 247-54.

[220] Buckner JD, Zvolensky MJ, Schmidt NB. Cannabis-related impairment and social anxiety: the roles of gender and cannabis use motives. Addict Behav 2012;37(1):1294-7.

[221] Carroll KM, Nich C, Lapaglia DM, Peters EN, Easton CJ, Petry NM. Combining cognitive behavioral therapy and contingency management to enhance their effects in treating cannabis dependence: less can be more, more or less. Addiction 2012;107(9):1650-9.

[222] Hendriks V, van der Schee E, Blanken P. Matching adolescents with a cannabis use disorder to multidimensional family therapy or cognitive behavioral therapy: treatment effect moderators in a randomized controlled trial. Drug Alcohol Depend 2012;125(1-2):119-26.

[223] Gates PJ, Sabioni P, Copeland J, Le Foll B, Gowing L. Psychosocial interventions for cannabis use disorder. Cochrane Database Syst Rev 2016;5:CD005336.

[224] Gates PJ, Norberg MM, Copeland J, Digiusto E. Randomised controlled trial of a noval cannabis use intervention delivered by telephone. Addiction 2012;107(12):2149-58.

[225] Hargraves D, White C, Frederick R, Cinibulk M, Peters M, Young A, et al. Implementing SBIRT (Screening, Brief intervention and Referral to Treatment) in primary care: lessons learned from a multi-practice evaluation portfolio. Public Health Rev 2017 Dec 29;38:31.

[226] Ryan S, Pantalon MV, Camenga D, Martel S, D'Onofrio G. Evaluation of a pediatric resident skills-based screening, brief intervention and referral to treatment (SBIRT) curriculum for substance use. J Adolesc Health 2018;63(3):327-34.

[227] Marshall K, Gowing L, Ali R, Le Foll B. Pharmacotherapies for cannabis dependence. Cochrane Database Syst Rev 2014;12:CD008940.

[228] Vandrey R, Haney M. Pharmacotherapy for cannabis dependence: how close are we? CNS Drugs 2009;23(7):543-53.

[229] Hjorthøj C, Fohlmann A, Nordentoft M. Treatment of cannabis use disorders in people withschizophrenia spectrum disorders-a systemic review. Addict Behav 2009;34(6-7):520-5.

[230] Vink JM. Genetics of addiction: future focus on gene x environment interaction? J Stud Alcohol Drugs 2016;77(5):684-7.

[231] Crippa JA, Derenusson GN, Chagas MH, Atakan Z, Matin-Santos R, Zuardi AW, et al. Pharmacologic interventions in the treatment of the acute effects of cannabis: A systemic review of literature. Harm Reduct J 2012;9(1):7.

[232] Bonnet U, Preuss UW. The cannabis withdrawal syndrome: current insights. Subst Abuse Rehabil 2017;8:9-37.

[233] Zhand N, Milin R. What do we know about the pharmacotherapeutic management of insomnia in cannabis withdrawal: A systematic review. Am J Addict 2018;27(6):453-64.

[234] Haney M, Cooper ZD, Bedi G, Herrmann E, Comer SD, Reed SC, et al. Guanfacine decreases symptoms of cannabis withdrawal in daily cannabis smokers. Addict Biol 2019;24(4):707-16.

[235] Sherman BJ, McRae-Clark AL. Treatment of cannabis use disorder: Current science and future outlook. Pharmacotherapy 2016;36(5):511-35.

[236] Kleinloog D, Liem-Moolenaar M, Jacobs G, Klaassen E, de Kam M, Hijman R, et al. Does olanzapine inhibit the psychomimetic effects of {Delta} 9-tetrahydrocannabinol? J Psychopharmacol 2012;26(10):1307-16.

[237] Sloan ME, Gowin JL, Ramchandani VA, Hurd YL, Le Foll B. The endocannabinoid system as a target for addiction treatment: Trials and tribulations. Neuropharmacology 2017;124:73-83.

[238] Weinberger AH, Pacek LR, Wall MM, Zvolensky MJ, Copeland J, Galea S, et al. Trends in in cannabis use disorder by cigarette smoking status in the United States, 2002-2016. Drug Alcohol Depend 2018;191:45-51.

[239] Hemsing N, Greaves L. New challenges: Developing gendered and equitable responses to involuntary exposures to electronic nicotine delivery systems (ENDS) and cannabis vaping. Int J Environ Res Public Health 2018;15(10). pii: E2097.

[240] Cassidy RN, Meisel MK, DiGuiseppi G, Balestrieri S, Barnett NP. Initiation of vaporizing cannabis: individual and social network predictors in a longitudinal study of young adults. Drug Alcohol Depend 2018;188:334-40.

[241] Cho BY. Associations of father's lifetime cannabis use disorder with child's initiation of cannabis use, alcohol use, and sexual intercourse by child gender. Subst Use Misuse 2018;53(14): 2330-8.

[242] Baskerville TA, Douglas AJ. Dopamine and oxytocin interactions underlying behaviors: potential contributions to behavioral disorders. CNS Neurosci Ther 2010;16(3):e92-123.

[243] McGregor IS, Bowen MT. Breaking the loop: Oxytocin as a potential treatment for drug addiction. Horm Behav 2012;61(3):331-9.

[244] Gray KM, Carpenter MJ, Baker NL, Desantis SM, Kryway E, Hartwell KJ, et al. A double-blind randomized controlled trail of N-acetylcysteine in cannabis-dependent adolescents. Am J Psychiatry 2012;169(8):805-12.

[245] Weinstein AM, Gorelicki DA. Pharmacologic treatment of cannabis dependence. Curr Pharm Des 2011;17(14):1351-8.

[246] Bhardwaj AK, Allsop DJ, Copeland J, McGregor IS, Dunlop A, Shanahan M, et al. Randomised controlled trial (RCT) of cannabinoid replacement therapy (Nabiximols) for the management of treatment-resistant cannabis dependent patients: a study protocol. BMC Psychiatry 2018;18(1):140.

[247] Mooney LJ, Zhu Y, Yoo C, Valdez J, Moino K, Liao JY, et al. Reduction in cannabis use and functional status in physical health, mental health, and cognition. J Neuroimmune Pharmacol 2018;13(4):479-87.

[248] Peacock A, Leung J, Larney S, Colledge S, Hickman M, Rehm J, et al. Global statistics on alcohol, tobacco and illicit drug use: 2017 status report. Addiction 2018;113(10):1905-26.

[249] Zhao Q, Kim BKE, Li W, Hsiao HY, Rice E. Incarceration history, social network composition, and substance use among homeless youth in Los Angeles. J Addict Dis 2018;37(1-2):64-76.

[250] Gjersing L, Bretteville-Jensen AL, Furuhaugen H, Gjerde H. Illegal substance use among 1,309 music festival attendees: An investigation using oral fluid sample drug tests, breathalysers and questionnaires. Scand J Public Health 2019;47(4):400-7.

[251] Banks DE, Hershberger AR, Pemberton T, Clifton RL, Aalsma MC, Zapolski TCB. Poly-use of cannabis and other substances among juvenile-justice involved youth: variations in psychological and substance-related problems by typology. Am J Drug Alcohol Abuse 2019;45(3):313-22.

[252] Daeppen JB, Billieux J, Achab S, Etter JF, Bertholet N, Deligianni M, et al. Addictions. Rev Med Suisse 2019;15(632-633):14-6. [French]

[253] Beck F, Lermenier-Jeannet A, Nguyen-Thanh V. Lutte contre le tabagisme et autres addictions: état des lieux et perspectives [Monitoring and tackling smoking and other addictions: Current situation and perspectives]. Bull Cancer 2019;106(7-8):656-664. [French]

[254] De Aquino JP, Sherif M, Radhakrishnan R, Cahill JD, Ranganathan M, D'Souza DC. The psychiatric consequences of cannabinoids. Clin Ther 2018;40(9):1448-56.

[255] Ford TC, Hayley AC, Downey LA, Parrott AC. Cannabis: An overview of its adverse acute and chronic effects and its implications. Curr Drug Abuse Rev 2017;10(1):6-18.

[256] Satre DD, Borsari B, Tompkins DA, Ramo D. Psychiatric disorders and comorbid cannabis use: When should we be concerned and what can we do about it? J Clin Psychiatry 2018;79(6): 18ac12268.

[257] Hiemstra M, Nelemans SA, Branje S, van Eijk KR, Hottenga JJ, Vinkers CH, et al. Genetic vulnerability to schizophrenia is associated with cannabis use patterns during adolescence. Drug Alcohol Depend 2018;190:143-50.

[258] deShazo RD, Parker SB, Williams D, Ingram JB, Elsohly M, Rodenmeyer K, et al. Marijuana's effects on brain structure and function: What do we know and what should we do? A brief review and commentary. Am J Med 2019;132(3):281-85.

[259] Lowe DJE, Sasiadek JD, Coles AS, George TP. Cannabis and mental illness: a review. Eur Arch Psychiatry Clin Neurosci 2019;269(1):107-20.

[260] Heinbockel T, Csoka AB. Epigenetic effects of drugs of abuse. Int J Environ Res Public Health 2018;15(10):2098.

[261] Banducci AN, Felton JW, Bonn-Miller MO, Lejuez CW. An examination of the impact of childhood emotional abuse and gender on cannabis use trajectories among community youth. Transl Issues Psychol Sci 2018;4(1):85-98.

[262] Wilson J, Freeman TP, Mackie CJ. Effects of increasing cannabis potency on adolescent health. Lancet Child Adolesc Health 2019;3(2):121-8.

[263] Freeman TP, Groshkova T, Cunningham A, Sedefov R, Griffiths P, Lynskey MT. Increasing potency and price of cannabis in Europe, 2006-16. Addiction. 2019;114(6):1015-23.

[264] Lenton S, Frank VA, Barratt MJ, Potter GR, Decorte T. Growing practices and the use of potentially harmful chemical additives among a sample of small-scale cannabis growers in three countries. Drug Alcohol Depend 2018;192:250-6.

[265] Dryburgh LM, Bolan NS, Grof CPL, Galettis P, Schneider J, Lucas CJ, et al. Cannabis contaminants: sources, distribution, human toxicity and pharmacologic effects. Br J Clin Pharmacol 2018;84(11):2468-76.

[266] Sullivan N, Elzinga S, Raber JC. Determination of pesticide residues in cannabis smoke. J Toxicol 2013;2013:378168.

[267] Stone D. Cannabis, pesticides and conflicting laws: the dilemma for legalized States and implications for public health. Regul Toxicol Pharmacol 2014;69(3):284-8.

[268] No Authors listed. Standard method performance requirements (SMPRs®) 2018.011: Identification and quantitation of selected pesticide residues in dried cannabis materials. J AOAC Int 2019;102(1):349-52.

[269] Cook JL, Blake JM. Cannabis: Implications for pregnancy, fetal development, and longer-term health outcomes. J Obstet Gynaecol Can 2018;40(9):1204-7.

[270] Godleski SA, Shisler S, Eiden RD, Heustis MA. Co-use of tobacco and marijuana during pregnancy: Pathways to externalizing behavior problems in early childhood. Neurotoxicol Teratol 2018;69:39-48.

[271] Metz TD, Borgelt LM. Marijuana use in pregnancy and while breastfeeding. Obstet Gynecol 2018; 132(5):1198-210.

[272] McDonnell BP, Keogan S, Clancy L, Regan C. Smoking cessation support and obstetrical outcomes in an Irish maternity hospital. Eur J Obstet Gynecol Reprod Biol 2019;232:1-4.

[273] Romano E, Torres-Saavedra P, Voas RB, Lacey JH. Marijuana and the risk of fatal car crashes: What can we learn from FARS and NRS data? J Prim Prev 2017;38(3):315-28.

[274] Pertwee RG. Cannabis and cannabinoids: pharmacology and rationale for clinical use. Foresch Komplementarmed 1999;Suppl 3:12-5.

[275] Beaulieu P, Rice AS. The pharmacology of cannabinoids derivatives: are there applications to treatment of pain? Ann Fr Anesth Rhanim 2002;21(6):493-508.

[276] Zheng Y, Smith PF. Cannabinoid drugs: will they relieve or exacerbate tinnitus? Curr Opin Neurol 2019;32(1):131-6.

[277] Shannon S, Lewis N, Lee H, Hughes S. Cannabidiol in anxiety and sleep: A large case series. Perm J 2019;23:18-041.

[278] Rajapakse T, Davenport WJ. Phytomedicines in the treatment of migraine. CNS Drugs 2019; 33(5):399-415.

[279] Alsherbiny MA, Li CG. Medicinal cannabis-potential drug interactions. Medicines (Basel) 2018; 6(1):3.

[280] Wang GC, Davies SD, Halmo LS, Saas A, Mistry RD. Impact of marijuana legalization in Colorado on adolescent emergency and urgent care visits. J Adolesc Health 2018;63(2):239-41.

[281] Wang GS, Hoyte C, Roosevelt G, Heard K. The continued impact of marijuana legalization on unintentional pediatric exposures in Colorado. Clin Pediatr (Phila) 2019;58(1):114-6.

[282] Chow RM, Marascalchi B, Abrams WB, Peiris NA, Odonkor CA, Cohen SP. Driving under the influence of cannabis: A framework for future policy. Anesth Analg 2019;128(6):1300-8.

[283] Karbakhsh M, Smith J, Pike I. "Where does the high road lead?" Potential implications of cannabis legalization for pediatric injuries in Canada. Can J Public Health 2018;109(5-6):752-5.

[284] Hasin DS. US Epidemiology of cannabis use and associated problems. Neuropsychopharmacology 2018;43(1):195-212.

[285] Hines L, Glick J, Bilka K, Lantos JD. Medical marijuana for minors may be considered child abuse. Pediatrics 2018;142(4):e20174310.

[286] Danovitch I, Gorelick DA. State of the art treatments for cannabis dependence. Psychiatr Clin North Am 2012;35(2);309-26.

[287] Forray A, Sofuoglu M: Future pharmacologic treatments for substance use disorders. Br J Clin Pharmacol 2014;77(2):382-400.

[288] Lévesque A, Le Foll B. When and how to treat possible cannabis use disorder. Med Clin North Am 2018;102(4):667-81.

[289] Hill KP, George TP. Cannabis legalisation in Canada: a crucial trial balloon. Lancet Psychiatry 2019;6(1):5-6.

[290] D'Souza DC, Cortes-Briones J, Creatura G, Bluez G, Thurnauer H, Deaso E, et al. Efficacy and safety of a fatty acid amide hydrolase inhibitor (PF-04457845) in the treatment of cannabis withdrawal and dependence in men: a double-blind, placebo-controlled, parallel group, phase 2a single-site randomised controlled trial. Lancet Psychiatry 2019;6(1):35-45.

[291] Lee DC, Schlienz NJ, Peters EN, Dworkin RH, Turk DC, Strain EC, et al. Systematic review of outcome domains and measures used in psychological and pharmacological treatment trials for cannabis use disorder. Drug Alcohol Depend 2019;194:500-17.

[292] Perron BE, Holt KR, Yeagley E, Ilgen M. Mental health functioning and severity of cannabis withdrawal among medical cannabis users with chronic pain. Drug Alcohol Depend 2019;194:401-9.

[293] Jacobs-Brichford E, Manson KF, Roitman JD. Effects of chronic cannabinoid exposure during adolescence on reward preference and mPFC activation in adulthood. Physiol Behav 2019;199: 395-404.

[294] Bogaty SER, Crouse JJ, Hickie IB, Hermens DF. The neuropsychological profiles of young psychosis patients with and without current cannabis use. Cogn Neuropsychiatry 2019;9:1-14.

[295] Winningham RD, Banks DE, Buetlich MR, Aalsma MC, Zapolski TCB. Substance use disorder and posttraumatic stress disorder symptomatology on behavioral outcomes among juvenile justice youth. Am J Addict 2019;28(1):29-35.

[296] Goodman S, Leos-Toro C, Hammond D. Methods to assess cannabis consumption in population surveys: Results of cognitive interviewing. Qual Health Res 2019;29(10):1474-82.

[297] Palace ZJ, Reingold DA. Medical cannabis in skilled nursing facility: A novel approach to improving symptom management and quality of life. J Am Med Dir Assoc 2019;20(1):94-8.

[298] Shackleton N, Milne BJ, Jerrim J. Socioeconomic inequalities in adolescent substance use: Evidence from twenty-four European countries. Subst Use Misuse 2019;54(6):1044-9.

[299] Campbell ANC, McCarty D, Rieckmann T, McNeeley J, Rotrosen J, Wu TL. Interpretation and integration of the federal substance use privacy protection rule in integrated health systems: A qualitative analysis. J Subst Abuse Treat 2019;97:41-6.

[300] Greydanus DE. Substance abuse disorders in adolescents: Pharmacologic management. In: Greydanus DE, Calles Jr JL, Patel DR, Nazeer A, Merrick J, eds. Clinical aspects of psychopharmacology in childhood and adolescence, second edition. New York: Nova Science, 2017:261-76.

[301] Pattnaik F, Nanda S, Mohanty S, Dalai AK, Kumar V, Ponnusamy SK, Naik S. Cannabis: Chemistry, extraction and therapeutic applications. Chemosphere. 2022 Feb;289:133012. doi: 10.1016/j.chemosphere.2021.133012.

[302] Bannigan P, Evans JC, Allen C. Shifting the Paradigm on Cannabis Safety. Cannabis Cannabinoid Res. 2022 Feb;7(1):3-10. doi: 10.1089/can.2020.0003.

[303] Hamid MA, Shaikh R, Gunaseelan L, Salim J, Arulchelvan A, Tulloch T. Recreational Cannabis Legalization in Canada: A Pediatrics Perspective. Subst Use Misuse. 2022;57(3):481-483. doi: 10.1080/10826084.2021.2012689.

[304] Rømer Thomsen K, Thylstrup B, Kenyon EA, Lees R, Baandrup L, Feldstein Ewing SW, Freeman TP. Cannabinoids for the treatment of cannabis use disorder: New avenues for reaching and helping youth? Neurosci Biobehav Rev. 2022 Jan;132:169-180. doi: 10.1016/j.neubiorev.2021.11.033.

[305] Hill KP, Gold MS, Nemeroff CB, McDonald W, Grzenda A, Widge AS, Rodriguez C, Kraguljac NV, Krystal JH, Carpenter LL. Risks and Benefits of Cannabis and Cannabinoids in Psychiatry. Am J Psychiatry. 2022 Feb;179(2):98-109. doi: 10.1176/appi.ajp.2021.21030320.

Chapter 11

Psychosocial treatments for substance use disorders

Muhammad Ather[1,*], MRCPsych, Nehdia Hashemi[2], MD, Ahsan Nazeer[1], MD and Muhammad Waqar Azeem[1], MD

[1]Department of Psychiatry, Sidra Medicine, Doha, Qatar

[2]Department of Clinical Academic Sciences, Qatar University School of Medicine, Doha, Qatar

Abstract

Worldwide use of illicit drugs is increasing, and substance use disorders (SUDs) have become a significant mental health problem in the West. Although the majority of young people do not use illicit drugs and of those who do use illicit substances, only a minority will develop serious problems; however, substance misuse can still be damaging to the developing brain. Continued use of illicit drugs can trigger or exacerbate developmental problems, particularly in those who are at risk or have a pre-existing developmental, physical or mental health conditions. The increased recognition of SUDs, its changing patterns, the impairment it causes and its cost to the society has promoted the interest to evaluate the effectiveness of available treatments. During the last thirty years, numerous pharmacological as well as psychosocial treatments have been developed and validated. Pharmacological treatments usually target withdrawal symptoms while psychosocial treatments are directed at drug use behaviors in general. There is a significant and growing evidence in support of psychosocial therapies on its own as well as in combination with pharmacological treatments for SUDs. In this discussion, we have described the various psychosocial treatments as well as reviewed the available evidence for such treatments and recommendations.

Introduction

Drugs have always been part of our society, some considered *legal* while others listed as *illegal*; most commonly used substances are alcohol and tobacco. These drugs can be addictive, trigger mental health problems, and cause impairments in day-to-day functioning of the user (1). Epidemiological trends for substance use disorders (SUDs) in children and adolescent vary

* ***Correspondence:*** Muhammad Ather, MRCPsych, Assistant Professor of Clinical Psychiatry, Weill Cornell Medical College, Consultant Child and adolescent psychiatrist, Sidra Medicine, Doha, Qatar. Email: mather@sidra.org.

In: Behavioral Pediatrics III
Editors: Donald E. Greydanus, Dilip R. Patel, Ahsan Nazeer et al.
ISBN: 979-8-88697-060-9

from country to country. Findings from the studies of nationally representative samples of the United States youth reveal that the lifetime prevalence of alcohol use disorders is approximately 8%, and illicit drug use disorders are 2–3% (2).

During 14-17 years of age, rates of illicit use are equal in both sexes; however, after age 17 rates are higher in males (11%) and lower in females (5.6%) (3). Substance use varies by age and also depends on the availability of the specific drug. SUDs are rare before the age of 10 and peak around age 20 years of age. In the United States (US), each year nearly 6% of adolescents start using illicit drugs while 10% begin drinking alcohol. Within Europe, the United Kingdom (UK) has the highest rates of binge drinking and cannabis use in young people; also, there are approximately 13,000 hospital admissions each year linked to young people's drinking (4).

There are a number of reasons why young people use these substances, and some of them are listed in Table 1. Other than alcohol, tobacco, and cannabis, youth also commonly experiment with inhalants in glue, cleaning agents, and medications that are prescribed to family members. Also common in some countries is use of lysergic acid diethylamide (LSD), amphetamine, and ecstasy (3-4 methylenedioxymethamphetamine [MDMA]); in addition, the difficulty in accessing cocaine, opioids and other injectable drugs limit their use in this population.

Table 1. Factors leading to substance use

1.	Issue of experimentation
2.	Need to feel inclusive in peer groups
3.	Avoidance of feelings of unhappiness
4.	Need for coping strategy to overcome depression
5.	Need to overcome anxious moods
6.	Others (see text)

SUDs are one of the most prevalent psychiatric disorders among young people aged 9 to 21 years (5). Young people with SUDs have high rates of comorbidity; for example, 60-80% have conduct disorder, up to 50% have attention-deficit/hyperactivity disorder (ADHD) and up to 25% have major depression as well as anxiety disorder (6). SUD is also very common among young people with bipolar disorder and psychosis. In addition, studies have noted the association of SUDs with antisocial and risk-taking behaviors (7).

Millions of adolescents all over the world meet one or more criteria of SUDs from the American Psychiatric Association's DSM-5 (Diagnostic and statistical manual of mental disorders, 5th edition) and/or World Health Organization's ICD-10 (International statistical classification of diseases and related health problems, 10th edition). Factors that influence the longitudinal course of substance misuse include those listed in Table 2. Drug use at an early age is an important predictor of the development of substance use disorder (SUD); also, the majority of individuals who are at risk of developing a SUD begin to use in their teenage years.

During the last decade, many prevention and treatment programs have been developed and implemented through the services for young people with SUDs. These programs play an essential role in reducing the problem as they aim to strengthen various protective factors including skills for self-control and improved parental monitoring. Also important is reducing SUD risk factors including contact with peers using substances, academic struggles, social adversity and early screening as well as treatment of mental health problems. There is consistently growing evidence that psychosocial interventions improve outcome for those with substance use disorders (7).

Table 2. Factors influencing course of substance use

1.	Pharmacological effects of various drugs
2.	Availability of drugs
3.	Acceptance of the drug taken
4.	Age of onset
5.	Comorbid mental health conditions
6.	Genetic disposition
7.	Social adversity
8.	Social rewards from other drug users
9.	Others

Psychosocial treatment of substance use disorders is a broad term that includes numerous non-pharmacological modalities with the goal of achieving and sustaining abstinence, or change patterns of use to avoid harm as well as improve functioning. The long-term goal of maintaining abstinence lies at the heart of effective SUD treatment programs, and psychosocial interventions are considered to be the key to success in achieving this goal.

Implementation and results of these interventions may differ as the efficacy of these modalities usually is influenced by various factors as noted in Table 3. Despite the individualized nature of these programs, common and critical elements of these modalities include the long-term goals of making positive lifestyle changes and maintaining a drug-free lifestyle or a life free of drug-related harm.

Table 3. Factors influencing efficacy of substance use treatment

1.	Patient characteristics
2.	Nature of drugs involved
3.	Types of pharmacological interventions that are being used
4.	Psychiatric comorbidities
5.	Psychosocial stressors that may be unique to a particular individual
6.	Others (see text)

Failure to engage adolescents in effective treatment for substance use disorders is one of the principal reasons for adult substance use disorders, since most substance use behavior begins during childhood and adolescence. While experimentation with getting high (euphoric) via drug use typically begins in the adolescent years, those who find this practice most captivating will progress over time into chronic substance dependence and their entire life existence is infused with drug use as a significant goal. Demonstrating the chronicity of SUD is the extent to which many require multiple SUD treatments and the number of consequences that must accumulate before they achieve recovery. Behavioral therapies have long been known to be an effective treatment option for common psychiatric disorders; indeed, since the 1990's, the National Institute on Drug Abuse (NIDA) has been supporting research and implementation of these approaches in community settings. The following is a brief review of these commonly used psychosocial interventions.

Primary prevention programs

Primary prevention programs constitute education about harmful substances, why as well as how to avoid such substances, and how to access help if needed. These interventions can be delivered universally (i.e., to all the children in their schools) or can be selective for those at risk of developing substance misuse. Following the identification of "the vulnerable group," specific skills training to this group of vulnerable youth and their families are given to reduce the risk factors and to strengthen the protective factors.

Assessment as an intervention

The National Institute of Clinical Excellence (NICE) has acknowledged that a comprehensive assessment of drug use is a consistent part of effective intervention (8). NICE compared an assessment-only arm with assessment plus intervention or no intervention. However, it was perceived that if comparator groups were offered assessment, improved outcomes were consistently reported. The NICE committee also concluded that the evidence was weak from reviews that assessments of substance use and other risky behaviors may prompt reductions in drug use.

An important literature review has been published of several electronic databases and journals that publish psychosocial issues, assessment, guidelines and treatment in substance use disorders; it reported an overall effectiveness of psychological interventions while some psychosocial interventions are effective for many forms of drug abuse and these interventions are cognitive behavioral therapy (CBT), motivational interviewing (MI) and relapse prevention (9). For opiate abuse, combined interventions (i.e., psychosocial and substitute prescription) are more effective than any single intervention.

Motivational treatments

Motivational interviewing

Effectiveness of *motivational interviewing* (*MI*) is mostly studied in alcohol use disorders. A meta-analysis found that MI was an effective intervention for reducing hazardous drinking, particularly in short-term and was more effective in young people with an occasional binging pattern of drinking (10). A Cochrane review compared MI with no intervention and found MI was effective in reducing the extent of drug abuse (11). There is evidence that MI is more effective if offered in combination with other psychosocial interventions. These authors recommend MI to be used in combination with other interventions where possible even though it can be used on its own as an effective intervention (11).

Motivational treatments are aimed at helping individuals act and make a change with the long-term goal of abstinence from substances. Young people may or may not show any motivation to change their substance-taking habit as this may be the only source of their pleasure. MI techniques accept the ambivalence that occurs in achieving change. This process of change occurs during therapy sessions and is characterized by moving through the stages noted in Table 4 (12).

On the basis of this process, *motivational interviewing* (MI) is designed to reduce ambivalence and to promote change. In this process, the therapist expresses empathy through listening and identifies discrepancies between the patient's goals and current behaviors while avoiding arguments as well as confrontations in addition to supporting self-efficacy and optimism. Individuals may cycle through "stages of readiness to change" numerous times before adopting a recovery-oriented lifestyle. The MI approach may motivate the individuals for total abstinence or to reduce the intake of substances in a manner that leads to no harm or reduced harm. These stages of change are now considered (see Table 4).

Table 4. Stages of change in substance use management (12)

1.	Pre-contemplation (denial)
2.	Contemplation (ambivalence)
3.	Preparation
4.	Action
5.	Maintenance
6.	Termination

Pre-contemplation stage

This stage identifies the individuals who are not ready to change and are not consciously aware of their negative behaviors nor the consequences of their behaviors. The young person will deny the relationship between the problem behavior and the consequences that have occurred, as well as the future risks anticipated by their parents or caregivers. They are not concerned about the current intensity or frequency of their use. They may react with surprise or hostility if their drug use is described as a problem by various family members. They may externalize their substance taking habits onto those around them (e.g., parents, the police, and teachers) who seen intolerant of their substance use. At times, these individuals remain in a pre-contemplation stage for years while rarely thinking about change. Research has identified that at least 80 percent of individuals with substance abuse disorders are currently in a pre-contemplation or contemplation stage.

Adolescents usually display less motivation to change, in part because they may have faced fewer significant adverse consequences than adults due to the shorter period of abuse. Besides, still developing cognitive processes in the adolescent may cause difficulty in recalling the details of the intoxication episode(s) (13). The most common defense mechanisms used by young substance users during the pre-contemplation stage include these: a) minimizing the risk and severity of adverse consequences of substance misuse; b) blaming others for their habit; and c) comparing their positive attributes with non-substance users to justify their habit of substance misuse.

Numerous social or legal situations might result in a call to the treatment facility, either by the youth or by the loved ones who have stated that the substance use is risky and harmful to self or others. The youth's response depends on their perception of the problem as well as the manner in which the facts are presented. They will be much more willing to engage if the relevant information is provided in a supportive and empathic manner. Being judgmental, dismissive, or confrontational will lead to further denial, anger, and defensiveness.

Assessing the emotional state in which the patient comes to treatment is an integral part of therapy. Youth referred to treatment will exhibit a range of emotions associated with the experiences that brought them to counseling. They may be feeling angry, withdrawn or guilty and may be displaying all of these feelings at the same time. These emotions can be managed through reflective listening.

The therapist must engage the youth in this phase while remaining neutral, avoiding confrontation, and trying to understand the world from the patient's point of view. The therapist provides feedback and explores the patient's perspective. In the therapy sessions, the patient's hopes are discussed, connections between choices and the consequences of those choices are made, and the discrepancy between actions and goals is highlighted. At times, involving families during this phase promote engagement with the patient by helping the patient to connect the substance use behaviors with identifiable consequences; indeed, family members are often able to provide useful examples of risky behaviors and subsequent consequences. Various themes may arise during these sessions as outlined in Table 5.

Table 5. Themes that typically arise during therapy sessions (see text)

1.	Youth may lack sufficient knowledge of the impact of substance use on self or the family. Providing feedback in an empathetic manner and supportive demeanor usually is helpful.
2.	Youth may be afraid of losing control of their lives. Shifting the energy and reframing personal control works well with these individuals.
3.	Youth may feel hopeless to change. This can happen in the face of previous treatment failures and when they do not feel that they have any energy left to engage in treatment in a meaningful way. Understanding barriers to recovery are helpful in these circumstances.
4.	Youth may have a complete lack of insight. They rationalize and feel that the drug use is a problem for everyone except for them. Self-reflection and patience in building rapport are essential to working with these individuals.

Contemplation stage

The *contemplation* stage follows the pre-contemplation and is characterized by the patient considering making a positive change in the future. The patient begins to become aware of his addictive behavior and its causal relationship to consequences. However, at the same time, the patient also values certain aspects of the substance use positively (e.g., relief of social anxiety, fitting in with peers, improving performance), and shows some reluctance to abstain while wanting to change. The challenge at the beginning of this phase of treatment is to create a safe and supportive environment in which the youth can feel comfortable about engaging in productive dialog. Adolescents are particularly prone to rebellion against adults, so confrontational approaches are more likely to promote defensive resistance. Without adequate support, patients will procrastinate deciding to change which can lead to chronicity of the disorder and accumulation of adverse consequences.

During this phase, by examining the pros and cons of continued substance use along with benefits of recovery, the therapist helps the patient to resolve ambivalence. During the contemplation phase, the decisional balance between pros and cons is reasonably even; however, by thoughtful evaluation, this balance gradually shifts in favor of non-use of substances in which benefits outweigh the risks of abstaining from substance use. On the other hand, if the perception of the patient is another way around – i.e., benefits outweighs the risks of taking the substance – it will lead to a return to pre-contemplation, relapse or continuing substance abuse with dropping out of the treatment program.

During this stage, the therapist does not advise nor seek action, but patiently waits until the patient is ready for the change. The therapist also makes clear the discrepancies between values and actions in addition to asking about positive and negative aspects of past periods of abstinence. Listening is key to moving on to the next stage. When the patient expresses a genuine desire to change, the therapist validates this statement and summarizes the patient's comments on substance use as well as abstinence; also, the therapist explores new behaviors including better decision-making, and participation in treatment as well as recovery support activities.

Those with dependence may do better when things in their environment are going well, but they may resume former heavier drinking patterns when under stress (14). The brain reward center is a single entity, triggered by a wide variety of addictive drugs; thus, it makes sense to recommend staying away from all drugs that have addictive potential or can trigger a relapse of drug behavior. However, the goal of abstinence from drugs that are socially accepted (such as alcohol and cannabis) and prescribed medications (such as opioids, anxiolytics, and stimulants) may not be readily acceptable for adolescents.

In the individual work with a teenage patient, the therapist looks at the reasons for the use of intoxicants. If reasons are relief of unpleasant feelings (e.g., anxiety, depression, pain, boredom), these might need to be addressed to facilitate the patient's decision making in giving up substance use. If the patient is using substances due to social pressure of the peer group, encouraging and helping them to change the peer group may be critical in the process of change; this may be challenging depending upon various factors including where one lives, the school that is attended, and patterns of substance use among current peers. Adolescents usually have little influence over these matters other than choices of friends. A realistic understanding of the process of one's substance use behavior, including the frequency and amount consumed, may be helpful to tackle the fantasy of becoming a non-problem substance user.

Preparation stage

The *preparation* stage is significant for the patient's intentions to act "shortly." Such individuals make an action plan at this stage and work actively with the therapist to execute their plans shortly. During this stage, the therapist clarifies the specific goals with them and provides support as well as guidance to succeed. In this stage, it is appropriate to counsel family members to curtail expressions of negativity in exchange for recovery of supportive expressions.

In this phase, the therapist clarifies this patient's own goals of and strategies for change. The significance of the decision to change is acknowledged. He/she works with this youth to strengthen the commitment while caution is provided that the road ahead is challenging but very important, and that relapse should not disrupt the patient-clinician relationship. A menu of options for change or treatment is provided which usually includes inpatient treatment, outpatient treatment and the 12-step program; also, help is provided to decide on a suitable and achievable action plan. With the youth's permission, expertise and advice are offered, and barriers to change are addressed. Social support is elicited, and the information is gathered about what has worked in the past either for him or for his other peers in the treatment.

Action stage

The *action* is the stage during which the individual makes specific changes in his /her behavior. Complete abstinence from some psychoactive substances may be attempted by some, while others may attempt to control the amount or frequency of substance use. For some patients, entry into a formal substance abuse treatment program may be necessary to support and maintain abstinence. Peer interactional group therapy may be useful for adolescents, but this may be counterproductive if the therapist is unable to curb unhealthy crosstalk between group members, within or outside of group sessions; indeed, such discussions may glorify drug use or result in different or additional substance use. Dishion and colleagues reported on two experimental studies that demonstrated increased substance use and deviant behavior among low-risk youth who participated with high-risk youth in therapy groups (15).

Neurobiological research on individuals with drug use reveal that both cortical gray matter and white matter in frontal lobes sustain widespread volume loss (16). These changes are more pronounced in those with alcoholism but are also seen in those with other drugs of abuse. In individuals with one month of cocaine abstinence, researchers have noticed higher gray matter density and lower subcortical gray matter density that correlated with performance on memory and reaction time tasks (17).

Some of these neurobiological changes explain the impaired decision making with poor impulse control in these youth that may be manifested by difficulties in attention, concentration, memory and learning new material during treatment. In practical terms, this may mean that youth may not have enough cognitive flexibility or sound mental structures in place to enable them to make the difficult decisions that they will face during the *action* stage of treatment.

In this phase, a youth requires help executing an action plan and may have to work on skills to maintain sobriety. The therapist should acknowledge the youth's feelings and experiences as a normal part of recovery. Brief interventions could be applied throughout this stage to prevent relapse. In this phase, the therapist avoids passive therapy and is more actively engaged in behavior change-oriented treatments. Specific suggestions are given that include those listed in Table 6.

Table 6. Therapist's goals for the patient during the active phase of treatment

1.	Facilitate participation in self-help group meetings
2.	Change the unhealthy peer group
3.	Try alternative recreational activities
4.	Deal with underlying emotional problems
5.	Others (see text)

Important elements of treatment include offering patients help to identify craving and cues that trigger the urges to use substances and equipping them with strategies to cope with urges. Also, a patient's ability to share successful and unsuccessful attempts to avert relapses is critical. It is also important to encourage honesty in treatment sessions, so guilt and shame do not promote concealing these important slips from the therapist that reveal gaps in the treatment protocol. Frequent drug testing (i.e., saliva, urine) is critical in detecting slips and making it clear to the patient that lying to the therapist will not be effective; in outpatient settings missed visits may be in part, motivated by a desire to conceal slips and dodge shame.

Patients may also benefit from participation in self-help groups. In large cities, there are many options, but in rural communities and smaller towns, there may not be appropriate self-help groups for adolescents. Online recovery-oriented chat rooms exist that may be helpful but only if they have appropriate parental and professional oversight. Alcoholics Anonymous (AA) and Narcotics Anonymous (NA) have a strong focus on spiritual investment mentioning faith in "God" or a "higher power" in the literature and steps. Those with objections to religion may find themselves distracted from the healing elements of these groups. Other programs provide alternatives in which faith or religion is not promoted as an element in the recovery process;

these include SMART Recovery, Secular Organization for Sobriety (SOS), Women for Sobriety, Rational Recovery™, and Moderation Management (18).

Cognitive behavioral therapy (CBT) is the mainstay during the *Action* stage. Relapse prevention treatment is a variant of CBT that is aimed at maintaining abstinence. After the initial period of sobriety, patients are taught to identify and deal with high-risk situations including drug paraphernalia, peers who use drugs, and stressful life situations that may trigger urges to use substances. Use of coping strategies are typically effective that include distraction, disclosing the urge to a support person, or just waiting until it (the urge) passes. These strategies are also recommended at 12-step groups. "Slips" are identified and are processed in the treatment sessions as "learning experiences." Efforts are made to differentiate these brief incidents from complete loss of control or "relapses."

Maintenance stage

The *maintenance* stage is characterized by the patient's and therapist's working together to prevent the relapse and learning to anticipate and avoid tempting situations as well as triggers that set off renewed substance use. Patients may remain in this stage from months to years before relapsing, depending on the number of personal and environmental factors that are present. However, those patients who are not ready for the sustained effort that is needed to maintain sobriety do relapse during times of emotional distress. In these cases, the efforts to guard against relapse were not all in vain. Youth who return to substance abuse do so with a better understanding of the social and psychological hazards of continued drug use. With it, they may be able to acknowledge that some of the goals they set and certain strategies they attempted are ineffective. With better insight into the dynamics of their substance abuse, they are better equipped to make another attempt at recovery, and to succeed (19).

It is in this phase that significant underlying issues start emerging such as poor self-image/self-esteem, relationship problems, shame/guilt, and memories of past traumatic events. Many of these youth need support and treatment by qualified health professional to manage these psychological themes. Process-oriented group therapy may be appropriate for some youth who are finally able to confront the painful realities of being abused and traumatized. With gradual improvement, they begin to understand healthy mutuality and start getting more skilled in resolving conflicts without the maladaptive influence of drugs. If the underlying conflicts are left unresolved, there is always a risk that they will engage in other compulsive behavior, such as excessive exercise, overeating, gambling, or other risk-taking behaviors (20).

Contingency management and community reinforcement approaches

Contingency management (CM) intervention theories are based on the literature that regards drug use as a form of operant conditioning in which behavior is shaped by its consequences. The likelihood of drug use is influenced by the context in which use occurs; also, alternative non-drug reinforcers decrease substance use if they are available in sufficient magnitude and according to a schedule that is incompatible with drug use. These observations form the theoretical basis for contingency-management approaches in which the patient's environment is gradually reorganized, and drug reinforcements are systematically replaced with alternative neutral reinforcing activities (21, 22).

There are various forms of CM approaches and one commonly used type, popularized by Higgins and colleagues, is called voucher-based reinforcement therapy (VBRT) (23). VBRT has particularly shown success in individuals with cocaine use. In VBRT, individuals receive "vouchers" that have various monetary values for providing urine or breath samples that are negative for the tested drugs. These vouchers are withheld when there is laboratory evidence of recent drug use and increase in value when the results are negative. Once earned, vouchers are exchanged for items or services that are compatible with a drug-free lifestyle. A bonus is provided after three consecutive negative urine drug screens, in order to continue reinforcing continuous abstinence.

Another CM technique that was developed by Petry is called the "variable magnitude of reinforcement procedure" or "fish-bowl" (24, 25). In this technique, patients receive draws from the paper-slips kept in a fishbowl for providing a negative specimen. If the specimen indicates recent drug use, the draw is withheld. Each time when a draw is held, the patient has a chance of winning a "prize," the value of which varies. Similar to the VBRT technique, patients receive bonus draws after submitting a given number of consecutive negative specimens.

These approaches have good empirical support and have been known to be an effective management strategy from studies as early as the 1970s. In one study, alcoholic human volunteers were placed in residential facilities where they were allowed to purchase and consume ethanol at will. Numerous consequences to this behavior were applied with the goal to modify ethanol self-administration. Researchers noted an increase in abstinence when the volunteers were provided with monetary reinforcements and were given access to alternate reinforcements. Abstinence also increased when the amount of work required to access alcohol was increased and when periods of isolation were imposed (14). There is also a significant body of evidence from methadone clinics that support the notion that positive consequences (rewards) are more effective in maintaining these patients in treatment and managing long-term abstinence than negative consequences (26).

Community reinforcement approach (CRA)

Community reinforcement approach (CRA) provides a way to achieve abstinence by using the contingencies that are present in the individual's natural environment. In CRA, patients learn to recognize the antecedents and consequences of their behavior. Ongoing counseling is provided to help them change their daily activities as well as their social contacts and to pursue a healthier lifestyle. Therapists gradually help these patients receive their reinforcements from alternate recreational or other activities that do not rely on drugs to have fun. This phase usually lasts for 24 weeks after which patients are encouraged to be in contact with the counselors on a monthly basis for brief therapy sessions.

Individual therapy sessions focus on changing attitudes and learning skills such as anger management, problem-solving, and assertiveness. This approach is different to the voucher and coupon-based programs that are placed for the explicit reason to get a negative urine drug screening (UDS) specimen. Comprehensive treatment programs usually involve both strategies in which individuals gradually phase from voucher-based programs that provide initial abstinence to more naturalistic resources in their community to maintain long-term abstinence.

Researchers have found an important relationship between the length of time spent in the program and the treatment outcomes including longer abstinence as well as decreased legal troubles. In the Drug Abuse Treatment Outcome Study (DATOS), 10,000 users from 96 programs were evaluated for long-term outcomes; this study identified a minimum threshold of 90 days for the treatment to be effective on a longer-term basis (27).

Cognitive-behavioral approaches

Cognitive behavioral therapy (CBT) for substance use disorders is a time-limited and structured therapy that has been in use for a long time with good efficacy. These interventions are based on well-known learning principles and theorize that behavior is influenced by cognitive processes including thoughts and feelings. Patient use substances as a maladaptive coping mechanism and providing patients with healthy coping mechanisms will reduce the need for substance use. As with any other behavioral treatment, the CBT model relies upon the individual's motivation to change the existing behavior and to replace it with new healthy behavior. *Motivation* is a dynamic phenomenon, and numerous factors influence this state at a given time. Dissatisfaction with the old behaviors increases motivation to replace them with new behaviors (28).

Therapists conceptualize drug use as a learned behavior that is associated with certain internal or external triggers. Some of these triggers act as reminders for these youth to self-administer drugs. The triggers that led to the use of drugs are called *antecedents*. Drug use following these cues/triggers usually leads to desired rewarding effects such as "feeling high" or "becoming relaxed;" they are called *consequences* or rewards that further consolidate the behavior.

A central element of CBT is anticipating likely problems and enhancing patients' self-control by helping them develop effective coping strategies. Behavioral part of CBT treatment is based on 1) detailed analysis of the target behavior including identification of antecedents and consequences; 2) skills training; and 3) relapse prevention. The cognitive part includes addressing and changing those cognitions, thinking patterns, and beliefs which promote or maintain substance use.

Functional analysis

Functional analysis is the analysis of the target behavior and is an essential first step in the treatment process. According to classical conditioning, neutral stimuli can become associated with cravings and drug use. Such neutral triggers in a non-substance user do not elicit craving responses; however, in substance users these triggers become paired with each other, and as a result, a previously neutral stimulus becomes a trigger for drug use.

Structured and non-structured interviews can be conducted to identify the patterns of use, triggers, and consequences. These triggers are then organized in a hierarchical pattern according to their frequency of occurrence and the strength of association with the target behavior. Numerous behavioral strategies and techniques have been derived from the above theories. In *cue exposure*, an individual is exposed to the stimulus that is closely associated with drug use. In therapy, substance users are repeatedly exposed to triggers without being permitted to use the substance. The model of extinction is applied in this strategy with a goal to disrupt the cycle of antecedent leading to substance use behavior.

Drug refusal skills (DRS)

After the functional analysis of the behavior, the main goal of CBT is to teach the necessary drug refusal skills. Behavioral theorists believe that after motivation, specific sets of skills are needed in order to learn and sustain new behavior (29). Numerous factors threaten long-term abstinence including cravings, withdrawal symptoms, and social stressors. DRS training consists of numerous manual-based approaches that teach the necessary skills to overcome the above barriers in achieving and maintaining abstinence. These skills are listed in Table 7.

Table 7. Drug refusal skills (see text)

1.	Relaxation training to combat stress
2.	Using assertive skills instead of passivity or aggressiveness
3.	Techniques to say "no" to the invitations from peers
4.	Anger management skills
5.	Handling criticism and compliments gracefully without becoming upset
6.	Expressing feelings and emotions in intimate relationships
7.	Managing negative thoughts (e.g., resentments, negative self-talk)
8.	Selecting and engaging in pleasant non-drug activities to maintain a balance in daily life
9.	Decision-making training to foresee the consequences of the decisions
10.	Problem-solving (i.e., identification of the problem, reviewing alternative solutions, and choosing the best possible solution among these options)
11.	Expanding the social network to include peers who do not use drugs, and diminishing exposure to peers who do.

Relapse prevention (RP)

Relapse prevention treatment assumes that an individual's ability to maintain abstinence is directly related to his/her ability to successfully negotiate stressful situations without relying on drug use. Therapists help individuals identify high-risk situations such as mood dysregulations, triggers, and social situations where peers are promoting the use of substances. Specific areas of problems are evaluated in depth, and a plan of coping strategies is crafted for each of these situations. Decision-making and interpersonal skills that patients learn from therapy are helpful for individuals to make rational decisions that include avoiding risky situations as well as encounters. In this model, "slips" are considered part of the treatment process in which the motivational aspects of the individual are reevaluated, the situations that lead to the slips are analyzed, and strategies are discussed to prevent complete relapse (30).

Family interventions

Adolescent substance abuse has always been considered as a multidimensional problem with impaired interactions among individuals, family, and society. Family interventions have been one of the mainstays of successful substance abuse treatment for such adolescents. Research has shown that genetic factors play a significant role in the etiology of SUD. Parental SUD increases the youth's risk of substance misuse due to their role models using drugs, easy access to drugs (in the home) and lack of parental concern /supervision. Heritability estimates typically range from 50% to 60% constituting about half of the cause of substance abuse by adolescents while the environment explains the other half. Family studies have found higher rates of drug abuse among siblings, particularly those whose parents had SUD (31).

Traumatic life experiences associated with various factors or events, as listed in Table 8, increase the risk of SUD. The environment is also important in determining whether a youth will experiment with drugs based on ease of access and influences by others. Other than genetic and environmental factors, preexisting comorbid conditions may play a role in adolescent drug use; these include attention-deficit/hyperactivity disorder (ADHD), anxiety disorders, and mood disorders (32).

Table 8. Traumatic life experiences associated with increased SUD risks

1.	Accidents
2.	Domestic violence
3.	Child abuse or neglect
4.	Early loss of parents through death, incarceration, parental divorce
5.	Poverty
6.	Deprivation
7.	Untreated medical/psychiatric problems

During the treatment process, families are engaged in managing resistance and denial as well as identifying the early signs of recovery or relapse. Family psychoeducation and support groups, such as Al-Anon or Families Anonymous, frequently are helpful.

Multidimensional family therapy (MDFT)

MDFT is an intervention that focuses on identifying and changing adolescents' behaviors within the context of family relations and interactions. It is not unusual for youths with SUDs to have families marked by issues listed in Table 9. In MDFT therapists address all the aspects of family relations and interactions which may be affecting the young person; also, therapists serve as an advocate for the youth and the family liaising between the school, community resources, and the legal system.

Table 9. Characteristics of families of youth with SUDs (see text)

1.	More critical
2.	Emotionally unavailable
3.	Only respond to negative behaviors
4.	Have inconsistent rules
5.	Display a high level of conflict

During the initial phase of treatment, therapists work with the adolescents to engage them in therapy, to break through resistance and to establish a positive patient-therapist alliance. Factors that are evaluated include a pattern of drug use, personality style, quality of relationship with the parents, and their interactions with the broader group. As the treatment progresses, the family is gradually integrated into the sessions in which the emphasis is placed on reducing conflict and emotional detachment between the patient and the family. Families are provided help with housing, transportation, and medical care to engage them fully in the treatment plan and to work with the adolescent closely.

Research based on RCT (randomized control trial) methodology, comparing residential treatment with MDFT, suggests that MDFT is a promising alternative to residential treatment for youth with substance use and co-occurring mental disorders (33, 34). A study of 11-15-

year-old Hispanic and African American youth was conducted that randomly assigned them to MDFT or group-based CBT for 12-16 weeks. Outcomes were assessed during the treatment, at the end of treatment, and then six as well as twelve months after treatment. Adolescents in the MDFT showed more robust and longer-lasting abstinence than those in group therapy (54% as compared to 13%); researchers also noticed a decrease in the frequency of drug and delinquent behaviors (34).

Conclusion

During the past three decades, psychosocial treatments for substance use disorders have undergone substantial growth as scientific scrutiny of outcomes has generated new therapies that have been validated. Adolescents with SUDs present a challenge in the degree of their denial, influence accepted from peers, and resistance to authority in their quest for autonomy. Psychosocial treatments continue to be the mainstay of the broader treatment of SUD, and there is strong evidence of improved long-term outcomes with these interventions.

References

[1] Gilvarry E. Substance abuse in young people. J Child Psychol Psychiatry 2000;41(1):55-80.

[2] Merikangas KR, He JP, Burstein M, Swanson SA, Avenevoli S, Cui L, et al. Lifetime prevalence of mental disorders in U.S. adolescents: results from the National Comorbidity Survey Replication--Adolescent Supplement (NCS-A). J Am Acad Child Adolesc Psychiatry 2010;49(10):980-9.

[3] 2015 National Survey on Drug Use and Health, 2016. URL: https://www.drugabuse.gov/national-survey-drug-use-health.

[4] National Drug Prevention Alliance. Harm reduction including HIV. URL: drugprevent.org.uk/ppp/category/papers/harm-reduction.

[5] Copeland W, Shanahan L, Costello EJ, Angold A. Cumulative prevalence of psychiatric disorders by young adulthood: a prospective cohort analysis from the Great Smoky Mountains Study. J Am Acad Child Adolesc Psychiatry 2011;50(3):252-61.

[6] Riggs PD. Treating adolescents for substance abuse and comorbid psychiatric disorders. Sci Pract Perspect 2003;2(1):18-29.

[7] Hser YI, Grella CE, Hubbard RL, Hsieh SC, Fletcher BW, Brown BS, et al. An evaluation of drug treatments for adolescents in 4 US cities. Arch Gen Psychiatry 2001;58(7):689-95.

[8] National Institute for Health and Care Excellence. Drug misuse prevention: targeted interventions. London: NICE, NG64/3, 2017.

[9] Jhanjee S. Evidence based psychosocial interventions in substance use. Indian J Psychol Med 2014;36(2):112-8.

[10] Vasilaki EI, Hosier SG, Cox WM. The efficacy of motivational interviewing as a brief intervention for excessive drinking: A meta-analytic review. Alcohol Alcohol 2006;41(3):328-35.

[11] Smedslund G, Berg RC, Hammerstrøm KT, Steiro A, Leiknes KA, Dahl HM, et al. Motivational interviewing for substance abuse. Cochrane Database Syst Rev 2011;5: CD008063.

[12] Prochaska JO, DiClemente CC, Norcross JC. In search of how people change: applications to addictive behaviors. Am Psychol 1992;47(9):1102-14.

[13] Morrison MA, Rabbit MW. A doctors own story of addiction, survival and recovery. New York: Berkley Books, 1989.

[14] Bigelow G, Griffiths R, Liebson I. Experimental models for the modification of human drug self-administration: Methodological developments in the study of ethanol self-administration by alcoholics. Fed Proc 1975;34(9):1785-92.

[15] Dishion TJ, McCord J, Poulin F. When interventions harm: Peer groups and problem behavior. Am Psychol 1999;54(9):755-64.

[16] Kubota M, Nakazaki S, Hirai S, Saeki N, Yamaura A, Kusaka T. Alcohol consumption and frontal lobe shrinkage: study of 1,432 non-alcoholic subjects. J Neurol Neurosurg Psychiatry 2001;71(1):104-6.

[17] Connolly CG, Foxe JJ, Nierenberg J, Shpaner M, Garavan H. The neurobiology of cognitive control in successful cocaine abstinence. Drug Alcohol Depend 2012;121(1-2):45-53.

[18] Galanter M, Egelko S, Edwards H. Rational recovery: alternative to AA for addiction? Am J Drug Alcohol Abuse 1993;19(4):499-510.

[19] Norcross JC, Krebs PM, Prochaska JO. Stages of change. J Clin Psychol 2011;67(2):143-54.

[20] Connor JP, Haber PS, Hall WD. Alcohol use disorders. Lancet 2016;387(10022):988-98.

[21] Davis DR, Kurti AN, Skelly JM, Redner R, White TJ, Higgins ST. A review of the literature on contingency management in the treatment of substance use disorders, 2009–2014. Prev Med 2016;92:36-46.

[22] Petry NM, Alessi SM, Olmstead TA, Rash CJ, Zajac K. Contingency management treatment for substance use disorders: How far has it come, and where does it need to go? Psychol Addict Behav 2017;31(8):897-906.

[23] Lussier JP, Heil SH, Mongeon JA, Badger GJ, Higgins ST. A meta-analysis of voucher-based reinforcement therapy for substance use disorders. Addiction 2006;101(2):192-203.

[24] Petry NM, Martin B. Low-cost contingency management for treating cocaine- and opioid-abusing methadone patients. J Consult Clin Psychol 2002;70(2):398-405.

[25] Petry NM, Martin B, Cooney JL, Kranzler HR. Give them prizes and they will come: Contingency management for treatment of alcohol dependence. J Consult Clin Psychol 2000;68(2):250-7.

[26] Kidorf M, Stitzer ML. Contingent use of take-homes and split-dosing to reduce illicit drug use of methadone patients. Behav Ther 1996;27(1):41-51.

[27] Simpson DD, Joe GW, Broome KM, Hiller ML, Knight K, Rowan-Szal GA. Program diversity and treatment retention rates in the Drug Abuse Treatment Outcome Study (DATOS). Psychol Addict Behav 1997;11(4):279-93.

[28] Winters KC, Botzet AM, Stinchfield R, Gonzales-Castaneda R, Finch AJ, Piehler TF, et al. Adolescent substance abuse treatment: A review of evidence-based research. Adolescent Substance Abuse. Eds: CG Leukefeld, TP Gullotta. Springer; 2018:141-71.

[29] Velasco V, Griffin KW, Botvin GJ, Celata C, Lombardia GL. Preventing adolescent substance use through an evidence-based program: effects of the Italian adaptation of life skills training. Prev Sci 2017;18(4):394-405.

[30] Marlatt GA, Donovan DM. Relapse prevention: Maintenance strategies in the treatment of addictive behaviors, 2nd edition. New York: Guilford, 2005.

[31] Biederman J, Faraone SV, Monuteaux MC, Feighner JA. Patterns of alcohol and drug use in adolescents can be predicted by parental substance use disorders. Pediatrics 2000; 106(4):792-7.

[32] Liepman MR, Calles JL, Kizilbash L, Nazeer A, Sheikh S. Genetic and nongenetic factors influencing substance use by adolescents. Adolesc Med 2002;13(2):375-401.

[33] Liddle HA, Dakof GA, Rowe CL, Henderson C, Greenbaum P, Wang W, et al. Multidimensional Family Therapy as a community-based alternative to residential treatment for adolescents with substance use and co-occurring mental health disorders. J Subst Abuse Treat 2018;90:47-56.

[34] Liddle HA, Rowe CL, Dakof GA, Henderson CE, Greenbaum PE. Multidimensional family therapy for young adolescent substance abuse: twelve-month outcomes of a randomized controlled trial. J Consult Clin Psychol 2009;77(1):12-25.

Chapter 12

Substance use disorders in adolescents: Pharmacologic management

Donald E Greydanus*, MD, DrHC(Athens)
Department of Pediatric and Adolescent Medicine, Western Michigan University Homer Stryker MD School of Medicine, Kalamazoo, United States of America

Abstract

Substance use disorders are a major public health conundrum of adolescents and adults throughout the world. The major problem of addiction in the world has intensified since the unfortunate biochemical isolation of cocaine, heroin, and morphine in the 19th century. The role of pharmacologic agents in the management of substance abuse disorders in adolescents is secondary or adjunctive, with psychological (psychosocial) therapies serving as the primary methods of treatment. Medications may serve a more primary role in the transient issue of helping in acute management of drug intoxication or withdrawal states. This article discusses current pharmacologic management of specific illicit drugs in which research indicates drug treatment can be beneficial; these drugs include alcohol, heroin, and cocaine.

Introduction

Substance abuse is a major public health conundrum of adolescents and adults throughout the world (1-35). The major problem of addiction in the world has intensified since the unfortunate biochemical isolation of cocaine, heroin, and morphine in the 19th century. Research over the past decade has noted that addiction is not an illness that is simply inherited, but a complex illness in which various genes combine with each addict's environment that includes influences of peers and family. Addiction is a chronic disorder that involves using drugs that provide euphoric effects in diverse ways, including enhancing the neurotransmitter dopamine in the areas of the brain involved in reward and motivation – such as the mesocorticolimbic pathway (3, 14, 17, 36, 37).

* ***Correspondence:*** Donald E Greydanus, MD, Professor and Founding Chair, Department of Pediatric and Adolescent Medicine, Western Michigan University Homer Stryker MD School of Medicine, 1000 Oakland Drive, Kalamazoo, MI 49008-1284 United States. Email: Donald.Greydanus@med.wmich.edu.

In: Behavioral Pediatrics
Editors: Donald E. Greydanus, Dilip R. Patel, Ahsan Nazeer et al.
ISBN: 979-8-88697-060-9

The role of pharmacologic agents in the management of substance abuse disorders in adolescents is secondary or adjunctive, with psychological therapies serving as the primary methods of treatment (37-40). Medications may serve a more primary role in the transient issue of helping in acute management of drug intoxication or withdrawal states. Non-pharmacologic management of substance abuse disorders in adolescents include motivational interviewing, cognitive-behavioral therapy, behavior motivation therapy, family therapy, and group counseling. Adolescents may require outpatient treatment, partial hospitalization, inpatient management, detoxification management, acute residential management, and even management in long-term residential programs.

In this review we discuss current pharmacologic management of specific illicit drugs in which research indicates drug treatment can be beneficial; these drugs include alcohol, heroin and cocaine (1, 3, 5, 40-43). The literature on psychopharmacologic management of drug abuse mainly focuses on adults, and there are no medications that are FDA-approved for those with substance abuse disorder under 18 years of age. Many of these medications, however, are used by various clinicians dealing with adolescents who have drug withdrawal and dependence problems. Medications used to treat nicotine addiction are reviewed in another chapter (44-52).

DSM-5

In 2013 the American Psychiatric Association published the 5th edition of its diagnostic and statistical manual of mental disorders (1). Changes in this issue included that its previous multiaxial system was deleted. There is now only one axis where all disorders are coded (previously I and II for mental disorders, III for medical disorders, IV for stressors, and V for level of functioning). In the 2013 or the 5th edition system, medical and psychiatric diagnoses share same single axis. The psychosocial stress domains previously captured in Axis IV can now be represented by V codes and abuse codes. The severity of illness previously shown in Axis V now can be more accurately explained by various scales provided in the manual. The category "*not otherwise specified*" was deleted and replaced with "other disorder" or "unspecified disorder."

In the 2013 DSM-5 the term *substance use disorders* replaces the DSM-IV categories of substance *abuse* and substance *dependence* in order to promote clarity among researchers and clinicians (1). In the DSM-5 the specific substance used defines the specific disorder. In this system it is noted that dependence is often confused with "addiction" even though dependence does not necessarily indicate addiction. It is also noted in the DSM-5 that *tolerance* and *withdrawal* are normal responses to prescribed medications that affect central nervous system Substance Use and Related Disorders. Criteria are provided for substance use disorder, accompanied by criteria for intoxication, withdrawal, *substance/medication-induced* disorders, and unspecified substance-induced disorders if this is relevant for a specific substance (1).

The DSM-5 *substance use disorder* criteria are nearly identical to the DSM-IV substance *abuse* and *dependence* criteria combined into a *single* list, with two exceptions: early remission and sustained remission. In *early remission* from a DSM-5 viewpoint, substance use disorder is defined as at least 3 but less than 12 months without substance use disorder criteria (except craving). S*ustained* remission is defined as having at least 12 months without criteria (except craving). The DSM-5 specifiers include "in a *controlled* environment" and "on *maintenance* therapy" as the situation warrants. The DSM-IV *recurrent legal problems* criterion for substance abuse was deleted from DSM-5. In the DSM-5 a new criterion has been added:

craving or a strong desire/urge to use a substance (1). The threshold for *SUD* diagnosis in DSM-5 is set at two or more criteria in contrast to a threshold of *one* or more criteria in DSM-IV *abuse* and *three* or more for DSM-IV substance *dependence*. Cannabis withdrawal is *new* for DSM-5, as is *caffeine* withdrawal (which was in DSM-IV Appendix B, "Criteria Sets and Axes Provided for Further Study") (1, 5, 6, 15). The Criteria for DSM-5 tobacco use disorder are the same as those for other SUDs and is new to DSM-5 (44-52).

The DSM-IV did not have a category for tobacco abuse. DSM-5 added criteria for Gambling Disorder (activates brain reward system as does tradition SADs) (1, 17). The *severity* of the DSM-5 substance use disorders is based on the number of criteria endorsed; 2 to 3 criteria indicate a *mild* disorder, 4-5 criteria indicate a *moderate* disorder, and 6 or more indicate a *severe* disorder. The DSM-IV specifier for a *physiological* subtype has been eliminated in DSM-5 and the DSM-IV diagnosis of *polysubstance dependence* was also eliminated in DSM-5 (1). Comments about specific substances are now provided.

Alcohol

Treatment of acute alcohol consumption includes gastric emptying, intravenous fluids along with glucose, respiratory support, and, if necessary, dialysis (3, 5, 11, 12, 17). A number of medications have been used to treat alcohol withdrawal syndrome, as noted in Table 1; benzodiazepines are sedation-inducing drugs and include diazepam, chlordiazepoxide, and lorazepam that are given every 1-4 hours (depending upon the agent) until withdrawal symptoms cease (13, 36, 40-42).

Table 1. Medications for management of alcohol withdrawal syndrome

• Lorazepam
• Chlordiazepoxide
• Diazepam
• Clorazepate
• Various antipsychotics

Table 2. Drugs for management of adults with alcohol dependence

Approved
• Disulfiram
• Naltrexone
• Acamprosate
Used but not officially approved (off label)
• Buspirone
• Carbamazepine
• Oxcarbazepine
• Gabapentin
• Nalmefene (opioid antagonist)
• Ondansetron
• Quetiapine
• Selective serotonin reuptake inhibitors (e.g., fluoxetine, sertraline)
• Tiapride (Orphan drug status)
• Topiramate (anticonvulsant)
• Tricyclic antidepressants

Table 3. FDA medications approved for adult alcohol dependence (63)

Agent	Mechanism	Adverse Effects	Dosage	Comments
Disulfiram (Antabuse, others)	Interferes with alcohol metabolism by inhibition of acetaldehyde dehydrogenase.	Drinking alcohol while on disulfiram leads to flushing, headache, nausea, palpitations, chest pain, vertigo & hypotension. Side effects apart from alcohol ingestion: sedation, allergic dermatitis, headache, metallic or garlicky taste in mouth. Rare: peripheral neuropathy, optic neuritis, polyneuritis, cardiac arrhythmias & psychosis. Can be hepatotoxic with rare idiosyncratic fulminant hepatitis with death (Must monitor liver function tests). Caution use in hepatic cirrhosis / insufficiency.	500 mg a day for the first one to two weeks. Abstain from alcohol for at least 12 hours before initiating. Maintenance dose is 250 mg daily (125 to 500 mg).	Small amount of alcohol consumed while taking disulfiram, the concentration of acetaldehyde can be 5-10 x higher than if alcohol is consumed without the disulfiram. Not approved for age <18. Tolerance does not develop. Increased sensitivity to disulfiram may develop over time. Maintenance treatment may be required for months to years. Tablets may be crushed or mixed with water or juice. May block tetrahydrocannabinol (THC) to increase the psychoactive effects of marijuana. Avoid alcohol in cough medications, & foods including ciders, vinegars, etc
Oral naltrexone (ReVia; Depade) FDA approval: 1994 IM (intramuscular) naltrexone (Vivitrol)	Inhibits reward effects of alcohol and thus decreases desire for alcohol. Competitive antagonist at opioid receptor sites.	Nausea, emesis, dry mouth, insomnia, lethargy, anxiety, dyspepsia, dizziness, headache, syncope, diarrhea, decreased appetite, increased liver enzymes, depression, suicide, & eosinophilic pneumonia.	Oral form: Give 25mg and may repeat within 1 hour if no withdrawal symptoms. Maintenance regimen is flexible and can be individualized.	Can precipitate acute opioid withdrawal syndrome and should not be given until 7-10 days after opioid is discontinued. Confirm by urinalysis. Not indicated at age < 18 years. Administer with food to minimize GI upset.

Agent	Mechanism	Adverse Effects	Dosage	Comments
FDA approval: 2006	Blocks effects of opioids (including antidiarrheals and antitussives that are opioid-based).	Local injection site reactions include cellulitis, induration, hematoma, abscess & necrosis. Black box warning regarding hepatotoxic potential at ≥ 5 times recommended dose.	Doses can range from 50mg daily to 100-150 mg three times weekly. IM form: 380 mg monthly. Do not administer IV or SQ	Monitor liver enzymes (aminotransferase levels)
Acamprosate calcium (Campral) Used in France and other countries since 1989 and FDA-approved in 2004	It is a synthetic homotaurine derivative which is similar in structure to gamma-amino-butyric acid (GABA); reduces the desire for alcohol use; activates γ-aminobutyric acid type A receptors and blocks glutaminergic-N- methyl-D-aspartate receptors: decreases glutamatergic transmission and modulates neuronal hyperexcitability after withdrawal/cessation from alcohol ingestion to encourage abstinence.	Main side effect: diarrhea (dose-related and transient) Others: suicidal ideation and suicides (attempts and completed), nausea, emesis, headache, abdominal pain, drowsiness, dizziness, flatulence, rash, pruritus; syncope; peripheral edema; depression; insomnia; anxiety	666 mg (two 333-mg enteric coated tablets) three times a day with or without meals. Start as soon as possible after alcohol abstinence occurs. Lower doses may be effective for some patients. Can be continued with a relapse.	Not studied in those <18 years old. Does not reduce or eliminate symptoms of alcohol withdrawal. Efficacy rates are similar to naltrexone. Can be used with naltrexone or disulfiram. Avoid in severe renal failure; dose adjust in renal insufficiency. Teratogenic in animals. Does not lead to dependence or abuse.

Table 2 lists drugs approved for treatment of adults with alcohol dependence in the United States; there are no FDA approved medications for adolescents (3, 5, 12, 14). The United States Food and Drug Administration (FDA) approved the use of disulfiram for the management of adult alcohol dependence nearly a half century ago. In 1994, the FDA approved naltrexone (opioid-receptor antagonist) for management of adult alcohol dependence, followed in 2004 by acamprosate. Other drugs (see Table 2) have been used in adults with alcohol dependence but are not FDA-approved and not discussed here.

Table 3 reviews the mechanism, side effects, and dosages of disulfiram, naltrexone and acamprosate; liver function tests (aminotransferase levels) must be monitored when taking disulfiram or naltrexone.

Drug interactions

Disulfiram may interfere with the metabolism of certain medications, such as phenytoin (causing phenytoin intoxication), oral anticoagulants (can prolong prothrombin time), benzodiazepines that undergo oxidative metabolism (i.e., diazepam and chlordiazepoxide), and isoniazid (can induce mental status changes and unsteady gait) (3, 5).

Naltrexone blocks opioid effects and can precipitate an acute opioid withdrawal syndrome if given to someone taking opioids; the individual must be off opioids for at least 7-10 days before taking naltrexone. Combining naltrexone with acamprosate increases serum acamprosate levels, but dosage adjustments are not necessary. Naltrexone is hepatotoxic at higher than recommended levels. Acamprosate is a safe medication when added to other medications; serum levels are increased when added to naltrexone, but without known adverse consequences.

Amphetamines

Management of this powerfully addictive drug is very difficult and depends on a firm resolve on the addict’s part to recover (3, 5, 10-12). There is no pharmaceutical chemical that is effective in treating methamphetamine addiction. The ß-blockers are used to manage cardiac arrhythmias noted in acute methamphetamine intoxication, while a benzodiazepine (such as lorazepam or others) is used to manage irritability, agitation and seizures. An antipsychotic medication is used for psychotic symptoms, but CYP2D6 inhibitors (such as haloperidol) are avoided, since they may increase serum methamphetamine levels. Patients with methamphetamine addiction should be provided with intense psychological therapies, perhaps supplemented with an antidepressant. Limited evidence suggests that fluoxetine and bupropion may be beneficial in reducing methamphetamine cravings (3, 5).

Research is currently seeking a medication to block the euphoric effects of methamphetamine. The development of such an “antibody” to neutralize this drug is also being sought for other drug addictions, including cocaine, heroin, and others (33, 34). A current drug under investigation to reduce methamphetamine addiction is GVG (vigabatrin). Research has noted that nicotine and donepezil (acetylcholinesterase inhibitor) can reduce the craving for methamphetamine; both drugs stimulate nicotinic acetylcholine receptors which are part of the brain's reward system (3, 5).

Cocaine

Cocaine is a central nervous system stimulant that is known as one of the most addictive and dangerous drugs of abuse in the world. It is made from Erythroxylon coca, a plant found in South America (3, 5, 10-12, 14, 30-32).

Treatment of cocaine abuse is a difficult problem and as with many types of substance abuse disorders, prevention is preferable to management of overt addiction. There are no medications to effectively treat cocaine addiction. Therapy is generally supportive with pharmacotherapy to treat delusions or autonomic hyperactivity. Short-acting beta-blockers are helpful with cocaine-related tachycardia and hypertension; some clinicians do not use ß-blockers because of risk of reduced coronary perfusion and increased myocardial infarction in acute cocaine intoxication (3, 5). Benzodiazepines can be useful for extreme agitation, while the risk of cerebrovascular accidents may be hypothetically reduced with the use of a calcium channel blocker (dihydropyridine-type) by increasing cerebral blood flow. Health care professionals should avoid long-acting vasodilators, since cocaine intoxication does not usually last long. Naloxone, useful for opioid addiction, is not helpful for cocaine abuse.

Cocaine addicts who also have attention-deficit/hyperactivity disorder (ADHD) note that stimulants like methylphenidate (MPH) calms them down and may allow less cocaine use. Cocaine addicts who also have ADHD may benefit from 40 to 60 mg of sustained-release MPH in reducing pathological craving for cocaine (3, 5). Research is currently seeking drugs to block the effects of cocaine and prevent its euphoric effect on multiple brain sites (33, 34). A vaccine currently under investigation (TA-CD) produces anti-cocaine antibodies and suggests promise in treating cocaine addiction. Dopamine within the brain plays an important role in providing the rewarding effects of cocaine. Agents that increase GABA modulate the effects of the dopamine reward system. GVG (vigabatrin), which is an irreversible inhibitor of GABA transaminase, has shown promise in treating cocaine addiction.

Topiramate (an anticonvulsant) has been shown in research trials to help cocaine addicts stay off cocaine; it can exacerbate cocaine withdrawal and is not used until the addict has been off cocaine for three days or more (3). Topiramate has been used to prevent relapse in those with alcohol, nicotine, and cocaine addiction; it may help with opiate addiction as well (3, 5). N-acetylcysteine amide is under study as well (32). Drugs used to treat alcohol abuse may be of help to cocaine addicts who also abuse alcohol; these drugs include disulfiram and naltrexone.

Opioids

Table 4 lists various opiate narcotics that are abused by youth as well as adults. Comments in this section focus on heroin (diacetyl morphine hydrochloride), a powerful addictive drug available around the world that is snorted/snuffed, injected intravenously, or is smoked (3, 5, 6, 10-12, 14, 24, 26-29, 53-61). Research indicates that addiction, such as that noted with heroin, is a neurobiological condition of the central nervous system involving the endogenous opioid system. Drugs of abuse block the dopamine transporter in the brain's reward circuits, a process complicated perhaps by reduced numbers of CNS D_2 receptors in heroin addicts. These youth need acute detoxification measures followed by intense treatment of the addiction process, often in residential treatment facilities, if available. A variety of medications are used to manage opioid addiction (3, 5, 10-12, 14, 24, 26-29, 53-61).

Table 4. Narcotic opiates

Heroin
Codeine
Oxycodone
Fentanyl
Propoxyphene
Meperidine
Methadone
Morphine
Pentazocine
Hydrocodone

Naloxone hydrochloride is an opiate antagonist and is used to manage overdose due to opioids (such as heroin); intravenous (IV) administration is recommended in emergency situations, though it can be given intramuscularly (IM) or subcutaneously (SC) as well (3, 5, 10-12, 26). In cases of heroin overdose, it is given at a dose (adult) of 0.4 mg to 2 mg IV and repeated every 2 to 3 minutes until improvement in respiratory depression occurs; it is also used to improve sedation and hypotension noted in the overdose (3,5). If a total of 10 mg has been given, the overdose may not be due to an opioid. In children, a trial IV dose of 0.01 mg/kg body weight is given followed by an IV dose of 0.1 mg/kg body weight if necessary. A relapse of the heroin overdose symptoms may occur over the next 24 hours as the naloxone is metabolized. Naloxone can lead to hypertension, acute opioid withdrawal syndrome, tachycardia, emesis, sweating, and tremors. Management of the pregnant mother who is on heroin and is delivering includes the use of naloxone for the mother and the neonate as necessary; IV administration is recommended for the neonate (3, 5).

Clonidine hydrochloride is a central α_2 adrenergic agonist and while not approved by the FDA to treat opiate withdrawal, it has been extensively studied (3, 5). Clonidine is useful for treating withdrawal symptoms including nausea, vomiting, diarrhea, cramps, and sweating. It does not reduce symptoms of craving. Side effects that may limit its use include hypotension, sedation, dizziness, and dry mouth. It is initiated at a dose of 0.1 mg three times daily and titrated until withdrawal symptoms are reduced. Treatment usually last 4-6 days and should be gradually withdrawn over 2-4 days to avoid rebound hypertension (3, 5).

Lofexidine hydrochloride is another α_2 adrenergic agonist used in England and other countries to treat opiate withdrawal over a 7–10-day period. It is started at 0.2 mg twice daily and increased by 0.2-0.4 mg per day to a maximum daily dose of 2.4 mg. Side effects and treatment withdrawal are similar to clonidine as noted above.

Heroin dependence management

Intensive behavioral therapy is necessary to help heroin addicts recover and community programs like Narcotic Anonymous (NA) are helpful as well. Youth who are addicted to heroin or other narcotic opiates should be under the care of an addiction specialist well trained in these various anti-narcotic medications. Behavioral interventions are a major part of treatment for adolescents and adults addicted to heroin and other opiates.

A number of medications are used to help blunt the profound euphoric effects of heroin by serving as opioid replacement therapy; these medications include methadone hydrochloride, LAAM (levo-alpha-acetylmethadol or levomethadyl acetate), and buprenorphine hydrochloride (24, 53-59). Other medications used to help with the treatment of opioid addiction include buprenorphine/naltrexone, anti-depressant drugs (such as selective serotonin reuptake inhibitors) and anti-anxiety medications (such as buspirone). In a few countries (e.g., the United Kingdom), heroin is available as diamorphine and has been prescribed for several decades to a select group of those with severe, refractory heroin addiction. Anesthesia-assisted detoxification, using anesthesia for 4 to 6 hours on day 1 of opiate detoxification, is a method that is not FDA approved and is not supported by research to be an effective detoxification method for opioid addicts.

Naltrexone is an opioid-receptor antagonist that blocks μ-opioid receptors and is used to manage opioid dependence, though more research is needed to establish its actual efficacy in this situation. It is not given until a week or more after the addict is free of opioids (and verified by checking a urinalysis); if given sooner, opioid withdrawal symptoms may develop that are sudden and severe. The maintenance dose for naltrexone is 50 mg per day; some start at 12.5 mg, increase to 25 mg and then to 50 mg per day. Heroin overdose risks seem to be increased for those who stop taking naltrexone for heroin dependence treatment, more so than other medications that are used for sobriety and then stopped.

Methadone is a μ-opioid receptor agonist and has been available for over 40 years (see Table 5) (3, 5). Use of methadone to treat narcotic addiction has been a controversial treatment since its beginning in the 1960s. In the United States, methadone is reserved for the individual severely addicted to heroin, since naltrexone will precipitate an opiate withdrawal state. In the United Kingdom, other European countries, and Australia, methadone is provided to the less severely addicted individual and maintenance is the main goal of its use. In the United States, methadone for the treatment of opiate addiction can only be dispensed through approved treatment facilities.

A search for longer-acting treatment medications led to the current use of buprenorphine and levomethadyl acetate (LAAM). Buprenorphine is a partial opioid receptor agonist given as sublingual tablets and has a similar side effect profile to other opioid agonists. Compared to methadone, it is safer in overdose due to less respiratory depression (38). It was originally developed in the 1970s as an injectable pain medication. It can be prescribed by any physician who has taken an eight-hour course on the treatment or management of opioid dependence, has the ability to provide or refer patients to specialists as needed, and accepts to treat 30 or fewer patients at any given time within their own or group practice. The patient can obtain the medication from the trained physician in the office, or pick it up at a pharmacy, and preferably its administration should be supervised.

Table 5. FDA-approved medications used for heroin dependence treatment (63)

Agent	Mechanism	Adverse Effects	Dosage	Comments
Methadone (Dolophine, others)	µ-opioid receptor agonist that blocks narcotic effects while avoiding basic narcotic euphoria; can eliminate opiate withdrawal symptoms and lessen need for additional addictive drugs.	Anorexia; hypotension; bradycardia; QTc prolongation; syncope; hypokalemia; hypomagnesemia; sedation; confusion; nausea; vomiting; constipation; respiratory depression; pruritis May lead to physical or psychological dependence. Patient must obtain daily dose from opioid treatment centers in US. Preferred drug for pregnant heroin addict.	Detoxification initial dose: 20-30mg. Consider lower doses in patients with low tolerance at initiation. May give an additional 5-10mg if withdrawal symptoms reappear or not suppressed after 2-4 hours. Total daily dose on first day should not exceed 40mg. Maintenance therapy: usual 80-120 mg daily. Titrate to dosage which prevents craving & lessens euphoric effect of opiate abuse. Adjust dose in severe renal insufficiency.	Electrocardiogram monitoring May administer liquid & dispersible tablet in fruit juice or water. Avoid use with grapefruit juice. Metabolized by CYP 450 enzymes. Inhibits CYP 450 2D6 isoenzyme. For withdrawal: dose reductions should be <10% of maintenance dose every 10-14 days.

Agent	Mechanism	Adverse Effects	Dosage	Comments
Buprenorphine (Subutex; other) (sublingual tablets: 2, 8 mg)	Schedule III partial opioid receptor agonist used for detoxification treatment of heroin and other narcotics. Developed in the 1970s as an injectable analgesic. Suppresses withdrawal symptoms & opposes effects of heroin.	Insomnia, nausea, constipation, stomach pain, dizziness, nervousness, headache, sweating, anxiety, lacrimation, respiratory depression.	*Induction*: 8mg on day 1, followed by 16mg on day 2. Induction is continued over 3-4 days. Begin at least 4 hours after last use of heroin and when first signs of withdrawal appear. Titrate dose as quickly as possible to avoid unnecessary withdrawal symptoms & decrease risk for drop-out. *Maintenance*: Usual 16mg/day. Range of 4-24mg daily.	Substrate for CYP 450 3A4—inhibitors will increase drug effect Can be prescribed in physician's office after obtaining certification from SAMHSA. Patients should be switched to combination therapy for maintenance & unsupervised treatment to prevent abuse. Abrupt cessation produces milder withdrawal symptoms compared to other opioid agonists. Overdose with benzodiazepines (usually parenteral) has led to case fatalities. Not indicated for those < 16 years.
Buprenorphine/naloxone (Suboxone) Sublingual tablets: 2mg/0.5mg, 8 mg/2mg	Buprenorphine: partial opioid receptor agonist. Naloxone: pure opioid antagonist. Suppresses withdrawal symptoms & opposes effects of heroin.	Headache, nausea, constipation, stomach pain, shortness of breath, vomiting. Can precipitate intense withdrawal symptoms in patients taking opioids before the opioid effects have dissipated.	Usual dose (based on buprenorphine component): 16 mg/day. Range: 4-24 mg/day. Tablets should be placed under tongue and allowed to dissolve.	Indicated for maintenance therapy (not induction). Substrate for CYP 450 3A4—inhibitors will increase drug effect Can be prescribed in physician's office after obtaining certification from SAMHSA. Not indicated for those < 16 years.

The Drug Addiction Treatment Act of 2000 (DATA 2000) sets up how a physician can qualify to use Schedule III, IV and V narcotic medications in the United States to manage opioid addiction in facilities other than the methadone clinic. Certification is through the US Substance Abuse and Mental Health Services Administration (SAMHSA) and further information may be obtained at http://www.dpt.samhsa.gov. The purpose of the extended use of this medication is to allow the treatment of opioid addiction to be similar to that of other chronic illness in which primary care clinicians care for many of these addicts in their offices. This model is popular in Europe and is growing in interest in the United States.

Buprenorphine is typically utilized as induction therapy and should be given when clear signs of withdrawal are present to avoid precipitating withdrawal symptoms and at least 4 hours after last use of the opioid. Induction phase is typically 3-4 days and supervision of administration is recommended. Titration should be done as quickly as possible to prevent withdrawal effects and increased risk for patient drop-out. For maintenance, patients should be switched to buprenorphine/naloxone and supervision is not necessary (3, 5).

Both agents are available as sublingual formulations and both are clinically effective for maintenance but the combination product is preferred due to the addition of naloxone. Buprenorphine has a longer duration of action and induces less analgesic effects than methadone. Opioid withdrawal may develop if buprenorphine is given to someone with recent opioid use. Research suggests it is as effective as methadone for maintenance treatment of heroin addiction and better tolerated than methadone or clonidine for opioid withdrawal. Patients are typically stabilized on 16 mg of buprenorphine a day and 4 mg of naloxone a day (see Table 5).

Levomethadyl acetate (LAAM) is a synthetic opioid analgesic and is taken every other day or three times a week instead of the daily administration for methadone. Life-threatening cardiac rhythm disorders were reported with LAAM including QT interval prolongation and case reports of torsades de pointes. Due to the severity of the adverse events, LAAM was removed from the European market in 2001 and Roxane Laboratories removed ORLAAM® from the US market in 2003 (3, 5).

Conclusion

All clinicians must work with their pediatric and adolescent patients to teach them about the dangers of substance use disorders and help them get off the precipitous slide that drugs take our youth down (3, 5, 10-12, 14, 16, 19-21, 23, 61-65). It is important to appreciate the neurobiologic and genetic components to the complex issue of substance use disorders (17, 22). We must work with various elements of society to reduce this major threat to our children. Prevention of drug abuse is the key to this immense problem and behavioral therapies are the mainstay of drug dependence management (3, 5, 19-21, 23, 62). Medications are needed for treatment of various drug withdrawal syndromes and overdoses.

Psychopharmacologic management can also be helpful in selected cases, particularly for alcohol dependence and opiate addiction (3, 5). The dangers of marijuana for children and adolescents should be appreciated even in the current climate that seems favorable to cannabis (5, 6, 15). The use of e-cigarettes is an example of the constant battle that occurs between manufactures and public health officials seek to maximize the health of its population (63-65).

The establishment of drug-free zones in schools, sports arenas and other areas remains an important goal for society as it educates its youth for the future about life without drugs (66).

Caring for adolescents and young adults with chronic illness such as substance use disorders should remain an important aspect of efforts by researchers and clinicians (3, 5, 16). The impact of the 2019-2022 COVID-19 pandemic on substance use disorders continues to be studied (67). Research in the 21st century continues on the causes and management of substance use disorders in Homo sapiens (68-75).

Acknowledgments

This paper is a modified version of an earlier published paper with permission from: Greydanus DE, Calles JRJr, Patel DR, eds. Pediatric and adolescent psychopharmacology. Cambridge: Cambridge University Press, 2008:240-77.

References

[1] American Psychiatric Association. Diagnostic and statistical manual of mental disorders, fifth edition. Arlington, VA, American Psychiatric Association, 2013.

[2] Hibell B, Guttormsson U, Ahlström S, Balakireva O, Bjarnason T, Kokkevi A, et al. The 2011 ESPAD (The European School Survey Project on Alcohol and Other Drugs) report. Substance use among students in 36 European countries. Stockholm: Swedish Council Information Alcohol other Drugs (CAN), 2011.

[3] Greydanus DE, Kaplan G, Patel DR, Merrick J, eds. Substance abuse in adolescents and young adults: A manual for pediatric and primary care clinicians. Second edition. New York: Nova Science, 2019.

[4] Peiper NC, Ridenour TA, Hochwalt B, Coyne-Beasley T. Overview on prevalence and recent trends in adolescent substance use and abuse. Child Adolesc Psychiatr Clin North Am 2016;25(3):349-65.

[5] Greydanus DE, Feucht C, Patel DR. Substance abuse disorders in adolescents: Pharmacologic management. In: Greydanus DE, Calles Jr JR, Patel DR, Nazeer A, Merrick J, eds. Clinical aspects of psychopharmacology in childhood and adolescence. New York: Nova Biomedical, 2010:167-75.

[6] Greydanus DE, Kaplan G, Baxter LE Sr., Patel DR, Feucht CL. Cannabis: The never-ending, nefarious nepenthe of the 21st century. What should be clinician know? Dis Mon 2015;61(4):118-75.

[7] Johnston LD, O'Malley P M, Bachman, JG, Schulenberg JE, Miech RA. Monitoring the Future national survey results on drug use, 1975–2014: Volume 2, College students and adults ages 19–55. Ann Arbor, MI: Institute for Social Research, University of Michigan, 2015.

[8] Johnston L D, O'Malley PM, Miech RA, Bachman JG, Schulenberg JE. Monitoring the Future national survey results on drug use, 1975-2015: Overview, key findings on adolescent drug use. Ann Arbor, MI: Institute for Social Research, University of Michigan, 2016.

[9] Kann L, McManus T, Harris WA, Shanklin SL, Flint KH, Hawkins J, et al. Youth risk behavior surveillance—United States, 2015. MMWR Surveill Summ 2016;65(6):1-178.

[10] Greydanus DE, Patel DR. Substance abuse in adolescents: A complex conundrum for the clinician. Pediatric Clin North Am 2003;59(5):1179-23.

[11] Greydanus DE, Patel DR. Substance abuse in the adolescent. In: Greydanus DE, Patel DR, Pratt HD, eds. Essential adolescent medicine. New York: McGraw-Hill, 2006:695-713.

[12] Greydanus DE, Patel DR. The adolescent and substance abuse: Current concepts. Curr Probl Pediatr Adolesc Health Care 2005; 35(3):1-21.

[13] Schydlower M, ed. Substance abuse: A guide for health professionals. Elk Grove Village, IL: American Academy Pediatrics, 2000.

[14] Greydanus DE, Pratt HD, Patel DR, Calles JR, Merrick J, eds. Behavioral pediatrics, 4th edition. New York: Nova Science, 2015.
[15] Greydanus DE, Hawver EK, Greydanus MM, Merrick J. Substance abuse and marihuana. In: Merrick J, ed. Child and adolescent health yearbook 2014. New York: Nova Biomedical, 2015:323-56.
[16] Apple RW, Greydanus DE. Caring for youth with chronic illness in the 21st century: the clinician's duty. J Comm Med Health Educ 2016;3(6):1000e127.
[17] Sharma A, Morrow JD. Neurobiology of adolescent use disorders. Child Adolesc Psychiatr Clin North Am 2016;25:367-75.
[18] Haughwout SP, Harford TC, Castle IJ, Grant BE. Treatment utilization among adolescent substance users: findings from the 2002-2013 National Survey on Drug use and Health. Alcohol Clin Exp Res 2016;40(8):1717-27.
[19] Harris SK, Louis-Jacques J, Knight JR. Screening and brief intervention for alcohol and other abuse. Adolesc Med State Art Rev 2014;25(1):126-56.
[20] Winters KC. Brief interventions for adolescents. J Drug Abuse 2016;2(1). pii: 14.
[21] Folayan MO, Adeniyi AA, Oziegbe EO, Fatusi AO, Harrison A. Integrated oral, mental and sexual health management for adolescents: a call for professional collaboration. Int J Adolesc Med Health. 2016 Aug 9;30(3):/j/ijamh.2018.30.issue-3/ijamh-2016-0060/ijamh-2016-0060.xml.
[22] Tawa EA, Hall SD, Lohoff FW. Overview of the genetics of alcohol use disorder. Alcohol Alcohol 2016;51(5):507-14.
[23] Harrop E, Catalano RF. Evidence-based prevention for adolescent substance use. Child Adolesc Psychiatr Clin North Am 2016;25:387-410.
[24] Buprenorphine implants for opioid dependence. Med Lett Dr Ther 2016;58:94-95.
[25] Veliz P, Boyd CJ, McCabe SE. Nonmedical prescription opioid and heroin use among adolescents who engage in sports and exercise. Pediatrics 2016;138(2): e20160677.
[26] Aboujaoude E, Salame WO. Naltrexone: A pan-addiction treatment? CNS Drugs 2016;30(8):719-33.
[27] Gunderson EW, Hjelmström P, Sumner M; 006 Study Investigators. Effects of a higher-bioavailability buprenorphine/naloxone sublingual tablet versus buprenorphine/naloxone film for the treatment of opioid dependence during induction and stabilization: a multicenter, randomized trial. Clin Ther 2015;37(10): 2244-55.
[28] Buprenorphine/naloxone versus methadone for the treatment of opioid dependence: A review of comparative clinical effectiveness, cost-effectiveness and guidelines. Ottawa, ON: Canadian Agency for Drugs and Technologies in Health, 2016.
[29] Bjarnadottir GD, Magnusson A, Rafnar BO, Sigurdsson E, Steingrimsson S, Johannsson M et al. Intravenous use of prescription psychostimulants; a comparison of the pattern and subjective experience between different methylphenidate preparations, amphetamine and cocaine. Eur Addict Res 2016;22(5):259-67.
[30] Davidson C. Developing treatments for simulant abuse: a brief overview. East Asian Arch Psychiatry 2016;26(2):52-9.
[31] Dürsteler KM, Vogel M. Effective drug therapy for cocaine dependence: a milestone. Lancet 2016;387(10034):2171-3.
[32] Jastrzębska J, Frankowska M, Filip M, Atlas D. N-acetylcysteine amide (AD4) reduces cocaine-induced reinstatement. Psychopharmacology (Berl) 2016; 233(18):3437-48.
[33] Pravetoni M. Biologics to treat substance use disorders: Current status and new directions. Hum Vaccin Immunother 2016;12(12):3005-19.
[34] Ohia-Nwoko O, Kosten TA, Halile CN. Animal models and the development of vaccines to treat substance use disorders. Int Rev Neurobiol 2016;126:263-91.
[35] Schydlower M, Arredondo RM, eds. Substance abuse among adolescents. Adolesc Med Clin 2006;17(2):259-505.
[36] Ross S, Hayden F. Study guide to substance abuse treatment: A companion to the American Psychiatric Publishing textbook of substance abuse treatment, Third edition. Washington, DC: American Psychiatric Publications, 2006.
[37] Bukstein OG, Bernet W, Arnold V. Practice parameter for the assessment and treatment of children and adolescents with substance abuse disorders. J Am Acad Child Adolesc Psychiatry 2005; 44:609-21.

[38] American Academy of Child and Adolescent Psychiatry. Practice parameter for the assessment and treatment of children and adolescents with substance use disorders. J Am Acad Child Adolesc Psychiatry 2005;44:609-21.

[39] Sofuoglu M, Kosten TR. Pharmacologic management of relapse prevention in additive disorder. Psychiatr Clin North Am 2004:27:624-8.

[40] Galanter M, ed. Alcohol problems in adolescents and young adults: Epidemiology, neurobiology, prevention and treatment. New York: Springer, 2006.

[41] Kranzler HR. Evidence-based treatments for alcohol dependence: new results and new questions. JAMA 2006;295(17):2075-6.

[42] Williams SH. Medications for treating alcohol dependence. Am Fam Phys 2005;72: 1775-80.

[43] Boyd CJ, McCabe SE, Cranford JA, Young A. Prescription drug abuse and diversion among adolescents in a Southeast Michigan school district. Arch Pediatr Adolesc Med 2007;161:276-81.

[44] Upadhyaya H, Deas D, Brady K. A practical clinical approach to the treatment of nicotine dependence in adolescents. J Am Acad Adolesc Psychiatr 2005;44(9):942-6.

[45] Fiore MC, Jaén CR, Baker TB. Treating tobacco use and dependence. Clinical practice guideline. Rockville, MD: Department Health Human Services, Public Health Services, 2008.

[46] National Institute on Drug Abuse. National Institutes of Health: Cigarettes and other nicotine products. URL: www.nida.nih.gov.

[47] Lancaster T, Stead LF. Individual behavioral counseling for smoking cessation: Cochrane review. Cochrane Database Syst Rev 2005;2:CD001292.

[48] Lancaster T, Stead LF: Self-help interventions for smoking cessation: Cochrane review. Cochrane Database Syst Rev 2000;2:CD001118.

[49] Cahill K, Lindson-Hawley N, Thomas KH, Fanshawe TR, Lancaster T. Nicotine receptor partial agonists for smoking cessation. Cochrrane Database Syst Rev 2016;5:CD006103.

[50] Benipal S, Budhram DR, Bilimoria K, Woods H, Wang R, Persaud N. Essential tobacco dependence medicines in 137 countries. Addiction 2021;116(6):1606-9.

[51] Harvey J, Chadi N. Strategies to promote smoking cessation among adolescents. Pediatr Child Health 2016;21(40):201-8.

[52] Nahvi S, Adams TR, Ning Y, Zhang C, Arnsten JH. Effect of varenicline directly observed therapy versus varenicline self-administered therapy on varenicline adherence and smoking cessation in methadone-maintained smokers: a randomized controlled trial. Addiction 2021;116(4):902-13.

[53] Kirchmayer U, Davoli M, Verster A. Naltrexone maintenance treatment for opioid dependence. Cochrane Database Syst Rev 2003;2:CD001333.

[54] Cozzolino E, Guglielmino L, Vigezzi P, Marzorati P, Silenzio R, De Chiara M, et al. Buprenorphine treatment: A three-year prospective study in opioid-addicted patients of a public out-patient addiction center in Milan. Am J Addict 2006;15(3):246-51.

[55] Johnson RE, Chutuape MA, Strain EC, Walsh SL, Stitzer ML, Bigelow GE. A comparison of levomethadyl acetate, buprenorphine, and methadone for opioid dependence. N Engl J Med 2000;343:1290-7.

[56] Oviedo-Joekes E, Brissette S, March DC, Lauzon P, Guh D, Anis A, et al. Diacetylmorphine versus methadone for the treatment of opioid addiction. N Engl J Med 2009;361:777-86.

[57] Berridge V. Heroin prescription and history. N Engl J Med 2009; 361:820-1.

[58] March LA. Comparison of pharmacological treatments for opioid-dependent adolescents: A randomized controlled trial. Arch Gen Psychiatry 2005;62:1157-64.

[59] Dydyk AM, Jain NK, Gupta M. Opioid use disorder. In: StatPearls. Treasure Island, FL: StatPearls Publishing, 2021 Jan–.

[60] Jones CM, Houry D, Han B, Baldwin G, Vivolo-Kantor A, Compton WM. Methamphetamine use in the United States: epidemiological update and implications for prevention, treatment, and harm reduction. Ann NY Acad Sci 2021 Sep 24.

[61] Kleber H, Weiss R, Anton R. Treatment of patients with substance abuse disorders, 2nd edition. Am J Psychiatry 2007;164(4 Suppl):5-123.

[62] Harvey J, Chadi N; Canadian Paediatric Society, Adolescent Health Committee. Preventing smoking in children and adolescents: recommendations for practice and policy. Paediatr Child Health 2016;21(4):209-21.
[63] McRobbie H, Kwan B. Tobacco use disorder and the lungs. Addiction 2021; 116(9):2559-71.
[64] No authors listed. E-cigarettes and smoking cessation. Similar efficacy to other nicotine delivery devices, but many uncertainties. Prescrire Int 2015; 24(165):271-6.
[65] Cobb NK, Sonti R. E-cigarettes: The science behind the smoke and mirrors. Respir Care 2016;61(8):1122-8.
[66] Koh H. Place matters for tobacco control. JAMA 2016;316(7):700-1.
[67] Ignaszewski MJ. The Epidemiology of Drug Abuse. J Clin Pharmacol 2021; 61(Suppl 2):S10-7.
[68] Cadet JL, Jayanthi S. Epigenetics of addiction. Neurochem Int 2021;147: 105069.
[69] Ahearn OC, Watson MN, Rawls SM. Chemokines, cytokines and substance use disorders. Drug Alcohol Depend 2021;220:108511.
[70] Connor JP, Stjepanović D, Le Foll B, Hoch E, Budney AJ, Hall WD. Cannabis use and cannabis use disorder. Nat Rev Dis Primers 2021;7(1):16.
[71] Strout TD, Baumann MR, Wendell LT. Understanding ED buprenorphine initiation for opioid use disorder: A guide for emergency nurses. J Emerg Nurs 2021;47(1):139-54.
[72] Azevedo K, Johnson M, Wassermann M, Evans-Wall J. Drugs of abuse-opioids, sedatives, hypnotics. Crit Care Clin 2021;37(3):501-16.
[73] Hadland SE, Bagley SM, Gai MJ, Earlywine JJ, Schoenberger SF, Morgan JR, Et al. Opioid use disorder and overdose among youth following an initial opioid prescription. Addiction 2021;116(10):2790-800.
[74] Komrowski MD, Sekhri NK. A history of opioid abuse: Why buprenorphine is superior for the management of opioid use disorder and pain. J Opioid Manag 2021;17(7):43-50.
[75] Fairley M, Humphreys K, Joyce VR, Bounthavong M, Trafton J, Combs A, et al. Cost-effectiveness of treatments for opioid use disorder. JAMA Psychiatry 2021; 78(7):767-77.

Chapter 13

Use of pharmacologic agents for smoking cessation

Dilip R Patel*, MD, MBA, MPH, Danielle Hirsch, MD, MPH and Kimberly Wells, MD

Department of Pediatric and Adolescent Medicine, Western Michigan University Homer Stryker MD School of Medicine, Kalamazoo, Michigan, United States of America

Abstract

Tobacco use has been clearly demonstrated to have negative health consequences. Smoking cigarettes is the predominant method of tobacco use. The tar contained within cigarettes and other similar products is also harmful. Other tarless tobacco containing products do exist but carry no significantly decreased risk. While nicotine is considered to be principally responsible for tobacco addiction, other chemicals in the cigarette smoke including acetaldehyde may contribute to the addictive properties of tobacco products. The adverse health consequences of tobacco use have been well documented. Studies have shown that a combined behavioral and pharmacological approach is more effective in smoking cessation than either approach alone. Pharmacotherapy can achieve 50% reduction in smoking. With pharmacotherapy the estimated 6-month abstinence rate is about 20%, whereas it is about 10% without pharmacotherapy. The first-line of drugs for smoking cessation are varenicline, bupropion sustained release, and nicotine replacement drugs, which are approved for use in adults. Data are insufficient to recommend their use in adolescents. This article reviews the pharmacological agents used for smoking cessation.

Introduction

Tobacco plant is native to South America, Mexico, and the West Indies (1). The American Indians used various forms of tobacco for its medicinal properties, for hundreds of years before the discovery by Christopher Columbus of the New World (1). The common tobacco, *Nicotiana tabacum*, is named after Jean Nicot, the French ambassador to Lisbon, who is believed to have sent its seeds to Catherine de Medicis, the queen consort and regent of France in 1566 (1).

* ***Correspondence:*** Dilip R Patel, MD, MBA, MPH, Professor and Chair, Department of Pediatric and Adolescent Medicine, Western Michigan University School of Medicine, 1000, Oakland Drive, Kalamazoo MI, United States. Email: Dilip.patel@med.wmich.edu.

In: Behavioral Pediatrics
Editors: Donald E. Greydanus, Dilip R. Patel, Ahsan Nazeer et al.
ISBN: 979-8-88697-060-9

Nicotine was first extracted in its crude form in 1571, purified form in 1928, and synthesized in a laboratory in 1904 (1). Over the decades, the causative role of smoking and other forms of tobacco use in cancer has been well-established. This article reviews the health effects of smoking and pharmacological agents used for smoking cessation in adolescents and young adults.

Table 1. Main forms of tobacco used

Cigarettes	Cigarette brands are categorize based on their tar content: Ultra-light 1-6 mg tar Light 6-15 mg tar Full-flavor > 15 mg tar Of all cigarettes sold in the United States, 84% are either light or ultra-light. Low-yield cigarettes and cigarette-like products are examples of a classification of products referred to as "potentially reduced-exposure products" (PREPs).
Cigars	Cigars contain the same toxic and carcinogenic compounds found in cigarettes. The three major types of cigars sold in the United States are large cigars, cigarillos, and little cigars.
Bidis	Bidis are small, thin hand-rolled cigarettes imported to the United States primarily from India and other Southeast Asian countries. They consist of tobacco wrapped in a tendu or temburni leaf (plants native to Asia), and may be secured with a colorful string at one or both ends. They have higher concentrations of nicotine, tar, and carbon monoxide than conventional cigarettes sold in the United States.
Kreteks	Kreteks (clove cigarettes) imported from Indonesia, typically contain a mixture consisting of tobacco, cloves, and other additives. Kreteks deliver more nicotine, carbon monoxide, and tar than conventional cigarettes.
Smokeless tobacco	Chewing tobacco comes in the form of loose leaf, plug, or twist. Snuff is finely ground tobacco that can be dry, moist, or in sachets (tea bag-like pouches). Although some forms of snuff can be used by sniffing or inhaling into the nose, most smokeless tobacco users place the product in their cheek or between their gum and cheek. Users then suck on the tobacco and spit out the tobacco juices, which is why smokeless tobacco is often referred to as spit or spitting tobacco.
Betel quid with tobacco (Gutka)	Gutka (*ghutka* or *gutkha*) is a dry, relatively nonperishable commercial preparation that consists of betel leaf (*Piper betle*), tobacco, areca nut (*Areca catechu*), catechu (extract of the *Acacia catechu* tree), and slaked lime (calcium hydroxide). Gutka is available in sachets and tins. It is consumed by placing a pinch of the mixture in the mouth between the gum and cheek and gently sucking and chewing. The excess saliva produced by chewing may be swallowed or spit out. *Gutka* is primarily consumed in the Indian subcontinent (India, Pakistan, and Bangladesh). In the Indian subcontinent, nonperishable, commercially manufactured preparations of betel quid without tobacco are known as *pan masala,* and freshly prepared betel quid (with or without tobacco) is known as *pan*.

Based on data from: Centers for Disease Control and Prevention. Smoking and tobacco use: fact sheets. URL: http://www.cdc.gov/tobacco/data_statistics/fact_sheets.

Epidemiology

Cigarette smoking is the most popular method of using tobacco; other forms of smoking and tobacco use are summarized in Table 1 (2-4). Worldwide, tobacco use causes more than 7 million deaths per year – more than HIV/AIDS, malaria, and tuberculosis combined (5). Despite a 67% reduction in the number of adult cigarette smokers in the United States since 1965, cigarette smoking remains the leading preventable cause of death in the United States, responsible for about one in five or half-million deaths every year (4, 6). Exposure to environmental tobacco smoke (ETS) results in an estimated 41,000 annual deaths in the United

States (2). Smoking and use of other forms of tobacco by youth is of particular significance, with 9 out of 10 adult cigarette smokers being under the age of 18 when they first smoked a cigarette and 98% being under the age of 26 at the time of their first cigarette (7).

Despite an approximately 20% reduction in youth tobacco use since 2011, more than 3.5 million American adolescents (aged 12–17 years) in 2017 reported using a tobacco product in the month prior to the survey and rates of electronic cigarette use among youth has increased (2, 8). Tobacco use by adolescents is influenced by multiple psychosocial and biological factors that increase adolescents' vulnerability for nicotine use (2, 9, 10). Studies show that adolescents are more sensitive to the reinforcing effects of nicotine and other chemicals found in cigarettes, further increasing their susceptibility to tobacco addiction. Intermittent smoking, such as over the weekends or at parties, has also been shown to result in tobacco addiction in adolescents. Tobacco use, especially the smokeless forms, is of special concern in athletes (11-20).

Chemistry and pharmacology

Approximately 4,000 chemicals are found in the smoke of tobacco products, of which nicotine is primarily responsible for tobacco addiction (2, 9, 10). The chemistry and neuropharmacology of nicotine has been extensively studied (21-24). Other main constituents of smoke that result in adverse health consequences include ammonia, benzene, carbon monoxide, cyanide, formaldehyde, acetaldehyde, phenols, and tar. Approximately 90% of the constituents of the smoke are in the form of vaporized chemicals, while rest are in the particulate form (2, 4 25).

Cigarettes are categorized (see Table 1) based on their tar content (total particulate matter in smoke, excluding water and alkaloid compounds), which is measured using a standardized protocol on a smoking machine (2-4). In filtered cigarettes (99% of cigarettes currently on the market), the filter vents dilute the smoke with air, reducing standard yields of tar, nicotine, and carbon monoxide. Many smokers block the vents or compensate with increased inhalations when smoking low-yield cigarettes. By doing so, they typically get as much tar and nicotine from cigarettes with low-yield ratings as those with higher yields. On an average a cigarette contains between 13 mg and 19 mg of nicotine and smoking of 1 cigarette typically delivers 1–2 mg of nicotine (2, 9, 10). The nicotine content of tobacco smoke is 1–2% and each inhalation delivers approximately 0.05–0.15 mg (2, 10).

Smoke is produced by incomplete combustion of tobacco. The fate of the cigarette smoke is depicted in Figure 1 (25). Mainstream smoke—the smoke inhaled by the smoker directly through the mouthpiece of the cigarette—constitutes approximately 45% of the total smoke; whereas, side stream smoke, which is the smoke emitted by smoldering tobacco between puffs and the smoke diffusing through the lit cigarette paper and escaping from the burning cone during smoking, constitutes 55% of the total smoke (25).

Nicotine, whose chemical structure resembles that of the neurotransmitter acetylcholine, acts on stereospecific nicotinic cholinergic receptors (nAChRs) in the brain and other organs (10, 24). The chemical structure and metabolic pathway of nicotine is depicted in Figure 2. It also has direct and indirect effects on the neuroendocrine system. The initial phase of stimulation of the central nervous system (CNS) by nicotine is typically followed by a phase of CNS depression (10, 23). The action of nicotine on nAChRs stimulates the release of various neurotransmitters and hormones including acetylcholine, norepinephrine, dopamine, vasopressin, serotonin, and beta-endorphins (2, 9, 10, 22). Research shows that smoking is associated with a marked decrease in monoamine oxidase (MAO) levels in the brain (10). It is postulated that this decrease in MAO is caused by chemicals in the smoke other than nicotine. Decreased levels of MAO-A and MAO-B in the brain result in a higher level of dopamine. The action of nicotine on the CNS increases alertness, improves memory, improves concentration, and decreases anxiety. The pharmacokinetic properties of nicotine are summarized in Table 2 (2, 4, 10, 11, 24).

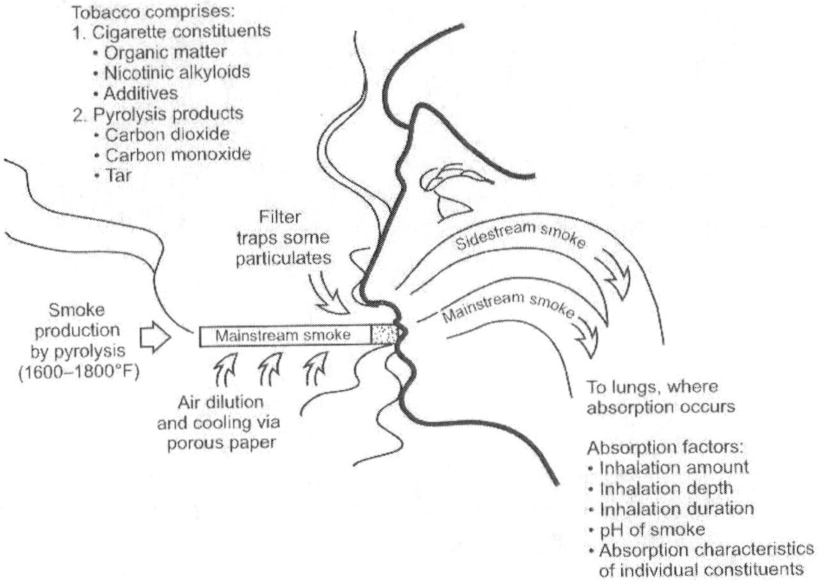

Figure 1. Fate of cigarette smoke. (From U. S. Department of Health and Human Services: The Health Consequences of Smoking. Nicotine Addiction: A Report of the Surgeon General. Washington, DC, 1988).

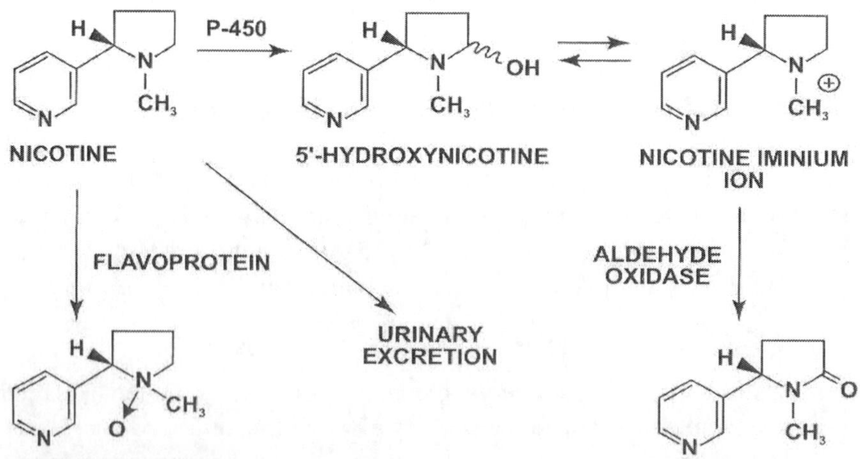

Figure 2. Chemical structure and metabolic pathway of nicotine. (From U. S. Department of Health and Human Services: The Health Consequences of Smoking. Nicotine Addiction: A Report of the Surgeon General. Washington, DC, 1988).

Table 2. Pharmacokinetics of nicotine (2, 4, 10, 11, 24)

Absorption	• 10–50% of available nicotine is absorbed during puffing; 80% during deep inhalation • Readily and completely absorbed via mucous membranes and skin
Distribution	• Readily distributed in all body tissues • Reaches brain within 10 s • Acute spike in arterial nicotine level occurs • Steady state volume of distribution is approximately 2.6 times the body weight in kg
Metabolism	• 80% is metabolized in the liver to continine by enzyme CYP2A6 (and to a lesser extent by CYP2B6 and CYP2E1) • Rest is metabolized in the lungs and kidneys
Elimination	• Average elimination half-life is 2 h • Average elimination half-life of nicotine metabolite cotinine is 16 h • Cotinine is not detectable in urine after complete abstinence of 1 wk • Unaltered nicotine and its metabolites excreted by kidneys

Effects on health

The wide-ranging adverse effects of tobacco use have been well-established and well-documented (2, 4, 9, 25-31). The numerous health consequences of smoking are summarized in Table 3. Nicotine activates reward pathways in the brain that regulate feelings of pleasure (10). These effects of nicotine are mediated by dopamine. Nicotine increases levels of dopamine mainly by its action on the mesolimbic dopamine system (10, 24). Chronic use of nicotine results in an increase in the number of nicotine receptors in the brain (9, 10, 22). Consequently, more nicotine is required to achieve the desired effect, eventually resulting in tolerance and dependence. Regular tobacco use results in nicotine accumulation in the body, exposing the user to the effects of nicotine throughout the 24 hours. Nicotine levels in the brain and the associated feelings of pleasure and reward peak within 10 seconds of inhalation (2, 4, 10).

However, the acute effects of nicotine dissipate rapidly. This causes the smoker to continue to smoke to maintain the effects of the nicotine and prevent withdrawal symptoms. The significant neurochemical changes in the brain that result from chronic nicotine use make it very difficult for the smoker to quit. Animal studies have shown that acetaldehyde, a chemical found in tobacco smoke, dramatically increases the reinforcing properties of nicotine and may also contribute to tobacco addiction (2, 4, 10). Adolescent animals show far more sensitivity to this reinforcing effect, suggesting increased vulnerability of adolescents to tobacco addiction.

Abrupt cessation of smoking results in withdrawal symptoms primarily due to decreased nicotine levels. Symptoms of nicotine withdrawal include irritability, craving, depression, anxiety, cognitive as well as attention deficit, sleep disturbances, and increased appetite (9, 25). The withdrawal symptoms, in most cases, begin within a few hours after the last cigarette, peak within the first few days of smoking cessation, and usually subside within a few weeks. In some cases, however the symptoms may persist for months (4, 9).

Table 3. Adverse health effects of smoking and tobacco use

Disease	
Cancer	• Bladder cancer • Cervical cancer • Esophageal cancer • Kidney cancer • Laryngeal cancer • Leukemia • Lung cancer • Oral cancer • Pancreatic cancer • Stomach cancer
Cardiovascular diseases	• Abdominal aortic aneurysm • Acute and episodic increase in blood pressure • Acute increase in peripheral vascular resistance and blood pressure • Atherosclerosis • Cerebrovascular disease • Coronary heart disease • Decreased coronary blood flow (due to constriction of coronary arteries) • Decreased oxygen carrying capacity of the hemoglobin • Hypertension • Increased baseline heart rate • Increased oxygen demands of the myocardium (due to increased heart rate and blood pressure) • Increased risk for thromboembolism • Increased risk of ventricular arrhythmias and sudden death (due to increased platelet adhesiveness, releasing catecholamines causing acute thrombosis and promoting ventricular arrhythmias) • Peripheral vascular disease
Respiratory diseases	• Bronchiolitis • Bronchitis • Chronic cough • Chronic obstructive pulmonary disease • Chronic obstructive pulmonary disease • Decreased forced expiratory volume (FEV1) • Decreased peak expiratory flow rate (PEFR) • Development and exacerbation of asthma Dyspnea • Eosinophilic granuloma • Halitosis • Hoarseness • Idiopathic pulmonary fibrosis • Impaired lung growth • Impaired respiratory immunity • Increased respiratory allergies • Interstitial lung disease • Laryngitis • Otitis media and middle ear effusions • Pneumonia • Pulmonary hemorrhage • Pulmonary hypertension • Rhinitis • Sinusitis • Snoring • Spontaneous pneumothorax • Upper respiratory infections

Disease	
Reproductive effects	• Fertility • Fetal death and stillbirths • Low birth weight • Pregnancy complications • Premature menopause
Musculoskeletal	• Decreased bone mineral density • Increased risk for fractures • Increased spinal disk disease
Gastrointestinal	• Decreased appetite • Gastroesophageal reflux disease • Impaired glucose tolerance • Increase insulin resistance • Peptic ulcer disease
Mental health and psychosocial	• Addiction • Anxiety, palpitations, tremors • Nervousness, depression • Tolerance and dependence • Withdrawal symptoms
Effects on offspring of maternal smoking during pregnancy	• Certain childhood cancers • Increased cotinine in breastfed infants if mother smokes • Increased incidence of conduct disorders • Increased probability of female children to be smokers • Low birth weight • Miscarriage • Prematurity • Sudden infant death syndrome
Specific effects of smokeless tobacco use	• Excess salivation • Gingivitis, gingival recession • Halitosis • Leukoplakia • Oropharyngeal cancers • Periodontal disease • Staining of teeth
Other effects	• Altered lipid profile • Altered metabolism of therapeutic drugs • Anorexia and weight loss • Cataracts • Decreased exercise performance • Diminished health status/increased morbidity • Esophagitis • Gastroesophageal reflux disease • Hip fractures • Low bone density • Macular degeneration • Nicotine addiction (tolerance dependence, withdrawal symptoms) • Osteoporosis • Peptic ulcer disease • Spinal disk disease

Sources: U.S. Department of Health Education, and Welfare 1964, 1967, 1979; U.S. Department of Health and Human Services 1980, 1982, 1983, 1984, 1989, 1990, 1994, 2001. Data from: (1) U.S. Department of Health and Human Services: The Health Consequences of Smoking. Nicotine Addiction: A Report of the Surgeon General. Washington, DC, 1988.

U. S. Department of Health and Human Services; (2) The Health Consequences of Smoking: A Report of the Surgeon General. Atlanta, GA: U.S. Department of Health and Human Services, CDC, National Center for Chronic Disease Prevention and Health Promotion, Office of Smoking and Health, 2004. URL: http://www.cdc,gov/tobacco/data_statistics/sgr_2004/index.htm.

Behavioral approaches to smoking cessation

Behavioral treatment is integral to smoking cessation—studies have shown that a combination of behavioral and pharmacological treatment is more effective than either approach alone (3, 32-35). In addition to the neurochemical effects of nicotine, behavioral factors also affect the severity of withdrawal symptoms. For some people, the feel, smell, and sight of a cigarette and the ritual of obtaining, handling, lighting, and smoking a cigarette are all associated with the pleasurable effects of smoking. Consequently, this can worsen withdrawal symptoms or cravings. Behavioral therapies can help smokers identify environmental triggers of craving so they can employ strategies to prevent or circumvent these symptoms and urges.

Table 4. Factors to be considered in the use of smoking cessation drugs

Practical considerations	Health insurance coverage, out-of-pocket costs, likelihood of adherence, dentures when considering the gums, or dermatitis when considering the patch.
Patient's prior experience with a medication	Prior successful experience (sustained abstinence with the medication) suggests that the medication may be helpful to the patient in a subsequent quit attempt, especially if the patient found the medication to be tolerable and or easy to use. However, it is difficult to draw firm conclusions from prior failure with a medication.
Heave users or smokers Light users or smokers	The higher-dose preparations of nicotine gum, patch, and lozenge have been shown to be effective in highly dependent smokers. Combination nicotine replacement therapy (NRT) may be particularly effective in suppressing tobacco withdrawal symptoms. NRT combinations are especially helpful for highly dependent smokers or those with a history of severe withdrawal. Cessation medications generally not beneficial to light smokers. If NRT is used with light smokers, consider reducing the dose of the medication. No adjustments are necessary when using bupropion SR or varenicline.
Gender	NRT can be effective with both sexes; however, evidence is mixed as to whether NRT is less effective in women than men. This may encourage the clinician to consider use of another type of medication with women, such as bupropion SR or varenicline.
Weight gain concern	Bupropion SR and nicotine replacement therapies, in particular 4-mg nicotine gum and 4-mg nicotine lozenge, delay—but do not prevent—weight gain.
Depression	Bupropion SR and nortriptyline appear to be effective, but nicotine replacement medications also appear to help individuals with a history of depression.
History of cardiovascular disease	The nicotine patch has been demonstrated safe for patients with a history of cardiovascular disease.
Long-term use	Long-term use is helpful with smokers who report persistent withdrawal symptoms during the course of medications, who have relapsed in the past after stopping medication, or who desire long-term therapy. A minority of individuals who successfully quit smoking use ad libitum NRT medications (gum, nasal spray, inhaler) long-term. The use of these medications for up to 6 months does not present a known health risk and developing dependence on medications is uncommon. The FDA has approved the use of bupropion SR, varenicline, and some NRT medications for 6-month use.
Combination therapy	Combining the nicotine patch long-term (> 14 weeks) with nicotine gum or nicotine nasal spray, the nicotine patch with the nicotine inhaler, or the nicotine patch with bupropion SR, increases long-term abstinence rates relative to placebo treatments. Combining varenicline with NRT agents has been associated with higher rates of side effects (e.g., nausea, headaches).

Modified from: Fiore MC, Jaen CR, Baker TB, et al. Treating Tobacco Use and Dependence 2008 Update. Clinical Practice Guideline. Rockville, MD: U. S. Department of Health and Human Services. Public Health Service. May 2008.

Pharmacological agents

Factors which should be considered when prescribing pharmacological agents for smoking cessation are summarized in Table 4 (3). Patients who smoke may be on therapeutic drugs for other chronic diseases. The effective dosages of these therapeutic drugs reflect the adjustments made because of concomitant exposure to nicotine. With smoking cessation and elimination of nicotine from the body, a new state of metabolic homeostasis will result that may necessitate adjusting dosage of therapeutic drugs (3).

Tobacco dependence should be considered a chronic disease and as such its management requires on-going patient education, counseling, and use of medications as indicated (3). Relapses are common during smoking cessation and patients require long-term monitoring and treatment. Long-term pharmacotherapy, combination therapy, and re-use of drugs previously used (recycling) should be considered in relapse prevention and treatment. In some patients who are not able to quit completely, pharmacotherapy has been used to reduce smoking, with some achieving a 50% reduction in smoking (3, 10). With pharmacotherapy, the estimated 6-month abstinence rate is about 20%, compared to approximately 10% without pharmacotherapy (3, 9, 10). All pharmacologic agents have been shown to be effective in smoking cessation with odds ratios between two and four when compared to placebo treatment (3, 9). Absolute smoking cessation rates vary depending on the particular pharmacologic agent used and the intensity of concomitant counseling; rates vary in range from 5% to 35% (3, 9, 10).

The first-line drugs for smoking cessation approved by the US Food and Drug Administration (FDA) are varenicline, bupropion sustained release (SR), and nicotine replacement drugs (3, 36-48). These drugs are approved by the FDA for use in adults and data are insufficient to assess their efficacy in adolescents (3). Pharmacotherapy has not been shown to be effective in light smokers and in those who use smokeless tobacco.

Varenicline

Varenicline acts by selective binding at α4β2 neuronal nicotinic acetylcholine receptors, which results in agonist activity, while simultaneously preventing nicotine binding to α4β2 receptors (7, 42–44). The FDA recommendation for varenicline product label includes a warning that serious neuropsychiatric symptoms have been reported in patients being treated with this drug. It is not uncommon for patients to experience feelings of depression, anxiety, irritability, and sleep disturbances during smoking cessation. Although some of these symptoms may be associated with nicotine withdrawal, symptoms have occurred in patients who continued to smoke.

Patients on varenicline should be monitored for agitation, depressed mood, and changes in behavior that are not typical for the patient. The patient also must be assessed for suicidal ideation or suicidal behavior. Varenicline is reported to be well-tolerated for up to 1 year and may reduce the incidence of relapse (44). Varenicline has been found in randomized controlled trials to be more effective than both buproprion and nicotine replacement monotherapy, and as effective as combination nicotine replacement therapy (nicotine patch plus rapid-onset formulation) (48). Prescribing information for varenicline is summarized in Table 5.

Table 5. Varenicline[Rx]

Product	Chantix® (Pfizer, Inc., New York City, NY) • 0.5 mg, 1 mg tablet
Precautions	Pregnancy • May worsen pre-existing psychiatric illness • Dosage adjustment required in patients with kidney disease (creatinine clearance less than 30 ml/min) or who are on dialysis • WARNING: Can cause depressed mood, agitation, change in behavior, suicidal ideation, suicide. Reported in patients attempting to quit smoking while using varenicline. Monitor closely.
Dosage	Recommended: 1-week titration: Days 1–3: 0.5 mg tablet daily Days 4–7: 0.5 mg tablet BID (AM and HS) Days 8+: 1 mg tablet BID (AM and HS) • Set quit date • Start one week before quit date • Take after eating and with a full glass of water • Nausea is dose related; if persistent and troubling, consider dose reduction Duration: 12 wk; if successful after 12 wk, an additional 12 wk is recommended for increased likelihood of long-term abstinence
Side effects	• Dose dependent nausea (most common) • Insomnia • Abnormal dreams • Headache • Dyspepsia • Constipation • Flatulence • Vomiting
Advantages	• Provides nicotine effects to reduce withdrawal symptoms and cravings • Blocks the nicotine effects from smoking and reduces reward of smoking • May be used in those with cardiovascular disease • No clinically meaningful drug interactions • Found to be more effective than bupropion SR
Disadvantages	• Not studied in combination with other therapies • Nausea associated with higher doses may be bothersome • Does not reduce weight gain • May cause impaired ability to drive or operate heavy machinery • May cause neuropsychiatric symptoms including behavioral changes, agitation, depressed mood, suicidal ideation, and suicidal behavior

Bupropion sustained release (SR)

The proposed mechanisms of action of bupropion sustained release (SR) include blockade of neuronal re-uptake of dopamine and norepinephrine (45). Similar to varenicline, bupropion SR also carries an FDA warning for neuropsychiatric adverse events. Bupropion SR is also anti-depressant and like other anti-depressant drugs, it carries a warning for increased risk of suicidal ideation. Patients on bupropion should therefore be closely monitored for emerging neuropsychiatric symptoms and signs of suicidal ideation. Buproprion has been found to be as effective as nicotine replacement therapy for smoking cessation (48). Prescribing information for bupropion SR for smoking cessation is summarized in Table 6.

Table 6. Bupropion SR[Rx]

Product	Zyban® (GlaxoSmithKline plc, Brentford, London, England, UK), Generic • 150 mg sustained-release tablet
Contraindications	• History of seizure disorder • History of stroke • History of brain tumor, brain surgery, or serious closed head injury • Eating disorders • Those taking another form of bupropion • Monoamine oxidase inhibitor therapy within previous 14 d • Abrupt discontinuation of alcohol or benzodiazepines at same time
Precautions	• Pregnancy • Concomitant therapy with medications known to lower the seizure threshold
Dosage	150 mg PO q AM × 3 d, then increase to 150 mg PO BID • Treatment should be initiated while patient is still smoking • Set quit date 1–2 weeks after initiation • DO NOT exceed 300 mg/d • Allow at least 8 h between doses • Avoid bedtime dosing to minimize insomnia • Can be used safely with NRT • If progression towards abstinence unsuccessful by week 7, discontinue Duration: 8–12 wk, maintenance up to 6 months
Side effects	• Insomnia most common (35–40%) • Dry mouth • Nervousness • Agitation • Anxiety • Weight loss • Constipation • Seizures (risk is 1/1000)
Advantages	• Bupropion can be safely used with NRT • Bupropion may be beneficial in patients with depression • No tapering required
Disadvantages	• Seizure risk is increased • May increase the risk of suicidal thinking in patients who have depression

Nicotine replacement therapies

Nicotine replacement therapy (NRT) drugs reduce craving and withdrawal symptoms by partially replacing lost nicotine intake. The main characteristics and prescribing information of available NRT products are summarized in Tables 7 through 11 (3, 32, 36-38, 46, 47).

Second-line medications

Clonidine and nortriptyline are second-line medications used for smoking cessation (3, 49). Although second-line medications have been shown to be effective in treating tobacco dependence, their use is limited mainly because of less favorable side-effect profile when compared to the first-line medications. Second-line medications are not approved by the FDA specifically for use in smoking cessation (3). Second-line medications should be considered for use on a case-by-case basis after first-line medications (either alone or in combination) have been used without success, or are contraindicated (3).

Table 7. Transdermal Preparations$^{OTC/Rx}$

Products		Nicotrol Patch® (McNeil Consumer Healthcare, Fort Washington, PA) • 5 mg • 10 mg, 15 mg (16 h)	Nicoderm® CQ (Sanofi-Aventis S.A., Paris, France); Generic nicotine patch • 7 mg • 14 mg, 21 mg (24 h)
Dosage	> 10 cigarettes/day	• 15 mg/d × 6 wk • 10 mg/d × 2 wk • 5 mg/d × 2 wk	• 21 mg/d × 6 wk • 14 mg/d × 2 wk • 7 mg/d × 2 weeks
	≤ 10 cigarettes/day	• 10 mg/d × 6 wk • 5 mg/d × 2 wk	• 14 mg/d × 6 wk • 7 mg/d × 2 wk If < 100 lbs or cardiovascular disease: • 14 mg/d × 4–6 wk • 7 mg/d × 2–4 wk
Commentsa		• Remove before bedtime • Nicotine released over 16 h	• May wear patch for 24 h • Remove at bedtime if patient experiences sleep disturbances.
Contraindications		• Pregnancy • Recent (2 or less wk post-myocardial infarction) • Unstable angina pectoris • Serious underlying arrhythmias	
Side effects		• Local skin reactions: erythema, pruritis, burning • Headache • Sleep disturbances: insomnia, vivid dreams	
Advantages		• Provides consistent nicotine levels over 16–24 h • Easy to use and conceal • Fewer adherence issues • Available without prescription	
Disadvantages		• Patients cannot titrate the dose • Allergic reactions to adhesive • Patients with certain skin conditions cannot use patch • Patch may contain aluminum	

[a]Patch should be applied in the morning when patient wakes on the quit day. Apply on relatively hairless areas between the neck and waist.

Table 8. Gum^{OTC}

Product	Nicorette® (GlaxoSmithKline plc, Brentford, London, England, UK), Nicorette DS® (GlaxoSmithKline plc, Brentford, London, England, UK), Generic • 2 mg, 4 mg; regular, mint, orange
Contraindications	• Pregnancy • Recent (≤ 2 weeks) myocardial infarction • Serious underlying arrhythmias • Serious or worsening angina pectoris • Temporomandibular joint disease

Dosage	≥ 25 cigarettes/day: 4 mg < 25 cigarettes/day: 2 mg Week 1–6: 1 piece q 1–2 h Week 2–4: 1 piece q 2–4 h Week 10–12: 1 piece q 4–8 h • Chew each piece slowly until peppery or flavored taste emerges • Park between cheek and gum when tingling sensation appears • Resume chewing when tingle fades • Repeat chew/park steps until most of the nicotine is gone (taste or tingle does not return; generally 30 min) • Park in different areas of mouth • No food or beverages 15 min before or during use (acidic beverages reduce buccal absorption) If there are strong or frequent cravings, may use a 2nd piece within the hour Max: 24 pieces/d Duration: Up to 12 wk
Side effects	• Mouth soreness • Throat irritation • Jaw pain • Hiccups • Dyspepsia • Hypersalivation • Flatulence • Nausea and vomiting • Unpleasant taste • Lightheadedness
Advantages	• Might satisfy oral cravings • May delay weight gain • Patients can titrate therapy to manage withdrawal symptoms • Available over the counter
Disadvantages	• Gum chewing may not be socially acceptable • Difficult to use with dentures • May cause loosening of dental fillings • Patients must use proper chewing technique to minimize adverse effects

Table 9. Lozenge^{OTC}

Product	Commit® (GlaxoSmithKline plc, Brentford, London, England, UK) • 2 mg, 4 mg
Contraindications	• Pregnancy • Recent (≤ 2 weeks) myocardial infarction • Serious underlying arrhythmias • Serious or worsening angina pectoris
Dosage	1st cigarette ≤ 30 min after waking up: 4 mg 1st cigarette > 30 min after waking up: 2 mg Week 1–6: 1 lozenge q 1–2 h; minimum 9 per d Week 7–9: 1 lozenge q 2–4 h Week 10–12: 1 lozenge q 4–8 h • Allow lozenge to dissolve slowly (20–30 min) • Nicotine release may cause a warm or tingling sensation • Do not chew or swallow the lozenge • Rotate the lozenge to different areas of the mouth • No food or beverages 15 min before, during or after use • Do not use more than 1 lozenge at a time Max: 5 lozenges every 6 h; 20 lozenges/d Duration: up to 12 wk

Table 9. (Continued)

Adverse Events	• Nausea • Hiccups • Cough • Heartburn • Headache
Advantages	• Might satisfy oral cravings • May delay weight gain • Patients can titrate therapy to manage withdrawal symptoms • Provides ~25% more nicotine than gum • Available over the counter
Disadvantages	• Gastrointestinal side effects might be bothersome • Contains phenylalanine

Table 10. Nasal Spray[Rx]

Product	Nicotrol NS® (Pfizer, Inc., New York City, NY) • Metered spray (0.5 mg nicotine/actuation) aqueous nicotine
Contraindications	• Pregnancy • Recent (≤ 2 weeks) myocardial infarction • Serious underlying arrhythmias • Serious or worsening angina pectoris
Dosage	1–2 doses/h (8–40 doses/d) One dose: 2 sprays (one in each nostril); each spray delivers 0.5 mg of nicotine to the nasal mucosa. • Patients should not sniff, swallow, or inhale through the nose as the spray is administered • For best results, initially use at least 8 doses/d • DO NOT exceed 5 doses/h and 40 doses/d • Gradually decrease usage Duration (maximal): 3 mo
Side effects	• Nasal and throat irritation (hot, peppery, or burning sensation) • Transient change in sense of smell and taste • Rhinitis • Tearing • Sneezing • Cough • Headache • Nausea
Advantages	• Patients can easily titrate therapy to rapidly manage withdrawal symptoms • Fastest acting nicotine product
Disadvantages	• Nasal/throat irritation may be bothersome • Dependence can result • Patients must wait 5 minutes before driving or operating heavy machinery • Patients with chronic nasal disorders (allergy, rhinitis, nasal polyps, or sinusitis) or severe reactive airway disease should NOT use the spray • No optimal tapering schedule • Prescription only

Table 11. Oral inhaler[Rx]

Product	Nicotrol Inhaler® (Pfizer, Inc., New York City, NY) • 10 mg cartridge delivers 4 mg inhaled nicotine vapor
Contraindications	• Pregnancy • Recent (≤ 2 weeks) myocardial infarction • Serious underlying arrhythmias • Serious or worsening angina pectoris
Dosage	6–16 cartridges/d; individualize dosing • Initially, use at least 6 cartridges/d for first 3-6 wk • Best effects with continuous puffing for 20 min • Nicotine in cartridge is depleted after 20 min of active puffing (oral inhalation) • Patients should inhale deeply into back of throat or puff in short breaths • Open cartridge retains potency for 24 h • Each cartridge delivers 4 mg of nicotine over 80 inhalations • Avoid eating or drinking for 15 min before and after use (acidic beverages reduce absorption) Duration: Treat for 3 mo and then taper over next 3 mo
Adverse Events	• Mouth and throat irritation (40%) • Unpleasant taste • Cough (32%) • Rhinitis (23%) • Dyspepsia • Headache
Advantages	• Patients can easily titrate therapy to rapidly manage withdrawal symptoms • The inhaler mimics hand-to-mouth ritual of smoking
Disadvantages	• Initial throat or mouth irritation can be bothersome • Dependence can occur • Cold temperatures (< 60 °F) reduce amount of nicotine delivered • Avoid hot environments (> 77 °F) and protect from light • Patients with underlying bronchospastic disease must use with caution • No definitive tapering schedule • Prescription only

Clonidine is contraindicated in pregnant women and in those who engage in potentially hazardous activities. The most common side effects of clonidine include dry mouth (40%), drowsiness (33%), dizziness (16%), sedation (10%) and constipation (10%) (3). As its abrupt discontinuation can result in severe rebound hypertension, clonidine should be tapered. Conidine is available as 0.1 mg, 0.2 mg, and 0.3 mg scored tablets and 0.1 mg/24h, 0.2 mg/24h, and 0.3 mg/24 transdermal patches. The usual dosage is 0.2 mg – 0.6 mg per day in divided doses (3, 49). Specific dosage of clonidine for smoking cessation has not been established.

Nortriptyline is a tricyclic antidepressant and therefore carries an FDA warning about increased suicide risk (3). The most serious side effects of nortriptyline are arrhythmias and impairment of myocardial contractility. More common and less serious side effects include sedation, dry mouth, blurred vision, urinary retention, lightheadedness, and shaky hands (3). Nortriptyline is available as 10 mg, 25 mg, 50 mg, and 75 mg capsules and 10 mg/5 ml liquid. The dosage of nortriptyline in smoking cessation studies ranges between 25 mg per day and 100 mg per day (3, 49, 50). Therapeutic drug level and cardiovascular monitoring, including electrocardiogram (ECG), is recommended.

Vaccine

Some of the latest research for smoking cessation is coming in the form of a vaccine. The principal behind this idea is that after the vaccine enters the systemic circulation, a substantial proportion of nicotine can bind with antibodies and then once bound can no longer cross the blood-brain barrier (51). The pathophysiological mechanism underlying smoking are the addictive properties within it by the impact nicotine has on the locomotion, cognition, affect, pain sensitivity, arousal and most importantly the increase it has on the reward stimuli in the brain (1).

In regular smokers studies have shown an almost complete saturation of the receptors, which may serve to prevent occurrences of withdrawal symptoms; thus, further developments in pharmacotherapy for smoking cessation should focus on reducing the rewarding effects of smoking that includes the development of vaccinations. Basically, an immunogenic substrate that causes T and B cell activation leads to the formation of specific antibodies that bind to a drug and thus disable that drug from crossing the blood-brain barrier. This idea was first tested in an animal model of heroin addiction and what the five reports of phase I-II trials have shown is therapeutic antibody levels are only established several weeks after the first vaccine injection (51, 52).

Vaccination for the treatment of nicotine or even other substances of abuse has various attractive features. However, efficacy of vaccination is largely related to subjects achieving the highest serum antibody concentration. Immunization can be achieved in two ways: actively through vaccination or passively via the administering a drug-specific monoclonal antibody. The clinical trials have focused on vaccination because of the safety profile, low cost and long duration of action (52). Passive immunization achieves higher serum antibody concentrations but is more costly than vaccines. Vaccination, although promising, is still at a very experimental stage and not currently available as a treatment option.

E-cigarettes

As of this writing, electronic cigarettes (e-cigarettes) were marketed legally in the United States without any clinical trials (53, 54). E-cigarettes are a battery-operated device that contains a cartridge that is generally filled with nicotine, flavor, and other chemicals (53). They do not burn tobacco thus they do not emit smoke. The nicotine contained in the refill bottles can contain more than 500mg, which is approximately 10 times the lethal dose. E-cigarettes are promoted with claims of reducing toxins in the mainstream and secondhand smoke as well as help smokers quit (53). The FDA and other health agencies are concerned about the marketing to the public about e-cigarettes because it can promote nicotine addiction, delay or derail serious quit attempts and even encourage youth to try them (53). The chemical propylene glycol is what is used to make the "vapor" emitted from e-cigarettes and this chemical has the potential to generate acute and chronic respiratory effects as well as reduced lung function with increased proximity and cumulative exposure (53).

The US Surgeon General has made statements repeatedly that there is no safe level of exposure to tobacco smoke; however, no clear-cut scientific research is available on the safety of the vapor from e-cigarettes. Despite this lack of research, the sales of e-cigarettes continue to increase with e-cigarettes being the most commonly used tobacco product among American adolescents (8). Since the FDA's determination in 2016 that the regulation of e-cigarettes falls under its authority, the agency has recognized the epidemic of youth e-cigarette use and is working to limit their sale to minors (55, 56). Although electronic nicotine delivery systems (ENDS) are often marketed as a tool to achieve smoking cessation, there is limited evidence that ENDS are an effective smoking cessation aid (58). A prospective cohort study of adult smokers in the United States did not find increased rates of smoking cessation among ENDS users, including those specifically using ENDS as a tool to quit smoking (57).

Conclusion

Tobacco use remains a great public health concern, especially in adolescents. The significant health hazards of smoking and other forms of tobacco use are well-documented. Smoking can also adversely affect exercise and sports performance. Tobacco addiction is primarily caused by nicotine, though other chemicals contained within tobacco products are now believed to play a secondary role in addiction.

A combined behavioral and pharmacological approach has been found to be more effective for smoking cessation than either approach used alone. A range of pharmacological agents and behavioral therapies are available for smoking cessation. Varenicline, bupropion SR, and nicotine replacement therapies are recommended as first-line drugs for smoking cessation. In selected cases the first-line drugs may also be used in combination with each other to improve outcomes. Treatment interventions have been shown to double the rate of smoking cessation when compared to quit attempts without intervention. Tobacco dependence should be considered a chronic disease with anticipated relapses requiring long-term monitoring and treatment.

Acknowledgments

Adapted with permission from Patel DR, Feucht C, Reid L, Patel ND. Pharmacologic agents for smoking cessation: A clinical review. Clin Pharmacol 2010;2:17-29.

The authors thank Kim Douglas for assistance with the preparation of this manuscript. Data in Tables 5 to 11 are derived from: 1) Fiore MC, Jaen CR, Baker TB, et al. Treating tobacco use and dependence 2008 update. Clinical practice guideline. Rockville, MD: US. Department of Health and Human Services. Public Health Service. May 2008; 2) Food and Drug Administration product information available at www.fda.gov; 3) Drug manufacturer product labels available at manufacturer web sites; including following web sites:

Chantix http://www.accessdata.fda.gov/drugsatfda_docs/label/2008/021928s007lbl.pdf;

Zyban http://www.fda.gov/Safety/MedWatch/SafetyInformation/ucm176815.htm;

Nicotrol inhaler http://media.pfizer.com/files/products/uspi_nicotrol_inhaler.pdf;

Nicotrol NS http://media.pfizer.com/files/products/uspi_nicotrol.pdf; Nicoderm CQ http://www.nicodermcq.com/; Commit http://www.commitlozenge.com/; Nicorette http://www.nicorette.com/

References

[1] Encyclopaedia Britannica. URL: http://www.britannica.com.

[2] Centers for Disease Control and Prevention. Smoking and tobacco use: Fact sheets. URL: https://www.cdc.gov/tobacco/data_statistics/fact_sheets/fast_facts/index.htm.

[3] Fiore MC, Jaen CR, Baker TB. Treating tobacco use and dependence 2008 update. Clinical Practice Guideline. Rockville, MD: US Department of Health and Human Services. Public Health Service, 2008.

[4] US Department of Health and Human Services. National Institute on Drug Abuse. Research Report Series: Tobacco, nicotine, and E-cigarettes. URL: https://www.drugabuse.gov/publications/research-reports/tobacco-nicotine-e-cigarettes/introduction.

[5] World Health Organization: WHO report on the global tobacco epidemic, 2017. Geneva: WHO, 2017.

[6] Wang TW, Asman K, Gentzke AS, Cullen KA, Holder-Hayes E, Reyes-Guzman C, et al. Tobacco product use among adults - United States, 2017. MMWR 2018;67(44):1225-32.

[7] Centers for Disease Control and Prevention. Youth and tobacco use: fact sheets. URL: https://www.cdc.gov/tobacco/data_statistics/fact_sheets/youth_data/tobacco_use/index.htm.

[8] Wang TW, Gentzke A, Sharapova S, Cullen KA, Ambrose BK, Jamal A. Tobacco product use among middle and high school students — United States, 2011–2017. MMWR 2018;67(22):629-33.

[9] Hatsukami DK, Stead LF, Gupta PC. Tobacco addiction. Lancet 2008;371(9629):2027- 38.

[10] Benowitz NL. Pharmacology of nicotine: addiction, smoking-induced disease, and therapeutics. Annu Rev Pharmacol Toxicol 2009;49:57–71.

[11] Walsh MM, Ellison J, Hilton JF, Chesney M, Ernster VL. Spit (smokeless) tobacco use by high school baseball athletes in California. Tob Control 2009;9(Suppl 2):II32–9.

[12] Melnick MJ, Miller KE, Sabo DF, Farrell MP, Barnes GM. Tobacco use among high school athletes and nonatheletes: results of the 1997 youth risk behavior survey. Adolescence 2001;36(144):727–47.

[13] Green GA, Uryasz FD, Petr TA, Bray CD. NCAA study of substance use and abuse habits of college student-athletes. Clin J Sport Med 2001;11(1):51–6.

[14] Alaranta A, Alaranta H, Patja K, Palmu P, Prättälä R, Martelin T, et al. Snuff use and smoking in Finnish Olympic athletes. Int J Sports Med 2006;27(7):581–6.

[15] Peretti-Watel P, Guagliardo V, Verger P, Pruvost J, Mignon P, Obadia Y. Sporting activity and drug use: alcohol, cigarette and cannabis use among elite student athletes. Addiction 2003;98(9):1249–56.

[16] Walsh MM, Hilton JF, Ernster VL, Masouredis CM, Grady DG. Prevalence, patterns, and correlates of spit tobacco use in a college athlete population. Addict Behav 1994;19(4): 411–27.

[17] Davis TC, Arnold C, Nandy I, Bocchini JA, Gottlieb A, George RB, et al. Tobacco use among male high school athletes. J Adolesc Health 1997;21(2):97–101.

[18] Epps RP, Lynn WR, Manley MW. Tobacco, youth, and sports. Adolesc Med 1998;9(3): 483–90.

[19] Rainey CJ, McKeown RE, Sargent RG, Valois RF. Patterns of tobacco and alcohol use among sedentary, exercising, nonathletic, and athletic youth. J Sch Health 1996;66(1):27–32.

[20] Yusko DA, Buckman JF, White HR, Pandina RJ. Alcohol, tobacco, illicit drugs, and performance enhancers: a comparison of use by college student athletes and nonathletes. J Am Coll Health 2008;57(3):281–90.

[21] Fletcher PJ, Lê AD, Higgins GA. Serotonin receptors as potential targets for modulation of nicotine use and dependence. Prog Brain Res 2008;172:361–83.

[22] Gamberino WC, Gold MS. Neurobiology of tobacco smoking and other addictive disorders. Psychiatr Clin North Am 1999;22(2):301-12.

[23] Rose JE. Disrupting nicotine reinforcement: from cigarette to brain. Ann NY Acad Sci 2008;1141:233–56.

[24] Taylor P. Agents acting at the neuromuscular junction and autonomic ganglia. In: Hardman JG, Limbird LE. Goodman and Gilman's The Pharmacologic Basis of Therapeutics, 9th ed. New York: McGraw-Hill, 1996:177–98.

[25] U.S. Department of Health and Human Services: The Health Consequences of Smoking. Nicotine Addiction: A Report of the Surgeon General. Washington, DC: DHHS, 1988.

[26] Aubry MC, Wright JL, Myers JL. The pathology of smoking-related lung diseases. Clin Chest Med 2000;21(1):11-35, vii.

[27] Fiore MC, Piaseck TH, Baker LJ, Decren SM. Cigarette smoking: the leading preventable cause of pulmonary disease. In Bone RC, ed. Pulmonary and critical care medicine. St Louis, MO: Mosby, 1998.

[28] Patel DR, Homnick DN. Pulmonary effects of smoking. Adolesc Med 2000;11:547-65.

[29] Sethi JM, Rochester CL. Smoking and chronic obstructive pulmonary disease. Clin Chest Med 2000;21(1):67-86, viii.

[30] U. S. Department of Health and Human Services. The health consequences of smoking: A report of the Surgeon General. Atlanta, GA: US Department of Health and Human Services, CDC, National Center for Chronic Disease Prevention and Health Promotion, Office of Smoking and Health, 2004. URL: http://www.cdc,gov/tobacco/data_statistics/sgr/sgr_2004/index.htm.

[31] U. S. Department of Health and Human Services: The health benefits of smoking cessation: A report of the Surgeon General. Washington, DC: DHHS, 1990. URL: http://www.cdc.gov/tobacco/data statistics/ sgr/index.htm.

[32] Burke MV, Ebbert JO, Hays JT. Treatment of tobacco dependence. Mayo Clin Proc 2008;83(4):479–83.

[33] Lemmens V, Oenema A, Knut IK, Brug J. Effectiveness of smoking cessation interventions among adults: a systematic review of reviews. Eur J Cancer Prev 2008;17(6):535–44.

[34] Patel DR, Greydanus DE. Office interventions for adolescent smokers. Adolesc Med 2000;11:577-88.

[35] Shah SD, Wilken LA, Winkler SR, Lin SJ. Systematic review and meta-analysis of combination therapy for smoking cessation. J Am Pharm Assoc 2008;48(5):659–65.

[36] Carrozzi L, Pistelli F, Viegi G. Pharmacotherapy for smoking cessation. Ther Adv Respir Dis 2008;2(5):301–17.

[37] Eisenberg MJ, Filion KB, Yavin D, Bélisle P, Mottillo S, Joseph L, et al. Pharmacotherapies for smoking cessation: a meta-analysis of randomized controlled trials. CMAJ 2008;179(2):135–44. Review. Erratum in: CMAJ 2008;179(8):802.

[38] Fant RV, Buchhalter AR, Buchman AC, Henningfield JE. Pharmacotherpay for tobacco dependence. Handb Exp Pharmacol 2009;192:487–510.

[39] Drugs for tobacco dependence. Treatment Guidelines. Med Lett Drugs Ther 2008;6(73): 61–6.

[40] Hajeck P, Stead LF, West R, Jarvis M, Lancaster T. Relapse prevention interventions for smoking cessation. Cochrane Database Syst Rev 2009;1:CD003999.

[41] Galanti LM. Tobacco smoking cessation management: integrating varenicline in current practice. Vasc Health Risk Manag 2008;4(4):837–45.

[42] Garrison GD, Dugan SE. Varenicline: a first-line treatment option of smoking cessation. Clin Ther 2009;31(3):463–91.

[43] Hays JT, Ebbert JO. Varenicline for tobacco dependence. N Eng J Med 2008;359(19): 2018–24.

[44] Lee JH, Jones PG, Bybee K, O'Keefe JH. A longer course of varenicline therapy improves smoking cessation rates. Prev Cardiol 2008;11(4):210–4.

[45] Paterson NE. Behavioural and pharmacological mechanisms of bupropion's anti-smoking effects: recent preclinical and clinical insights. Eur J Pharmacol 2009;603(1–3):1–11.

[46] Walsh RA. Over-the-counter nicotine replacement therapy: a methodological review of the evidence supporting its effectiveness. Drug Alcohol Rev 2008;27(5):529–47.

[47] Amodei N, Lamb RJ. Over-the-counter nicotine replacement therapy: Can its impact on smoking cessation be enhanced? Psychol Addict Behav 2008;22(4):472–85.

[48] Drugs for tobacco dependence. JAMA 2018;320(9):926-7.

[49] Stahl SM. Essential psychopharmacology: a prescriber's guide. New York: Cambridge University Press, 2006:53-58,353-60.

[50] Hughes JR, Stead LF, Lancaster T. Antidepressants for smoking cessation. Cochrane Database Syst Rev 2007;1:CD0000311.

[51] Raupach T, Hoogsteder PH, Onno van Schayck CP. Nicotine vaccines to assist with smoking cessation, current status of research. Drugs 2012;5(72):e1-16.

[52] Cornish KE, Harris AC, LeSage MG, Keyler DE, Brroughs D, Earley C, et al. Combined active and passive immunization against nicotine: Minimizing monoclonal antibody requirements using a target antibody concentration strategy. Int Immunopharmacol 2011; 11(11):1809-15.

[53] Riker CA, Darville LK, Hahn EJ. E-Cigarettes: promise or peril? Nurs Clin North Am 2012;47(1):159-71.

[54] McNeil JJ, Piccenna L, Ioannides-Demos LL. Smoking cessation-recent advances. Cardiovasc Drugs Ther 2010;24(4):359-67.

[55] Office of the Commissioner of Food and Drugs. Press Announcements - FDA takes new steps to address epidemic of youth e-cigarette use, including a historic action against more than 1,300 retailers and 5 major manufacturers for their roles perpetuating youth access.URL: https://www.fda.gov/NewsEvents/Newsroom/PressAnnouncements/ucm620184.htm.

[56] Voelker R. Stepped up e-cigarette enforcement. JAMA 2018;320(15):1528.

[57] Weaver SR, Huang J, Pechacek TF, Heath JW, Ashley DL, Eriksen MP. Are electronic nicotine delivery systems helping cigarette smokers quit? Evidence from a prospective cohort study of U.S. adult smokers, 2015–2016. Niaura R, ed. PLoS One 2018;13(7): e0198047.

[58] Eaton DL, Kwan LY, Stratton K, eds. Health practice; Committee on the Review of the Health Effects of Electronic Nicotine Delivery Systems. Public health consequences of e-cigarettes. Washington, DC: National Academies Press, 2018.

Section three: Selective concepts of management (editor: Ahsan Nazeer)

Chapter 14

Psychotherapeutic intervention with children and adolescents

Nehdia Hashemi[1], MD, Salma Malik[2], MD, Nazish Imran[3], FRPsych, Muhammad Zeeshan[4], MD and Ahsan Nazeer[5,*], MD

[1]Western Michigan University, Homer Stryker MD School of Medicine, Kalamazoo, Michigan
[2]Institute of Living/Hartford Healthcare, Hartford, Connecticut, United States of America,
[3]King Edward Medical University, Lahore, Pakistan, and [4]Rutgers New Jersey Medical School, Newark, New Jersey, The United States of America, [5]Sidra Medicine/Weill Cornell Medicine, Doha, Qatar

Abstract

In this chapter, the authors summarize psychotherapeutic interventions with pediatric persons, general principles, and categories of the psychotherapeutic and psychosocial interventions for various mental disorders. Also, a guide is given on the recommended interventions for specific diagnoses and problem areas in mental illnesses of children and adolescents. Interventions considered include supportive psychotherapy, behavioral therapy, parent management training (PMT), parent-child interaction training (PCIT), behavioral classroom management (BCM), play therapy, dialectical behavior therapy (DBT), cognitive-behavioral therapy (CBT), interpersonal therapy (IPT), dialectical behavior therapy (DBT), the early intensive behavioral intervention (EIBI), discrete trial training (DTT), applied behavior analysis (ABA), family-based treatment (FBT)-Maudsley method and group psychotherapy approaches.

Introduction

There is a substantial need for child and adolescent psychiatry services in the country; however, only a limited number of young people obtain mental health services at a given time. Services are unavailable for the families because the mental health resources lag behind the steep rise in the diagnosed mental health disorders. According to the World Health Organization (WHO),

* ***Correspondence:*** Email: anazeer@sidra.org.

In: Behavioral Pediatrics
Editors: Donald E. Greydanus, Dilip R. Patel, Ahsan Nazeer et al.
ISBN: 979-8-88697-060-9

approximately 10-20% of children and adolescents experience mental health disorders; this is a figure that is consistent with the prevalence rates in the United States (1, 2). In the primary care setting, the prevalence of mental health disorders is 12-22%, and these numbers reach a staggering 70% among the patients who visit the pediatric emergency department (3, 4). As providers of medical care for children and adolescents, primary care physicians (PCP's), especially pediatricians, are often the first to be consulted by parents about a child's behavioral, emotional, psychological, and developmental difficulties. It is estimated that one-third of the children receiving care for mental health conditions see only the primary care physicians (5).

During the outpatient visits, PCPs are frequently asked for advice on managing a child's medical and mental health problems, such as diabetes, obesity, non-adherence, depressed mood, irritability, self-harming, risk-taking behaviors, and overall life stressors. Even with the increasing use of medications, the importance of including psychotherapeutic and psychosocial interventions as an integral part of the treatment plan is getting increased recognition. In these situations, a primary care physician should understand different treatment modalities, including psychotherapies, to make appropriate referrals and enhance follow-through with referrals to the treating therapist during this process.

The American Academy of Pediatrics (AAP) has released guidelines on common psychiatric disorders during the last decade, including attention deficit hyperactive disorder and depressive disorders. It has encouraged PCPs to actively identify and manage psychiatric disorders (6, 7). During the last three decades, there has been an increasing acceptance of psychotherapies for child and adolescent mental health disorders. This acceptance has become possible because of the increased awareness of their efficacy, increased recognition of their use in early intervention, and a gradually developing evidence base of the manualized therapies. As a result, the range of available options is now broader in-depth, and more diverse; clinical use of these approaches is now more widespread, simultaneously offering greater flexibility and more precisely targeted applicability.

The following section of this review describes the general principles and categories of the psychotherapeutic and psychosocial interventions for children and adolescents. A guide is presented on the recommended interventions for specific diagnoses and problem areas.

General principles

As stated before, mental health issues impact the child's emotional, physical, and cognitive development and have long-term consequences. Primary care physicians are usually the first professionals to be consulted by a parent about a child's behavioral, emotional, or psychological issues. Briefly, the problems that make families seek help can be because of pathological behavior, disability/developmental deviances, a response to a traumatic or stressful event, abuse, or a psychological expression of a medical or neurological condition. In general, younger children present with developmental disorders, including attention deficit hyperactivity disorder, autism spectrum disorder, intellectual disability, learning disability, or disorders of genetic origin. On the other hand, adolescents usually present with anxiety, depression, bipolar disorder, the prodrome of psychosis, conduct disorder, or self-harming behaviors.

During these encounters, the initial task is always to determine what constitutes a "problem" in the family's opinion. The initial session also entails building a trusting relationship with the child and the family and identifying the presence, absence, and severity of the problem with the help of good history taking. Table 1 lists some of the items to consider during this process (8).

Table 1. General principles of assessment

• Initially, speak with the family as a whole unit;
• During the initial phase of evaluation, ask open-ended questions to let the family describe the problem in their own words;
• Keep evaluating nonverbal communication within the family along with parent-child interactions;
• Make time to speak with the child alone during the evaluation process. They need to know that they can discuss their problems in a trustworthy environment;
• During the middle to later evaluation phase, ask closed-ended questions to clarify the specific information. During this phase, keep the questions simple and concrete;
• For externalizing behaviors (hyperactivity, mood swings, temper tantrums, oppositional behaviors, etc.), rely on family members to get a thorough history as children are not good observers of their external behaviors;
• For internalizing behaviors (depressed mood, anxiety symptoms, hopelessness, feeling overwhelmed, etc.), rely on the children and adolescents to get more information as, in this case, parents are not good observers of the psychopathology;
• Assess the severity of the problem by focusing on its impact on the psychosocial functioning of the youth and the dysfunction within the family;
• As a general rule, psychotherapies are effective for mild severity of the symptoms, while psychopharmacology alone on in combination with psychotherapy works well for moderate to severe psychopathology;
• Use HEEADSSS (*H*ome–*E*ducation–*E*ating-*A*ctivity–*D*rugs–*S*exuality-*S*uicide/depression-*S*afety) as a clinical tool to access further vital areas (8);
• Do basic labs to rule out organic causes of mental health symptoms.

Treatment planning and referral

Table 2. Criteria for a referral to child and adolescent mental health specialist

• Thoughts of self-harm (cutting, burning) or harm to others;
• A sudden significant *change* in the psychosocial functioning (e.g., deterioration in academic functioning, social isolation in a previously well-functioning child);
• Mental health problems *causing* significant disruptions in psychosocial functioning;
• The inability of the family to provide adequate support to the child (e.g., symptoms of depression and hopelessness in a child of a mother with bipolar disorder);
• Recent discharge from the psychiatric inpatient unit;
• Unclear diagnosis, including multiple medical or psychiatric comorbidities;
• Lack of effectiveness of treatment after 6-8 weeks of interventions by the primary care;
• Partial response to the ongoing treatment;
• Suspicion of ongoing physical, emotional, or sexual abuse.

Because the assessment of behavioral problems and disorders can be complicated, situations may arise when intervention by a child and adolescent psychiatrist or a psychologist is needed.

This decision to seek help is based on numerous complex interrelating factors, as listed in Table 2. Families must be educated about decision-making and the referral to the specialist. The following is a brief description of the most commonly used psychotherapies.

Therapies for depressive disorders

Cognitive-behavioral therapy (CBT) and interpersonal therapy (IPT) are two primary evidence-based therapies that effectively treat depression. CBT is described below under "therapies for anxiety disorders."

Interpersonal therapy

Interpersonal therapy is a time-limited, structured, present-focused, empirically validated therapy that usually lasts about 12-16 sessions and is an effective treatment for mild to moderate depressive disorders (9, 10). Its success in depressive disorder is subsequently being used in eating disorders, post-traumatic stress disorder, panic disorder, and generalized anxiety disorder (11-17). IPT builds on the alliance of the therapist with the patient in which the patient feels understood and works on the life triggers that may be causing the current episode of depressed mood. During the therapy, the therapist emphasizes that depression is a medical illness and is not a patient's fault and that depressive symptoms and life stressors are related; thus, there is a linking of the current life events with the onset of the mood disorder. Table 3 lists the clinically relevant life events as the primary focus of IPT.

Table 3. Focus areas of Interpersonal therapy

Grief	Unresolved grief after the loss of a loved one
Role dispute	Conflicts in relationships
Role transition	Changing life circumstances, including geographical move, medical illness
Interpersonal deficit	Feelings of isolation and lack of support

Rather than focusing on the past, IPT takes a "here and now" approach. As a result, the focus is on the interpersonal problems considered to maintain and progress the depressive symptom. During the initial phase of the treatment, the therapist reviews the patient's relations and the ability to maintain those relationships. As listed in Table 3, the four problem areas are reviewed, and an "interpersonal inventory" is established. This "inventory" helps the therapist to focus on the central "crisis or predicament" in the patient's present life (18). After both the therapist and the patient agree on the treatment focus and "link" the depression to the patient's current life events, therapy proceeds to the "middle phase" of the treatment.

During the middle phase, the therapist is the patient's ally who, at times, assumes the "sick role." Both the therapist and the patient use specific strategies to manage ongoing problems. The time-limited nature of the therapy encourages the patient to take action and be more capable and independent in managing interpersonal problems (10). During the weekly sessions, the therapist helps the patient analyze the ongoing problem, offers support and role plays, and encourages the patient to test the new ideas. During this phase, the patient learns new interpersonal skills and gets more comfortable managing the conflicts in life. This process then leads to the termination phase of the therapy. The therapist discusses the termination process, reviews skills learned, and schedules the sessions from weekly to monthly to offer support for future problems.

For IPT to be successful, the patient should have sufficient motivation to develop a therapeutic alliance, the capacity to withstand internal and external stress (ego strength), a relatively secure attachment, and good social support.

Supportive psychotherapy

Supportive psychotherapy is a broadly defined therapeutic approach that can be effectively applied in the primary care physician's office. One of the guiding concepts in psychotherapy is that a supportive approach is beneficial when there is a high degree of impairment. It assists in channeling the acute expression of the emotional discomfort. At the core, supportive psychotherapy employs the techniques of comforting, encouraging, reassuring, attentive, and empathetic listening.

Through a directive approach, supportive therapy aims to reduce symptomatology and restore self-esteem (e.g., efficacy, confidence, hope, and self-concept), ego function (e.g., reality contact, affect, cognitive and impulse regulation), adaptive skills, and daily functioning. The above-listed goals are achieved by analyzing the symptoms, interactions and relationships, adaptive functioning, patterns of thinking, emotional reactions, and actions or behavior. Supportive psychotherapy approaches also can be beneficial in treating chronic medical conditions.

Therapies for anxiety disorders

According to the National Comorbidity Survey Replication-Adolescent Supplement (NCS-A), anxiety disorders are the most common (31.9%) mental health disorders in adolescents aged 13-18 years (19). The median age of onset of anxiety symptoms is six years of age. The long-term course of these disorders is variable as they may remit spontaneously or, at times, persist into adulthood.

Cognitive-behavioral therapy

Cognitive-behavioral therapy (CBT) is the most widely used psychotherapy to treat child and adolescent anxiety disorders. Table 4 lists some of the basic principles of CBT, and Table 5 lists the conditions in which CBT has been noted to be effective.

CBT is a short-term and focused therapy that aims to change patients' emotional responses by changing their thoughts and behaviors. Numerous therapeutic approaches are integrated under the rubric of CBT, including cognitive therapy (CT), behavioral therapy (BT), exposure therapy, cognitive-behavioral therapy (CBT), behavior modification (BM), and applied behavioral analysis (ABA). The discussion of all of the above approaches is out of the scope of this publication; however, it is essential to note that significant similarities exist between the above techniques, and therapists usually incorporate a combination of the above while treating anxiety disorders.

Table 4. Basic principles of CBT

CBT is a time-limited and evidence-based therapy;
CBT is problem-focused;
CBT focuses on the present, "here and now";
CBT is manual-based and structured;
CBT requires strong motivation and active collaboration from the patient;
CBT teaches patients to understand their current way of thinking and acting;
CBT helps relieve stress by assisting patients in developing flexible thinking patterns and behaviors;
CBT requires patients to be flexible in learning new skills and changing cognitive patterns.

Table 5. Indications of CBT

Mild to moderate symptoms of depression;
Generalized anxiety disorder (GAD);
Panic disorder;
Post-traumatic stress disorders (PTSD). A particular form of CBT, called trauma-focused CBT; (TF-CBT), is used in these patients;
Obsessive-compulsive disorder (OCD);
Autism spectrum disorder by using applied behavioral analysis (ABA).

Cognitive therapy is based on the concept that thoughts, feelings, and behaviors are interrelated, as shown in Figure 1 (20). As a result, negative feelings and maladaptive behaviors can be changed by changing negative thoughts.

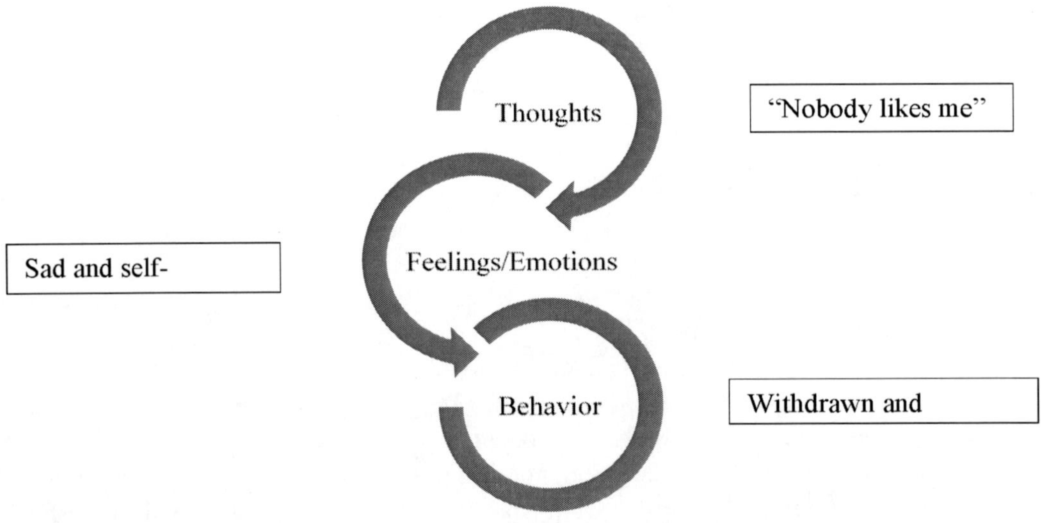

Figure 1. Information processing model (20).

During the therapy sessions, the therapist provides psychoeducation to the patient about the tri-part model, identifies negative thoughts and underlying schemas (catastrophizing, all or none thinking, etc.), challenges the maladaptive thoughts by examining the evidence against them, and in this process, alters the problematic behavior. The therapist also assigns the homework to the patient to identify the negative thoughts in different circumstances, challenging them while mastering the techniques. These cognitive techniques are usually employed with behavioral interventions, including exposure techniques (21).

Exposure therapy or techniques are simply a way to confront the patient's internal (thoughts) or external situations (e.g., stage fear) and feared stimuli without resorting to avoidant behaviors. The underlying premise of this method is that repeated exposure to a fearful stimulus will eventually reduce the patient's fearful reaction. At the start of the therapy, the therapist and the patient create an exposure hierarchy. An exposure hierarchy is a list in which fearful stimuli are ranked according to their tendency to generate fear. The goal is to start the therapy targeting the stimuli that generate only mild fearful responses and then gradually proceed to more strongly feared stimuli. Table 6 is an example of such an exposure hierarchy. Exposure therapy techniques have proven to be particularly useful in treating PTSD, GAD, panic disorder, and OCD (22-25).

Table 6. An exposure hierarchy

Anxiety provoking situations	Level of anxiety/fear (1-10)
Walking on the side path	3
Going into a shopping mall	4.5
Going into a store in the shopping mall	6
Going up an escalator	7
Going into an elevator	8

Therapies for childhood behavioral problems (ADHD, oppositional defiant disorder, and conduct disorder)

Parent management training (PMT)

PMT focuses on the parents as their children's primary teachers and coaches. When facing the child's oppositional behaviors, parents must regulate their thoughts and behaviors while assessing the situation to effectively respond to the child's problematic behavior (26). Harsh, coercive, and authoritative parenting increases the risk that the child will have sustained problems with aggression, conduct issues, academic difficulties, and depression. Parent management training aims to reinforce positive parenting methods while diminishing coercive tactics. The skill sets that the parents require change with the child's developmental age. For example, during infancy and early childhood, the focus is on providing the skills to facilitate healthy parent-child interactions.

During the school-age years and adolescence, parents need to expand their parenting skills by learning how to improve children's social, cognitive, and academic development and monitor adolescents while away from home to prevent experimentation with drugs and troubles with the law. However, it is essential to note that PMT is most frequently employed in treating pre-school and school-age children who struggle with aggression, temper tantrums, and oppositional behaviors in clinical practice. PMT focuses on five necessary parenting skills listed in Table 7 (27).

Table 7. Positive parenting skill sets

Encouragement	Promoting appropriate behaviors while rewarding the children during the process
Discipline	Establishing appropriate rules to target problematic behaviors and providing immediate short-term consequences, e.g., time out, removing electronics as a privilege, etc.
Monitoring	Ability to be aware of the child's whereabouts and activities
Problem-solving	Skills to help resolve disagreements and establishing positive and negative consequences
Positive engagement	Ways in which parents can be positively involved in their child's life

During the PMT, the therapist is the coach of the parents who teaches them healthy parenting strategies. At times, parents question being the focus of the therapy, as in their opinion, the problem is the child and not them. However, by reframing the objective that they are the "solution" to the problem, most parents buy into the process and get adequately engaged. The therapist then uses different techniques, including role-playing, didactics, video instructions, and homework assignments, to gradually build the rapport of parenting skills in a sequential and integrated fashion (27).

Behavioral therapy

Behavior therapy is an umbrella term for the techniques that are used to treat numerous disorders and have a common premise of promoting desirable behaviors and, at the same time, reducing unwanted behaviors. During behavior therapy, therapists encourage youth to try new behaviors, reward the desired behavior, and allow the unwanted behavior to fade away. The following are the most commonly used behavioral therapies for disruptive behaviors.

Parent-child interaction training (PCIT)

As the name implies, PCIT focuses on parents struggling to interact with their children positively. PCIT was developed for 2-7 years old children with disruptive behaviors and is also used in children who have autism spectrum disorder or have experienced trauma. PCIT is a combination of play and behavioral therapy in which parents learn specific skills to restructure the interactions with their children. In a typical clinic setup, the therapist provides training and guidance to the parents through a one-way mirror via earphones. Parents are encouraged to ignore negative behaviors and praise positive behaviors during the session. They also learn skills to improve their vocabulary by repeating their words and imitating their good behaviors.

By improving the interactions with the child, the family works toward better dynamics within the family members. When these skills are repeatedly used, they reduce anger and aggression within the children and improve the parents' confidence.

In contrast to PCIT, parent management training (PMT) focuses on the parents of 3-13 years old who are struggling with defiance, aggression, and temper tantrums. In PMT, parents' needs are more urgent, and they are usually seen alone without the child for the first five sessions, taught new skills, and encouraged to use those skills at home.

Behavioral classroom management (BCM)

Behavioral classroom management is a teacher-led approach with significant evidence of efficacy for managing children with ADHD (28, 29). The underlying concept of BCM is similar to other behavioral therapies in which positive behaviors are rewarded, and negative behaviors are discouraged.

Play therapy

Like other therapies, play therapy is also time-limited and is focused on a particular therapeutic goal. Play therapy was first utilized in the 1930s as a psychoanalytical approach to therapy with children and adolescents; currently, it falls under various theoretical conceptualizations, i.e., psychodynamic, cognitive, behavioral, interpersonal, client-centered, or integrationist. Play is utilized throughout the assessment, case conceptualization, and intervention during the sessions. At present, there are numerous applications of play therapy, including its use in abused children, victims of natural disasters, or the ones struggling with adjustment disorders; however, the most robust evidence of efficacy is in preoperative anxiety (for children facing medical procedures) and ADHD (30-32).

Therapies for youth with repeated self-harming behaviors

Dialectical behavior therapy (DBT)

DBT has numerous similarities with cognitive-behavioral approaches and has unique elements targeting self-harming and suicidal behaviors. Individuals with borderline personality disorder (BPD) and those who engage in repeated self-harm (non-suicidal self-injury-NSSI) usually feel invalidated and criticized by others. DBT is founded on the principle of self-acceptance and acceptance of the world surrounding the patient at a fundamental level. Table 8 highlights the essential components of DBT (33). A shorter version of DBT, dialectal behavior therapy for adolescents (DBT-A), has also proven effective in youth with depression, suicidal ideations, and repeated self-harming behaviors (34, 35).

Table 8. Essential components of DBT

Skill development	• How to regulate emotions; • How to tolerate distress and uncertainty; • How to be effective in interpersonal situations; • How to focus on the present; • How to accept themselves and the environment around them.
Skill generalization	• Generalizing the above skill set to the patient's natural environment. This is done by role-playing during the individual and group sessions, practicing in real life, troubleshooting in weekly sessions, re-learning, and reaching out to the therapist during the crisis.
Improving motivation to change	• Prioritizing the dysfunctional behaviors (e.g., self-harming behaviors) and reviewing the triggers that led to the behavior and the consequences of the target behavior. The patient and the therapist then find ways to replace the behaviors that are detrimental to the patient's life with healthy behaviors.
Modifying the environment	• Avoiding social circles that promote unhealthy behaviors and promoting a healthy lifestyle.

Therapies for children with autism spectrum disorder

Applied Behavior Analysis (ABA)

Several therapies, including speech therapy, occupational therapy, and social skill training, can help autistic children improve their abilities and reduce core deficits. Behavioral interventions for children with autism are designed to teach new skills, support families, and reduce inappropriate behaviors. ABA is the primary therapy used in most behavioral intervention programs and is considered most effective if started when children are younger than five years of age. ABA is an extensive 20-40 hours per week therapy that involves assessing behavior and implementing instructional modifications and systematic reinforcement to produce improvements in behavior. Discrete trial training (DTT) and early intensive behavioral intervention (EIBI) are the ABA's most commonly used techniques.

Discrete trial training (DTT)

DTT is a highly structured technique that involves breaking down the desired behaviors into small, achievable tasks that are then taught systematically. The DTT approach helps teach foundation skills such as attention, compliance, imitation, and discrimination.

Early intensive behavioral intervention (EIBI)

EIBI is a behavioral approach delivered before five years of age and usually over multiple years (2-3 years). However, it is essential to note conflicting evidence on the optimal age for early intervention. While in some studies, younger age at intake predicted better outcomes and gains in cognitive and language abilities, others found the absence of such influence (36-39).

Irrespective of the age at which the treatment is started, researchers agree that it is an effective treatment modality that improves intelligence quotient (IQ), adaptive behavior, daily living skills, socialization, and communication. Research indicates that the intensity of the interventions affected the outcome (40-42). For example, EIBI is very effective when provided for 25 hours per week, although increased program intensity above 25 hours did not produce better outcomes.

Therapies for eating disorders

Family-based treatment (FBT)-Maudsley method

Since the early 1960s, family dynamics have been recognized as an essential focus of intervention in the process of change. Consequently, family therapy aims to improve interfamilial relationships and interactional patterns within the family system and among family sub-systems. The effectiveness of family-based interventions is well documented in the literature in treating individuals with anorexia nervosa (AN). FBT for AN is a manual-based therapy, and the treatment consists of three phases, as listed in Table 9 (43).

It is essential to understand some of the basic tenants of this treatment modality. First, in the FBT, eating disorders are complex and multifactorial, and assumptions are not made on what caused the disorder. During the treatment, the focus is not to blame the adolescent or the family but instead on how to move forward with the recovery as soon as possible. Second, an eating disorder is "external" to the child and has "taken over" their thinking and behavior. Families are educated that their child is not "in control" of the disorder, and just as they did not choose the disorder, similarly, they cannot "start" or "stop" the disorder. This technique is called "externalizing" the disorder and is very helpful in reducing the parent's criticism of the child's behavior.

Table 9. Three phases of FBT for the treatment of anorexia nervosa

Rapid weight restoration	• Parents take control of the child's nutritional needs; • Parents monitor food intake and curtail physical activity.' • Phase 1 continues until a reasonably healthy weight is restored, the child starts eating without parental involvement, and the eating disorder begins to recede;
Reverting responsibility to the adolescent	• Done gradually to reduce the chances of relapse; • Adolescents start taking responsibility for choosing the food and portions of the meals; • Parental oversight is still maintained;
Healthy family life	• Family life reverts to normal; • The therapist works with the family and adolescent to anticipate future life challenges and ways to navigate through those challenges.

Third, in FBT, the therapist takes a nondirective approach to the child's care. Thus, instead of "telling" the family how to help the child, the therapist "guides" the family to make appropriate choices for their child. For example, families are told that they are in command of their child's nutritional status, but they are not told how to achieve this goal. In this way, parents who know how their family functions and their likes and dislikes can come up with a better plan for helping their child. The therapist empowers the parents and trusts them to overcome the eating disorder during this process.

Finally, the focus of the treatment is always to restore the physical health to normal, so during the early phases of the care, the comorbid disorders of depression, anxiety, and mood lability are not addressed directly. This helps to maintain focus on the weight restoration, and once the weight is restored, most of the secondary problems improve by themselves (43).

Group psychotherapy approaches

Group psychotherapy is a very effective form of intervention that has been applied to work with children and adolescents in outpatient, inpatient, and acute treatment settings. It has been used to treat depression, substance abuse, social anxiety, bipolar disorders, psychosis, eating disorders, children of alcoholics, and others. Group therapy can be problem-specific (e.g., social anxiety, children of divorce, grief). In acute mental health treatment settings and substance abuse treatment programs, multi-systemic treatment approaches and group therapy are consistently integrated into the treatment process. In group therapy approaches with children, play therapy, role-play, and other interactional processes are utilized. With adolescents, action-oriented and role-play techniques are customarily used.

Various situations can be role-played, such as conflicts between parents and adolescents, issues between friends, difficulties with expressing feelings or wishes (assertiveness), and appropriate use of social skills. The focus of group therapy is often on the various developmental issues of adolescence, such as individuation, independence, and autonomy, control problems or conflict with authority figures, uncertainty about the future, dealing with peer pressure, social effectiveness and self-concept, sexuality as well as coping with societal demands.

Another form of group intervention with children and adolescents involves *psycho-educational groups.* These groups tend to be issues, themes, or skills-focused. Examples of such groups include emotional regulation, aggression and anger control, self-esteem/self-concept, social skills, conflict resolution, coping skills, stress management, or dealing with a specific problem (i.e., depression, bipolar disorder, anxiety). Often, they are an integral component in acute treatment settings, such as inpatient and partial hospitalization programs, substance abuse inpatient or intensive outpatient treatment programs, and residential programs for the severely behaviorally disturbed. Participation in psychoeducational groups is also essential for many standard outpatient treatment plans.

Conclusion

During the last few decades, the field of psychotherapy has advanced significantly, and the research has moved beyond the point of "whether the psychotherapies are effective in children and adolescents" (44). Recently, practitioners have noted an improved number and quality of studies focusing on the outcomes, efficacy of manualized therapies, and reliability of treatments provided to the youth population. Nonetheless, understanding the available treatment options has lagged in general medical education; indeed, given the broad array of potential treatments, many of which are empirically supported, it behooves the primary care physician to understand their role in the overall treatment plan. Therefore, primary care physicians must identify mental health issues, utilize integrated health and behavioral health care models to address them, and have ready access to referral resources for assessment and treatment needs that require more specialized expertise.

References

[1] World Health Organization. Child and adolescent mental health, 2020. URL: https://www.who.int/mental_health/maternal-child/child_adolescent/en/.

[2] Merikangas KR, He JP, Burstein M, Swanson SA, Avenevoli S, Cui L, et al. Lifetime prevalence of mental disorders in U.S. adolescents: results from the National Comorbidity Survey Replication--Adolescent Supplement (NCS-A). J Am Acad Child Adolesc Psychiatry 2010;49(10):980-9.

[3] Sheldrick RC, Merchant S, Perrin EC. Identification of developmental-behavioral problems in primary care: a systematic review. Pediatrics 2011;128(2):356-63.

[4] Grupp-Phelan J, Delgado SV, Kelleher KJ. Failure of psychiatric referrals from the pediatric emergency department. BMC Emerg Med 2007;7:12.

[5] Anderson LE, Chen ML, Perrin JM, Van Cleave J. Outpatient visits and medication prescribing for US children with mental health conditions. Pediatrics 2015;136(5): e1178.

[6] Zuckerbrot RA, Cheung A, Jensen PS, Stein REK, Laraque D. Guidelines for Adolescent Depression in Primary Care (GLAD-PC): Part I. Practice preparation, identification, assessment, and initial management. Pediatrics 2018;141(3): e20174081.

[7] Wolraich ML, Hagan JF, Allan C, Chan E, Davison D, Earls M, et al. Clinical practice guideline for the diagnosis, evaluation, and treatment of attention-deficit/hyperactivity disorder in children and adolescents. Pediatrics 2019;144(4):e20192528.

[8] Goldenring JM, Rosen DS. Getting into adolescent heads: an essential update. Contemp Pediatr 2004;21(1):64-92.

[9] Cuijpers P, Geraedts AS, van Oppen P, Andersson G, Markowitz JC, van Straten A. Interpersonal psychotherapy for depression: a meta-analysis. Am. J. Psychiatry 2011; 168(6):581-92.

[10] Markowitz JC, Weissman MM. Interpersonal psychotherapy: principles and applications. World Psychiatry 2004;3(3):136-9.

[11] Wilfley DE, Welch RR, Stein RI, Spurrell EB, Cohen LR, Saelens BE, et al. A randomized comparison of group cognitive-behavioral therapy and group interpersonal psychotherapy for the treatment of overweight individuals with binge-eating disorder. Arch Gen Psychiatry 2002;59(8):713-21.

[12] Markowitz JC. IPT and PTSD. Depress Anxiety 2010;27(10):879-81.

[13] Rafaeli AK, Markowitz JC. Interpersonal psychotherapy (IPT) for PTSD: A case study. Am J Psychother 2011;65(3):205-23.

[14] Steinert C, Leichsenring F. No psychotherapy monoculture for anxiety disorders. Lancet 2017;389(10082):1882-3.

[15] Vos S, Huibers M, Diels L, Arntz A. A randomized clinical trial of cognitive behavioral therapy and interpersonal psychotherapy for panic disorder with agoraphobia. Psychol Med 2012;42(12):2661-72.

[16] Lipsitz JD, Gur M, Miller NL, Forand N, Vermes D, Fyer AJ. An open pilot study of interpersonal psychotherapy for panic disorder (IPT-PD). J Nerv Ment Dis 2006; 194(6):440-5.

[17] Carl E, Witcraft SM, Kauffman BY, Gillespie EM, Becker ES, Cuijpers P, et al. Psychological and pharmacological treatments for generalized anxiety disorder (GAD): a meta-analysis of randomized controlled trials. Cogn Behav Ther 2020; 49(1):1-21.

[18] Lipsitz JD, Markowitz JC. Mechanisms of change in interpersonal therapy (IPT). Clin Psychol Rev 2013;33(8):1134-47.

[19] Merikangas KR, He J-P, Burstein M, Swanson SA, Avenevoli S, Cui L, et al. Lifetime prevalence of mental disorders in US adolescents: Results from the National Comorbidity Survey Replication--Adolescent Supplement (NCS-A). J Am Acad Child Adolesc Psychiatry 2010;49(10):980-9.
[20] Beck AT, Clark DA. An information processing model of anxiety: Automatic and strategic processes. Behav Res Ther 1997;35(1):49-58.
[21] Kaczkurkin AN, Foa EB. Cognitive-behavioral therapy for anxiety disorders: an update on the empirical evidence. Dialogues Clin Neurosci 2015;17(3):337-46.
[22] Powers MB, Halpern JM, Ferenschak MP, Gillihan SJ, Foa EB. A meta-analytic review of prolonged exposure for posttraumatic stress disorder. Clin Psychol Rev 2010;30(6):635-41.
[23] Borkovec TD, Costello E. Efficacy of applied relaxation and cognitive-behavioral therapy in the treatment of generalized anxiety disorder. J Consult Clin Psychol 1993; 61(4):611-9.
[24] Mitte K. A meta-analysis of the efficacy of psycho- and pharmacotherapy in panic disorder with and without agoraphobia. J Affect Disord 2005;88(1):27-45.
[25] Sánchez-Meca J, Rosa-Alcázar AI, Marín-Martínez F, Gómez-Conesa A. Psychological treatment of panic disorder with or without agoraphobia: A meta-analysis. Clin Psychol Rev 2010;30(1):37-50.
[26] Lorber MF, O'Leary SG. Mediated paths to over-reactive discipline: mothers' experienced emotion, appraisals, and physiological responses. J Consult Clin Psychol 2005;73(5):972-81.
[27] Forgatch M, Martinez C. Parent management training: A program linking basic research and practical application. Tidsskr Norsk Psykologforening 1999;36:923-37.
[28] Fabiano GA, Pelham Jr WE. Improving the effectiveness of behavioral classroom interventions for attention-deficit/hyperactivity disorder: A case study. J Emot Behav Disord 2003;11(2):122-8.
[29] Cooper JT, Gage NA, Alter PJ, LaPolla S, MacSuga-Gage AS, Scott TM. Educators' self-reported training, use, and perceived effectiveness of evidence-based classroom management practices. Prev Sch Fail 2018;62(1):13-24.
[30] Ray DC, Schottelkorb A, Tsai M-H. Play therapy with children exhibiting symptoms of attention deficit hyperactivity disorder. Int J Play Ther 2007;16(2):95-111.
[31] Phillips RD. How firm is our foundation? Current play therapy research. Int J Play Ther 2010;19(1):13-25.
[32] Kool R, Lawver T. Play therapy: Considerations and applications for the practitioner. Psychiatry (Edgmont) 2010;7(10):19-24.
[33] Chapman AL. Dialectical behavior therapy: Current indications and unique elements. Psychiatry (Edgmont) 2006;3(9):62-8.
[34] Mehlum L, Tørmoen AJ, Ramberg M, Haga E, Diep LM, Laberg S, et al. Dialectical behavior therapy for adolescents with repeated suicidal and self-harming behavior: A randomized trial. J Am Acad Child Adolesc Psychiatry 2014;53(10):1082-91.
[35] Pochyly J, Walkup JT. Editorial: Dialectical behavior therapy and the function of self-injury. J Am Acad Child Adolesc Psychiatry 2021;60(9):1062-3.
[36] Granpeesheh D, Dixon DR, Tarbox J, Kaplan AM, Wilke AE. The effects of age and treatment intensity on behavioral intervention outcomes for children with autism spectrum disorders. Res Autism Spectr Disord 2009;3(4):1014-22.
[37] Harris SL, Handleman JS. Age and IQ at intake as predictors of placement for young children with autism: A four-to six-year follow-up. J Autism Dev Disord 2000;30(2): 137-42.
[38] Magiati I, Charman T, Howlin P. A two-year prospective follow-up study of community-based early intensive behavioural intervention and specialist nursery provision for children with autism spectrum disorders. J Child Psychol Psychiatry 2007;48(8):803-12.
[39] Eikeseth S, Smith T, Jahr E, Eldevik S. Outcome for children with autism who began intensive behavioral treatment between ages 4 and 7: A comparison controlled study. Behav Modif 2007;31(3):264-78.
[40] Strauss K, Mancini F, Fava L, Group S. Parent inclusion in early intensive behavior interventions for young children with ASD: A synthesis of meta-analyses from 2009 to 2011. Res Dev Disabil 2013;34(9):2967-85.

[41] Virues-Ortega J. Applied behavior analytic intervention for autism in early childhood: meta-analysis, meta-regression and dose-response meta-analysis of multiple outcomes. Clin Psychol Rev 2010;30(4):387-99.

[42] Makrygianni MK, Reed P. A meta-analytic review of the effectiveness of behavioural early intervention programs for children with autistic spectrum disorders. Res Autism Spectr Disord 2010;4(4):577-93.

[43] Rienecke RD. Family-based treatment of eating disorders in adolescents: current insights. Adolesc Health Med Ther 2017;8:69-79.

[44] Kazdin AE. Psychotherapy for children and adolescents. Annu Rev Psychol 2003; 54(1):253-76.

Chapter 15

Behavioral and cognitive behavioral therapies

Stephen McLearie[1], MRCPsych, Nehdia Hashemi[2], MD, Madeeha Kamal[1], FRCP, Nazish Imran[3], MRCPsych, Sadiq Naveed[4], MD, Muhammad Waqar Azeem[1], MD and Ahsan Nazeer[1,*], MD

[1]Sidra Medicine/Weill Cornell Medicine, Doha, Qatar, [2]Western Michigan University, Homer Stryker MD School of Medicine, Kalamazoo, Michigan,
[3]King Edward Medical University, Lahore, Pakistan and Institute of Living/Hartford Healthcare, Hartford, Connecticut, United States of America

Abstract

A summary of behavioral and cognitive behavioral therapies is provided regarding the children and adolescents receiving mental health care. The basis of behavioral therapy stems from the idea of conditioning that views responses and actions of human beings as results of environmental interaction. Cognitive behavioral therapy (CBT) is formed from social learning theory with treatment models based on operant and classical conditioning concepts. CBT is reviewed along with cognitive behavioral therapy for psychosis (CBTp). Other therapies that are discussed include applied behavioral analysis (ABA), exposure and response prevention (ERP), Maudsley method-family based treatment (FBT), and habit reversal therapy (HRT).

Introduction

Behavioral therapy is an umbrella term that encompasses numerous therapies. The therapist focuses on the maladaptive patterns of behaviors that a child/adolescent may knowingly, unknowingly, or unconsciously display in their settings. Behavioral therapy is based on the theory of conditioning, which focuses on the concept that the person's responses and actions result from their interaction with the environment. Behaviorists believe that any action can be

* ***Correspondence:*** Email: anazeer@sidra.org.

In: Behavioral Pediatrics
Editors: Donald E. Greydanus, Dilip R. Patel, Ahsan Nazeer et al.
ISBN: 979-8-88697-060-9

studied systematically and modified regardless of the person's inner state, personality, or life tendencies.

During these therapies, the therapist empowers the youth and family to reinforce the desired behavior and use strategies to eliminate the unwanted behavior. By connecting attitudes, rewards, and learning, therapists help the family and the youth to achieve their personal and family goals. Behavior therapies are often used to treat the mild to moderate symptoms of numerous psychiatric disorders, including depressive disorder, anxiety disorders, posttraumatic stress disorder (PTSD), attention-deficit/hyperactivity disorder (ADHD), eating disorders, obsessive-compulsive disorder (OCD), and self-harming behaviors, to name few (1-3).

Basic principles

The following is a brief review to help the reader understand the basic principles of behavior therapy, starting with concepts of classical conditioning and operant conditioning.

Classical conditioning

Classical conditioning is simply a pairing of two stimuli to elicit a response (4). Numerous classical conditioning examples are found in day-to-day life. For instance, in a routine well-child examination, it is noted that the child needs a vaccination shot. For the child, it is unexpected as he was promised "no shots" by the parents before the visit. The injection pain becomes associated with the doctor's office, and any future visits may elicit feelings of pain, distress, and anxiety. The teacher can pair verbal warning with clapping two times in the classroom to make the children quiet. In the beginning, she can give a verbal warning and pair it with clapping to elicit the response (be silent); however, after a few repetitions, an association is formed. Later, only clapping two times can elicit the same response, and children stay quiet.

Classical conditioning can also be understood as unconscious learning and is considered a reflex (5, 6). For example, after having a bout of food poisoning at a restaurant, the person may begin to associate all of the restaurant chains with feelings of nausea and vomiting. Similar is the case of someone having a panic attack in an elevator. That individual will start associating all the elevators with anxiety, distress, and panic and will begin avoiding the elevators.

A therapist can use this information about the association to unlearn or unconditioned the phobic behavior. One technique called *flooding* exposes the individual to the most fearful stimuli and prevents them from escaping. In the above example of the phobia of elevators, the therapist identifies that the fear of elevators is irrational; thus, with support and guidance, he then exposes the individual to fifty or more elevator rides to "unlearn" the behavior without negative outcome.

Systematic desensitization is another technique that is based on the concept of classical conditioning. In this technique, individuals make a hierarchical list of their fears, from the least fear-inducing to the most fear-inducing stimuli. They are then taught relaxation techniques, including deep breathing, gradual muscle relaxation, and meditation. The therapist then works with the individual in 6-8 sessions to gradually expose them to the least fearful stimuli and work their way up to the most anxiety-provoking stimuli. Patients move to the next stage of the fear hierarchy only when they master the stage before it. The goal of the therapy is to replace the fearful response to the stimuli with a more neutral or relaxing response. To illustrate the point, Table 1 lists a systematic desensitization program for an individual who has a phobia of flying.

Table 1. Desensitization program for a person with a fear of flying

Behavior	**Level of anxiety (1-100)**
Talking about flying	35
Looking at the planes	40
Driving by the airport	50
Booking a flight	65
Packing luggage in anticipation of the travel	70
Checking in and sitting in the airport lobby	75
Imagining boarding the plane	87
Flying a short inter-state trip	95

Operant conditioning

Operant conditioning is based on the theory that the consequences of behavior can change/modify our behavior (7). In other words, if a positive outcome follows a behavior, that behavior is more likely to be repeated in the future. However, if a negative outcome follows a behavior, it is less likely to be repeated by the individual. As an example, if a child tells a funny story in the class and other children laugh, it is more likely that he will tell the same story to others. This repetition is because the behavior (telling a funny story) was followed by the reinforcement (others laughing, which is a desirable outcome), thus strengthening the future behavior (re-telling the same account). On the other hand, if no one laughs, then the probability of the child repeating the same story is less in the future.

In operant conditioning, the therapist evaluates the observable causes of the behavior and tries to modify them using rewards or punishments. The reinforcement can be positive or negative. In *positive reinforcement,* something is *added* to encourage the behavior. For example, a child is praised after getting good grades in a subject. In this situation, praise is a positive reinforcement that will increase the probability of future good grades.

On the other hand, negative reinforcement takes something away to *encourage* the behavior. For example, ungrounding the child when he starts following the rules will increase the probability of continuing to follow the rules to avoid being grounded. In this example, ungrounding is negative reinforcement (grounding was taken away) to improve the behavior.

It is worth noting that reinforcement is a very complex phenomenon. Numerous factors, including "when and how" the behaviors are reinforced, dictate how often and how quickly the behaviors are learned. Some reinforcement schedules are continuous reinforcement, fixed ratio, fixed-interval schedules, variable-ratio, and variable-interval schedules. The detailed description of these processes is outside the scope of this publication, and the reader is advised to consult other resources for further study.

Types of behavioral therapies

The following is a brief description of some commonly used behavioral therapies in day-to-day practice beginning with applied behavioral analysis (ABA) and proceeding to cognitive behavioral therapy (CBT).

Applied Behavioral Analysis (ABA)

ABA is an umbrella term that encompasses numerous techniques and is the most commonly used evidence-based intensive behavioral therapy for children with autism spectrum disorder (ASD) (8). It promotes essential skills and minimizes undesirable behaviors, including aggression and self-harm. Because of the intensity of the work, ABA sessions for autism usually last 40 hours per week. Techniques of ABA include discrete trial training (DTT), treatment of the pivotal response (PRT), and the Denver early start model (ESDM).

Discrete Trial Training (DTT)

Discrete Trial Training is a technique used in ABA that Dr. Ivar Lovaas (University of California, Los Angeles) pioneered. In DTT, the desirable behaviors that need to be taught to the child are broken into small "discrete" steps. The therapist then guides the child through each stage multiple times and reinforces it with a reward or a consequence. The steps involved are clearly defined, the process is repetitive, and the child progresses to the next step after mastering the first one (9).

Treatment of the Pivotal Response (PRT)

PRT is another technique used in ABA. Instead of focusing on a single skill, the therapist focuses on the critical "pivotal" areas of development, including motivation, self-management, and initiation of social interactions. The goal is that by focusing on development, the child will make broader gains in areas of communication and social skills (10).

ESDM

The Denver Early Start Model (ESDM) belongs to a group of approaches called naturalistic developmental behavioral interventions (NDBIs) that are aimed toward very young children (12-48 months) with autism. NDBIs are techniques used in naturally occurring environments to teach content and strategies to children and families. The ESDM can be used in person or group sessions using play-based activities, like PRT (following child's lead), or by taking a more structured approach as in ABA to improve social deficits, communication, and cognition (11).

Cognitive Behavioral Therapy (CBT)

CBT is a manualized, evidence-based therapy for treating child and adolescent anxiety disorders, depressive illness, school refusal, obsessive-compulsive disorder (OCD), posttraumatic stress disorder (PTSD), and panic disorder, to name a few (12).

CBT is derived from social learning theory, and treatment models are based on operant and classical conditioning concepts. The underlying premise of CBT is that life events and memories impact the children, creating negative thoughts, maladaptive schema, and cognitive distortions. These thoughts, emotions, and actions become a part of the "cognitive loop" that interacts with each other and can turn into a 'vicious circle' type of negative thinking accompanied by physiological symptoms of hyperarousal. By the time the children reach early adolescent years, they have developed a negative attributional style of thinking, which creates stress, anxiety, and depression in their lives. By changing this negative, pessimistic style to a positive, optimistic style, the therapist can help the children to improve their mood and anxiety symptoms.

CBT is evidence-based, time-limited, manualized, and collaborative; some of its components include psychoeducation, in situ exposure-response avoidance approaches, and homework activities. As CBT asks for active participation from the patient, it is critical to consider cognitive ability and Piaget and Vygotsky's developmental stages while evaluating the children for the suitability for participation in CBT. In primary care and pediatric settings, resource availability can restrict the use of structured manualized cognitive behavioral therapy (CBT). However, having a basic understanding of the CBT process can be beneficial, especially when referring to psychiatric services. The following is an illustrative case.

CBT in an adolescent with social anxiety disorder-A clinical vignette

Elaine is a thirteen-year-old girl referred to the local child psychiatry clinic by her primary care physician with a six-month history of reluctance to socialize due to significant anxiety levels in social situations.

Pre-treatment assessment

The assessment was carried out over two sessions. Elaine and her parents were interviewed both separately and together.

Family background

Elaine is a thirteen-year-old middle school student who lives with her parents and two sisters. Her father is a 45-year-old lawyer with a history of depression. Mom is a 43-year-old homemaker with a history of social anxiety disorder and panic attacks.

Developmental history

Elaine's early development was normal; the pregnancy was planned, delivery was uncomplicated, and she reached all developmental milestones appropriately. She started school at five years of age and retrospectively had features of selective mutism. Elaine received no formal intervention at that time. By the age of six, she separated well from her mother, made friends, and was interacting and speaking much more in school.

History of presenting problem

Elaine presented with a six-month history of significant anxiety in social situations, particularly in family gatherings and during interactions with peers. The level of functional impairment had deteriorated over the previous few months, such that Elaine was refusing to attend family events and was withdrawn around peers. The precipitant for the current presentation appeared to be an incident several months previously when she overheard girls in her class commenting on her appearance.

Rating Scales
Elaine completed the following questionnaires:

1. Spence Children's Anxiety Scale (Spence, 1997).
2. Birleson Depression Scale (Birleson, 1981).

The *Spence Children's Anxiety Scale* is a 46-item self-report measure used to assess symptoms of anxiety disorder. Possible scores range from 0 to 118, with norms available for children between the ages of 8 and 12 years. Elaine had just turned thirteen years old at the time of assessment; however, the Spence seemed the most appropriate instrument, and scores were extrapolated. Elaine's score of 28 was within the normal range; however, her score on the social phobia subscale was significantly elevated. This suggests the presence of clinically significant symptoms of anxiety disorder with functional impairment.

The *Birleson Depression Scale* is an 18-item self-report measure used to assess depressive feelings in children and adolescents. Total scores range from 0 to 36, with a score of 17 or higher suggesting clinically significant depression. Elaine's total Score of 5 was well within the normal range.

Behavioral observations
Elaine was interviewed with her parents and alone. She presented as a well-kempt girl on a mental state examination in a school uniform. She was well orientated in time, place, and person, made poor eye contact initially, blushed slightly when spoken to directly, but was appropriate in her interactions. Elaine is of medium height and build, and her parents reported that she often receives compliments on her appearance. However, Elaine believes that her eyes are prominent and refers to a comment made by a classmate the previous year. There was no evidence of psychotic features or thoughts of deliberate self-harm.

Diagnostic impression
Elaine presented with a persistent, pervasive fear of negative evaluation. She had physiological anxiety symptoms in social situations, including blushing and sweating, accompanied by avoidance behaviors. She met the diagnostic criteria for a diagnosis of social phobia. A current mood disorder was excluded. There was no evidence of Asperger's syndrome, Fragile X syndrome, or paranoid/psychotic illness.

Treatment targets
In discussion with Elaine and her parents' therapist collaboratively agreed on three treatment goals for Elaine:

1. To be able to attend family functions without experiencing marked anxiety symptoms.
2. To be able to interact with peers without overwhelming fear of negative evaluation.
3. Increased enjoyment of family occasions/interactions with peers.

Monitoring of treatment targets

A variety of measures were used to monitor the treatment targets. These included:

1. Spence Children's Anxiety Scale (pre-treatment and post-treatment).
2. Birleson Depression Scale (pre-treatment and post-treatment).
3. Frequent ratings of Elaine's subjective units of distress in social situations.
4. Parental diaries recorded Elaine's behavior in social situations and their responses to her behavior (pre-treatment and post-treatment).
5. Dysfunctional thought records of anxiety-provoking situations, as listed in Table 2.

Table 2. Dysfunctional thought record

Situation	Being at the family party
Negative thought	People will think I look "stupid" / "my eyes stick out"
Bodily sensation	Abdominal discomfort, 'butterflies' (no other panic symptoms)
Behaviors	Blush, avoid eye contact, cover face with hands, and become oppositional until brought home
Consequences	When blushing/covering face/oppositional, others at the party look and pay more attention, parents bring her home, thus reinforcing her behavior

Description of treatment

Sessions 1–2: Decreasing self-focused attention

Self-focused attention is an essential maintaining factor in anxiety disorder. To modify excessive self-focus, Elaine had to learn to be externally focused by monitoring and observing the details of the external environment and those in it during feared social situations. Practicing this skill in the session involved the use of spontaneous conversational role-plays. Following the role-play, Elaine was asked to describe in detail the conversation, especially the comments made by her conversational partner (therapist). Elaine practiced this skill in everyday encounters at school as a homework exercise and monitored her anxiety pre- and post-conversation. At this stage of the intervention, Elaine was instructed to use dysfunctional thought records and was asked to keep a record of social situations, which could then be examined in the subsequent sessions. She quickly became adept at completing these records and, after several sessions, began to challenge her negative automatic thoughts (NATs) and spontaneously generate more balanced alternative thoughts.

Sessions 3-5: Social skills training

As therapy progressed and Elaine's interactional style became apparent, it was clear that her poor performance in social situations may not be solely anxiety-induced but may also be due to poorly developed social skills. This deficit was not apparent at assessment, and therefore it was necessary to re-formulate the development and maintenance of Elaine's social anxiety to incorporate this possibility. Various techniques were utilized to improve Elaine's understanding and application of appropriate social skills; these included modeling, role-play, and psychoeducation.

These skills included active listening, nonverbal communication, eye contact, and verbal communication, e.g., asking open-ended questions. Video feedback was also used to present

Elaine with an objective picture of how she interacted in the session. This was an invaluable tool as it enabled her to identify the kinds of messages she gives out in social situations via verbal and nonverbal communication channels.

Sessions 6-8: Constructing a more realistic image of self in social interactions
Closely related to the excessive self-focused attention that characterizes socially anxious individuals is the distorted impression they create of themselves. Elaine entered therapy with a deeply ingrained mental image of herself as "stupid-looking, ugly and boring" when interacting with others. This part of the intervention began with some education about the problems associated with self-processing, e.g., directing attention away from processing external social information that could modify negative beliefs. A thorough review of recent episodes of social anxiety revealed the strength of Elaine's belief in her mental image of herself. Also, video feedback methods were incorporated into the sessions to modify Elaine's distorted observer perspective.

Sessions 9-11: Exposure in vivo incorporating dropping safety behaviors
To prepare Elaine for the prospect of exposure to feared social situations, she was provided with some information about the self-defeating nature of safety behaviors. The next step involved drawing up a hierarchy of feared social situations. Homework exercises incorporated behavioral experiments to disconfirm negative beliefs and thoughts about anxiety-provoking situations. The experiment's first phase involved utilizing all of her typical safety behaviors, e.g., dropping her gaze, covering her face with her hands, avoidance of conversations with others, among others, in a feared social situation. Then, the second phase required her to drop all of these safety behaviors in the same situation.

Afterward, she recorded any differences in her subjective units of distress ratings between the two situations. With repeated practice over several weeks, Elaine could confront feared situations in vivo while redirecting her self-focused attention externally and dropping her safety behaviors. With practice, she was able to construct a more realistic image of herself in social situations and develop the skills to target those processes maintaining her anxiety.

Session 12: This was the final session
Elaine had a blueprint of materials, and she made a ten-minute PowerPoint presentation to her parents on what she had learned, the underlying CBT principles, and the goals achieved. Elaine's parents then described the significant improvements they had noticed in her over the preceding months, and her parent's feedback was positively reinforcing for Elaine.

Treatment outcome
By the end of treatment, Elaine had achieved all of the collaboratively agreed goals. She was socializing more easily, both subjectively and objectively. She had dropped the safety behaviors that perpetuated her social anxiety, attending less to what people may be thinking and generating alternative thoughts of what other people may be thinking.

This is an example of a complex case with multiple interacting factors in the context of a strong family history of anxiety and mood disorders. There is also an application of a structured, systematic cognitive behavioral approach to the management with an excellent treatment outcome.

Cognitive-behavioral therapy for psychosis (CBTp)

Cognitive behavioral therapy for psychosis (CBTp) is an evidence-based individual or group intervention shown to improve the distress and disability of individuals with psychotic disorders (13). It is recommended for individuals with early-onset psychosis or who are at risk of developing psychosis. CBTp as an adjunct to medication management improves functioning despite the patient's ongoing experience with positive symptoms, thought disturbances, and negative symptoms. In the CBTp, the therapist collaborates with the patient to explore the psychotic symptoms and disability. Research has shown that CBTp helps reduce the symptoms of psychosis and depression, changing the beliefs of self, improving coping skills, and improving functioning in individuals with psychotic disorders. CBTp progresses through five stages; as shown in Table 3, the three components below make the therapeutic model's core.

1. Collaborative identification of the problem that is troublesome to the patient.
2. Normalization of the psychotic experience.
3. Acceptance of the psychotic experiences to reduce the distress.

Table 3. Typical phases of CBTp

Engagement	Building the therapeutic relationship is an essential aspect of the therapy. In this phase, the therapist helps the patient identify the core issues and make a "problem list."
Assessment	This is a collaborative experience where the therapist works on understanding the experiences from the patient's perspective.
Formulation	The goal of the formulation is to develop a shared understanding of the problem's goals and identify the changes that need to take place for improvement.
Intervention	Based on the above formulation, cognitive and behavioral interventions are developed to help patients achieve their goals. The focus here is on functional recovery and maintaining this recovery. Functional recovery can be achieved even without a reduction in psychotic symptoms.
Consolidation and relapse prevention	In this phase, the aims are to have the patient test the newly learned skills in the real world, provide therapist feedback for problem-solving, and then work on strategies for relapse prevention.

Exposure and response prevention (ERP)

Exposure and response prevention is the gold standard for treating obsessive-compulsive disorders (14). ERP is based on the behavioral theory known as habituation. Habituation is a process in which an individual's maladaptive responses diminish over time due to prolonged exposure to anxiety-provoking stimuli. The habituation process is a phenomenon that we encounter in day-to-day settings. For example, it is difficult to focus on the work in a noisy environment; however, if a person stays in that environment for long, they get desensitized to the sound and can start focusing on the work with ease. Thus, gradual and controlled exposure to the fearful stimuli and abstaining from avoidance or escape also leads to habituation and learning, which helps overcome the compulsions.

For example, a patient who fears germs can confront their fear with the help of a therapist, starting from the exposure that causes the least anxiety and then gradually increasing the intensity of the exposure. In the above example, the patient can start by touching the surface of the table in the therapist's office. They let themselves experience the fear until it becomes manageable in this process. They then move to the next step of fear intensity, for example, touching the knob of the door. This gradual exposure to increasingly fearful situations can be conducted in real-life situations (in vivo exposure) or using the imagination until they feel comfortable facing the anxiety-producing stimulus. By repeatedly touching the doorknob, they unlearn and decouple the association between the doorknob and the fear. Thus, habituation leads to a diminished response, and ultimately the response gets extinguished (learning theory).

In obsessive-compulsive disorder (OCD), individuals usually develop ritualistic behaviors to "undo" the anxiety. These responses are rewarding (as they eliminate stress) and become an intrinsic component of the disorder. In the above example, hand washing after touching the doorknob can become a ritual, and it relieves the patient from the anxiety of touching the doorknob. Thus, for the treatment of OCD, exposure therapy is usually conducted with response prevention, which is based on the principle of learning theory.

Maudsley method-family based treatment (FBT)

The Maudsley method is an intensive outpatient-based treatment for eating disorders in which the parents play an active role in helping their child restore a healthy weight (15). They achieve this by promoting normal adolescent development and gradually handing over the food intake control. This manualized treatment usually happens in the outpatient setting and progresses through three phases, typically completed over 12 months.

Phase 1: Weight restoration

During this phase, the therapist assesses the family's interactions with each other eating habits and assists them in feeding their child. Families and adolescents are not blamed for the eating disorder (ED); instead, ED is considered a medical disease that has empowered their child and is beyond their control. Parents are encouraged to be supportive and understanding about their child's struggles with weight and eating, but at the same time maintain the notion that not eating is not a choice. The therapist supports the parents through this process and models an uncritical stance by addressing any overt or covert parental criticism of their child.

Phase 2: Return of control to the adolescent

This phase usually starts once the weight is restored to a relatively normal range, the adolescent is engaging in eating and accepts the parental insistence on adequate food intake, and when the family's conflicts and behaviors are manageable. During this phase, parents gradually relinquish the control to the adolescent, who is expected to return to eating habits in an age-appropriate manner. They can start eating meals without parental supervision; however, parents are encouraged to control food intake in relapse.

Phase 3: Establishing independence and identity

This phase is initiated when adolescents eat independently, maintain greater than 95% of the ideal body weight, and do not exhibit any ED behaviors. During this phase, the therapist works on the developmental issues of the adolescent, any comorbid disorders, and autonomy while at the same time encouraging parents to maintain appropriate boundaries. The therapist also helps the family come back to a normal lifestyle by improving the relationships.

Habit reversal therapy (HRT)

HRT is an effective treatment for tics, Tourette's disorder, and trichotillomania (16). The therapist focuses on building tic awareness (premonitory feeling) in the child during therapy. The premise of awareness training is that increased understanding of tic behaviors enables improved self-control which can be done by developing competing responses. A competing response is physically incompatible with the tic that is being targeted. Children are also taught skills to control their anxiety better via deep breathing and muscle relaxation as increases in stress increase the frequency of tics.

Conclusion

Behavioral therapies are time-limited, manual-based therapies with excellent scientific evidence to use alone or adjunct to medication management to treat common psychiatric problems. Primary care physicians need to identify mental health issues (as described in the above body of text) to make appropriate and timely referrals to specialist outpatient mental health services.

References

[1] Klein RG, Abikoff H. Behavior therapy and methylphenidate in the treatment of children with ADHD. J Atten Disord 1997;2(2):89–114.

[2] Smith P, Yule W, Perrin S, Tranah T, Dalgleish T, Clark DM. Cognitive-behavioral therapy for PTSD in children and adolescents: a preliminary randomized controlled trial. J Am Acad Child Adolesc Psychiatry 2007;46(8):1051-61.

[3] Bhatia SK, Bhatia SC. Childhood and adolescent depression. Am Fam Physician 2007; 75(1):73-80.

[4] Gormezano I, Moore JW. Classical conditioning. In: Sidowski JB, ed. Experimental methods and instrumentation in psychology. New York: McGraw-Hill, 1966:385-420.

[5] Clark RE, Squire LR. Classical conditioning and brain systems: The role of awareness. Science 1998;280(5360):77-81.

[6] Weinstein L. Classical conditioning with suitable controls in the classroom: a refinement. Psychol Rep 1987;61(1):15-8.

[7] Staddon JE, Cerutti DT. Operant conditioning. Annu Rev Psychol 2003;54(1):115-44.

[8] Axelrod S, McElrath KK, Wine B. Applied behavior analysis: Autism and beyond. Behav Intervent 2012;27(1):1-5.

[9] Smith T. Discrete trial training in the treatment of autism. Focus Autism Other Dev Disabil 2001;16(2):86-92.

[10] Koegel LK, Koegel RL, Harrower JK, Carter CM. Pivotal response intervention I: Overview of approach. J Assoc Pers Sev Handicaps 1999;24(3):174-85.

[11] Vismara LA, Rogers SJ. The Early Start Denver Model: A case study of an innovative practice. J Early Interv 2008;31(1):91-108.

[12] Albon T, Schneider S. Psychotherapy of childhood anxiety disorders: a meta-analysis. Psychother Psychosom 2007;76(1):15-24.

[13] Wood L, Burke E, Morrison A. Individual cognitive behavioural therapy for psychosis (CBTp): a systematic review of qualitative literature. Behav Cogn Psychother 2015; 43(3):285-97.

[14] Lindsay M, Crino R, Andrews G. Controlled trial of exposure and response prevention in obsessive–compulsive disorder. Br J Psychiatry 1997;171(2):135–9.

[15] Gelin Z, Cook-Darzens S, Simon Y, Hendrick S. Two models of multiple family therapy in the treatment of adolescent anorexia nervosa: A systematic review. Eat Weight Disord 2016;21(1):19-30.

[16] Himle MB, Woods DW, Piacentini JC, Walkup JT. Brief review of habit reversal training for Tourette syndrome. J Child Neurol 2006;21(8):719-25.

Chapter 16

Introduction to pediatric psychopharmacology

Muhammad Zeshan[1,*], MD, Fauzia Arain[2], MD, Aiman Tohid[3], MD, MPH, Muhammad Youshay Jawad[4], MBBS, Ali Imam Awan[5], MD and Haroon Arain[6], BS

[1]Department of Psychiatry, Rutgers New Jersey Medical School, Newark, New Jersey, Unites States of America
[2]Child and Adolescent Psychiatry, Icahn School of Medicine at Mount Sinai, BronxCare Health System, New York, United States of America
[3]Department of Psychiatry, University of Southern California, Los Angeles, California, United States of America
[4]King Edward Medical University, Lahore, Pakistan
[5]Department of Psychiatry, Services Institute of Medical Sciences, Lahore, Pakistan and [6]Columbia University, New York, United States of America

Abstract

The use of psychopharmacologic agents for pediatric persons with mental health conditions has undergone increasing research in the past few decades. Studies have shown that there are differences between children and adults in the efficacy and safety of these medications. Drugs that are reviewed include antidepressants, antipsychotics and medications used to manage attention-deficit/hyperactivity disorder, both stimulants and non-stimulants.

Introduction

Pharmacotherapy is used contrarily in different nations for children and adolescents with mental health disorders. Stimulant medication use is more prevalent in some countries, while the use of antidepressants or antipsychotics is notably more significant in other countries (1). Factors that contribute to the nationwide variation in usage and prescription include diagnostic systems, medication regulation, clinical practice standards, health-care organizations,

* ***Correspondence***: Muhammad Zeshan, MD, Clinical Assistant Professor of Psychiatry, Rutgers New Jersey Medical School, 601 Ewing Street, Suite C-12, Princeton NJ, United States.
Email: zeshan.muhammad@outlook.com.

In: Behavioral Pediatrics
Editors: Donald E. Greydanus, Dilip R. Patel, Ahsan Nazeer et al.
ISBN: 979-8-88697-060-9

availability of financial resources, and cultural attitudes regarding behavioral as well as emotional disorders in children (1). Likewise, a given cultural environment plays a vital role in the identification and treatment of mental health disorders. Cross-national surveys have shown that cultural or ethnic characteristics have been proven to be important predictors of patients' reactions to psychiatric medications in clinical trials (2). Additionally, dosage needs and the possibility of hazardous responses may differ between racial and ethnic groupings.

Background

Aside from stimulants, there are very few-line medications that are approved for use in children and adolescents. In this patient population, most antidepressants and atypical antipsychotics are more commonly used on an off-label basis. Tricyclic anti-depressants (TCAs), often prescribed as second-line medications for depression in adults, are not approved for children under 12.

Studies have shown that there are differences between children and adults in the efficacy and safety of medications (3-6). Compared to adults, children have a smaller body size, more body water, and less plasma albumin to bind drugs. These pharmacokinetic and pharmacodynamic differences result in a slower metabolism than when the same medication is used in adults. Moreover, in children and adolescents, many factors affect bioavailability, including a lesser volume of distribution, increased abstraction via the liver, a quicker metabolism, and faster elimination, all of which result in reduced bioavailability. Adolescent males have an amplified total body water content and a diminished fat percentage, whereas the reverse is true in females. This difference alone results in gender differences in pharmacokinetics. Most psychotropic medications act through neurotransmitters such as serotonin, dopamine, and norepinephrine; also, their receptors experience major variations during human development.

Like adults, before starting a medication, children should be given thorough information about their medications and the many other therapy choices available to them. Parent-child relationship dynamics have a substantial influence on the implementation of psychopharmacologic treatment. Parents are responsible for administering the exact prescribed dose of medicine as instructed by the clinician and reporting any adverse effects. Furthermore, parents have a natural tendency to refuse medical treatment for their children. This is partly due to the stigma associated with mental health treatment and a lack of infrastructure for mental health provision. Psychoeducation should be provided to both parents and the patient that should cover: course of the disease, risks, benefits, side effects, alternatives (pharmacological, non-pharmacological, therapies), prognosis (good, fair, poor, guarded), estimated length of treatment and significance of a follow-up. Medications should always be initiated after obtaining consent from the legal guardian. Instructions should be provided to monitor the side effects of medications.

In the last ten years, there has been a significant increase in research in pediatric psychopharmacology (3-6). Still, there is debate over the usefulness and safety of frequently used psychotropics and their role as a combined treatment with psychotherapy, highlighting the need for further in-depth and focused research.

Antidepressants

Due to a surge in efforts to destigmatize mental health treatment in the past two decades, there has been a robust response to psychopharmacological treatment. Health care professionals around the world have successfully used several medications for the management of mental health illnesses.

Selective serotonin reuptake inhibitors

Selective serotonin reuptake inhibitors (SSRIs) are a group of medications that are thought to treat depression by increasing serotonin levels in the central nervous system (7-10). Serotonin, or 5-hydroxytryptamine (5-HT), is a monoamine neurotransmitter responsible for modulating mood, reward, learning, memory, cognition, and numerous physiological processes. They inhibit the reuptake of serotonin and are called selective as they have little or no effect on norepinephrine or dopamine reuptake. SSRIs usually need 2 to 4 weeks before noticeable achievement of the therapeutic benefit.

SSRIs are the most widely prescribed medications for the treatment of depression, obsessive-compulsive disorder, eating disorders (including bulimia and anorexia nervosa), panic disorder, social anxiety, generalized anxiety disorder, and social phobia (7-10). Possible side effects of SSRIs may include sexual dysfunction, such as reduced sexual desire, difficulty reaching orgasm or inability to maintain an erection (erectile dysfunction), gastrointestinal symptoms, headache, insomnia, tremor, dizziness, and dry mouth. They also carry an FDA-issued black box warning for worsening suicidal ideation. A summary of the most common side effects of SSRIs is listed in Table 1.

Table 1. Side effects of selective serotonin reuptake inhibitors (SSRI)

- Black box warning: The FDA has issued a black box warning in 2004 for the use of all SSRIs in children and adolescents regarding increased risk of "suicidal thinking and behavior."
- Gastrointestinal side effects: nausea, decreased appetite, vomiting, diarrhea. Advise to take the medication with food or take in divided dosage.
- Insomnia/nightmares: more common with Fluoxetine. Advise to take the medication in the morning or add trazodone at night or switch to mirtazapine if necessary.
- Sexual side effects: decreased libido, erectile dysfunction, delayed ejaculation, anorgasmia. If severe, switch to Mirtazapine, Wellbutrin.
- Activation symptoms: irritability, agitation, emotional lability, akathisia (psychomotor restlessness, hypomania, mania. Activation symptoms happen early in the treatment. Discontinue the medication and switch to another SSRI or Mirtazapine)
- Serotonin syndrome: nausea, confusion, hyperthermia, autonomic instability, tremors, myoclonus, rigidity, seizure, coma, death. This syndrome occurs when SSRI is combined with MAOIs (Monoamine oxidase inhibitors).
- Teratogenic effects: All SSRIs are pregnancy Category C.
- Bleeding.
- Drug-drug interactions: SSRIs may increase the level of Warfarin via P450 interactions.
- Withdrawal symptoms: more common with short-acting SSRIs like Paroxetine and Fluvoxamine.

Serotonin and norepinephrine reuptake inhibitors

Serotonin and norepinephrine reuptake inhibitors (SNRIs) are another class of medications that are found to be effective in treating depression. As the name indicates, these act primarily upon serotonergic and noradrenergic neurons but have little to no effect on cholinergic or histaminergic receptors. An example is venlafaxine (11). SNRIs also treat other conditions, such as anxiety disorders and chronic pain, especially nerve pain like diabetic peripheral neuropathy, fibromyalgia, and chronic musculoskeletal pain. In addition, SNRIs can be used to treat obsessive-compulsive disorder, body dysmorphic disorder, posttraumatic stress disorder, and premenstrual dysphoric disorder. Other less common indications include menopausal hot flashes (vasomotor symptoms), urinary incontinence, and vulvodynia. Common adverse effects include the following:

- Nausea
- Dizziness
- Dry mouth
- Constipation
- Diaphoresis

Other adverse effects include the following:

- High blood pressure
- Headaches
- Sexual dysfunction including reduced libido, erectile dysfunction, delayed ejaculation, and anorgasmia.

Atypical antidepressants

Atypical antidepressants are frequently used in patients with major depression who have insufficient responses or worsening side effects with first-line agents such as SSRIs. However, in some patients, they can be used as the first-line treatment due to their specific notable characteristics (e.g., sexual side effects and weight gain occur less often with *bupropion* than SSRIs). Some undesirable side effects include seizures (bupropion), weight gain and sedation (mirtazapine), dry mouth, dizziness.

Monoamine oxidase inhibitors

Monoamine oxidase inhibitors (MAOIs) were the first class of antidepressants developed. Although they are effective, they have been replaced by antidepressants that are safer and have better side effects. They are primarily reserved for refractory episodes due to safety concerns rising from severe drug-drug and drug-food interactions. Their mechanism of action is not clear. One hypothesis is that MAOIs block monoamine oxidase, which is found in the brain and is involved in removing the neurotransmitters norepinephrine, serotonin, and dopamine from the brain. MAOIs thus increase their concentration within neuronal synapses. MAOIs can have serious interactions with certain foods (containing high levels of tyramine) and medications (affecting serotonin regulation), resulting in hypertensive crisis and serotonin syndrome.

Tricyclic antidepressants

Tricyclic antidepressants treat many other psychiatric disorders besides depression, including panic attacks, generalized anxiety disorder, post-traumatic stress disorder, bulimia nervosa, and smoking cessation. They are also used for a variety of chronic pain states, such as chronic headaches and neuropathy. They inhibit the reuptake of both serotonin and norepinephrine, which increases neurotransmitters in the synaptic cleft. This class of medications is not widely used as even therapeutic doses tend to have dose-related side effects.

Tricyclics block muscarinic M1, histamine H1, and alpha-adrenergic receptors. As a result, most TCAs commonly have cardiac, anticholinergic, and antihistaminic side effects. Other side effects include decreased seizure threshold, sexual dysfunction, diaphoresis, and tremors. In addition, cyclic antidepressants are lethal in overdose.

The serotonin modulators are distinct from other classes of antidepressants. They act by altering the activity of various post-synaptic serotonin (5-HT) receptors and inhibit the reuptake of postsynaptic serotonin. They can be used for depression, insomnia, premenstrual syndrome, and functional dyspepsia. Major side effects include nausea, sedation, hepatotoxicity (nefazodone), dry mouth, and dizziness. Table 2 lists the most used antidepressants and the recommended doses.

Antidepressants are commonly used in pediatric major depressive disorder (MDD), obsessive-compulsive disorder (OCD), and anxiety disorders; however, in most of these disorders, psychopharmacology is not recommended as a first line treatment. Psychosocial treatments that include cognitive-behavioral therapy (CBT), interpersonal psychotherapy (IPT), and dialectical behavior therapy (DBT) are usually the first-line strategy and, at times, used in conjunction with medications. Table 3 lists some of the commonly used psychotherapies that are also covered in detail in other sections of this book.

Antipsychotics

Antipsychotics medications are used to treat the symptoms of schizophrenia and other psychiatric disorders that cause agitation (12-28). These medications are also known as neuroleptics or major tranquilizers. FDA-approved indications for antipsychotics in children and adolescents include schizophrenia, bipolar I disorder, and autism spectrum disorders (23-28).

Antipsychotics are usually classified into first-generation antipsychotics and second-generation antipsychotics (SGAs). In first-generation antipsychotics, most of the dopamine receptor antagonists can be administered orally or parenterally; haloperidol and fluphenazine can be given in depot form. SGAs can be administered in oral or parenteral forms. Despite their widespread usage, atypical antipsychotics are not authorized by the FDA for children under the age of five. FDA-approved medications for children and adolescents include haloperidol (Haldol), thioridazine (Mellaril), risperidone (Risperdal), aripiprazole (Abilify), quetiapine (Seroquel), olanzapine (Zyprexa), and ziprasidone (Geodon).

For patients with psychomotor agitation, irritability, and mood dysregulation, these medications have a calming effect. This distinguishes SGAs from anxiolytics and hypnotics in two significant ways. To begin with, antipsychotics are not muscle relaxants and, in high doses, are not narcotics. Second, they treat the psychotic symptoms while also positively impacting mood dysregulation and irritable moods. It takes several days or weeks to achieve the therapeutic antipsychotic effects of these medications. The therapeutic effects of these medications include reducing symptoms of delusions, psychomotor agitation, catatonic symptoms, and symptoms of schizophrenia.

Table 2. Antidepressants and recommended doses

	Drug name	Formulations	Starting/Titration/ Maintenance dosage	Maximum dose	Indication	Common Side Effects:	
SSRI	Fluoxetine	Tablet and capsule: 10/20/40/60 mg Suspension: 20 mg/5 ml	Starting dose: 10 mg. Low-weight children should always be started on 10 mg. Titration: After 2 weeks, the dose may be increased to 20 mg once a day. Any dose increase above that should be done after several weeks and should be given in divided doses per day	The maximum licensed dose is 20 mg. Doses above this up to 60 mg are usually reserved for OCD and bulimia nervosa (both off-licensed indications). Dose > 20 mg given once daily or in two divided doses.	8-18 years old: MDD, 7-17 years old: OCD	Stomachaches, and/or diarrhea Sleep disturbance, Headaches Risk of serotonin syndrome when co-administered with triptans, linezolid, and methylene blue.	Black Box Warning common to all anti-depressants: Families and caregivers should be advised to closely monitor patients for clinical worsening, suicidality, or unusual changes in behavior. FDA safety communication warned regarding heart arrhythmic issues with fluoxetine, thus not recommended for patients on medication that can prolong the QT interval/ patients with a recent myocardial infarction, heart failure, congenital long QT syndrome, bradycardia, hypokalemia, or hypomagnesemia.
	Escitalopram	Tablet: 5/10/20 mg Suspension: 1 mg/1 ml	Starting dose: 2.5–5 mg or 10 mg Increased to 20 mg daily after 2-4 weeks or increased to 20 mg once a day after 3 weeks.	20 mg	12-17 years old: MDD		

	Drug name	Formulations	Starting/Titration/ Maintenance dosage	Maximum dose	Indication	Common Side Effects:	
	Citalopram	Tablet: 10/20/40 mg Suspension: 10 mg/5 ml	Starting dose: 10 mg and can be increased to 20 mg over 2-4 weeks.	40 mg	Off-label use in MDD & Impulsive Aggressive Behavior		
	Fluvoxamine	Tablet: 25/50/100 mg	Starting dose: 25 mg Increased by 25 mg every 4 to 7 days	200 mg per day (8-12 years old), 300 mg (12-17 years old)	8-17 years old: OCD		
	Paroxetine	Tablet: 10/20/30/40 mg Tablet CR: 12.5/25/37.5 mg Suspension: 10 mg/5 m	10–50 mg daily dosing		Not recommended in the pediatric population		
	Sertraline	Tablet: 25/50/100 mg Suspension: 20 mg/ml	Initial dose: 12.5-25 mg (6-12years old) 50 mg for >12 years old. Increase 50 mg daily at intervals of at least a week	200 mg	6-17 years old: OCD		
	Drug name	**Formulations**	**Initial dosage**	**Titration and Maintenance dosage**		**Maximum dose**	**Indication**
SNRI	Venlafaxine	Tablet: 25/37.5/50/75/100 mg Capsule and Tab ER 24 hrs: 37.5/75/150/225 mg	37.5 mg	150–300 mg			Generalized Anxiety Disorder (GAD)
	Duloxetine	Tablet: 20/30/40/60 mg	The initial dose maybe 20 mg or 30 mg	Dose increases should be in increments of 30 mg.		120 mg once a day	7-17 years old: GAD

Table 2. (Continued)

	Drug name	Initial dosage	Titration and Maintenance dosage	Maximum dose	Indication	Common side effects	Black box warning
TCA	Imipramine	25 mg once a day	The dose may be increased after 1 week.	6-11 years old: 50 mg 12-17 years old: 75 mg	6 years and older: Childhood enuresis	Drowsiness, dry mouth, urinary retention, blurred vision, constipation, decreased sexual drive, dizziness, increased risk of cardiac side effects in patients with congenital heart disorders. Tricyclics are also more cardiotoxic in young people than in adults. Baseline and on-treatment electrocardiograms (ECGs) should be performed.	Caution should be used when prescribing clomipramine to patients with a history of seizures. Increased risk of seizure with clomipramine depends on the duration of treatment or dose or both factors. It should not be used in children and adolescents with congenital long QT syndrome, and caution is advised in those with congenital heart disease or hepatic impairment.
	Clomipramine	25 mg	Dose increased gradually over the first 2 weeks to 3 mg per kg or 100 mg per day, whichever is lower. Further dose increases should occur gradually over several weeks.	3 mg per kg or 200 mg per day, whichever is lower	10-17 years old: OCD		
	Drug name	**Formulations**	**Initial dosage**	**Titration and Maintenance dosage**	**Maximum dose**	**Indication**	
OTHER DRUGS	Mirtazapine	Tablet: 7.5/15/30/45 mg Tablet disintegrating: 15/30/45 mg	The initial dose may be 15 mg	Increased after 2-4 weeks to 30 mg, further increase up to 45 mg done after several weeks	45 mg	Off-label use in Depression	

Table 3. Commonly used psychotherapies

Name of Therapy	Focus	Principle/Technique	Indication
Cognitive Behavioral Therapy	Identifying complex and repetitive patterns of thinking that are ingrained over the years and challenging cognitive distortions and behaviors, emotional dysregulation, and the development of personal coping strategies that target solving current problems	Education, coping skills training, relaxation exercises, and stress management	Depression, generalized anxiety disorder, panic disorder, Eating disorders, Schizophrenia, Bipolar disorder, Posttraumatic stress disorder, and Obsessive-compulsive disorder
Psychodynamic psychotherapy	Childhood experiences and past unresolved conflicts	Interpretation of psychological roots of unconscious patterns of interpersonal relationships, conflicts that begin in childhood	Depression, anorexia nervosa, and personality disorders
Interpersonal psychotherapy	Attachment-focused psychotherapy that centers on resolving interpersonal problems that can lead to psychological problems	Complicated grief, role disputes, role transitions, and interpersonal deficits.	Depression and eating disorders
Motivational interviewing	Changing maladaptive behaviors and helps people become motivated to change the behaviors that are preventing them from making healthier choices	Expressing empathy, helping the patient identify maladaptive behaviors, accepting the patient's resistance to change, and improving their confidence and self-efficacy.	Substance use disorders, promoting lifestyle changes (e.g., weight reduction, smoking cessation), improving medication compliance in heart failure self-management
Dialectical behavior therapy	Severe emotional dysregulation and curb self-harm behaviors, especially in people who have a borderline personality disorder	Skill training, Mindfulness	Borderline Personality Disorder, ADHD, PTSD, depression, anxiety, and OCD
Supportive psychotherapy	Improving self-esteem, ego functions, and adaptive skills.	Communication of interest and empathy, alliance building, esteem building, skill-building, expanding awareness, reducing and preventing anxiety	Schizophrenia, bipolar disorder, depression, anxiety disorders, personality disorders, substance use disorders, eating disorders, and postpartum depression.

Pharmacokinetics and pharmacodynamics

The majority of antipsychotics are highly lipophilic and freely cross lipoidal membranes (14-16). They are well absorbed and undergo significant pre-systemic elimination when administered orally. The primary route of elimination for most antipsychotics is via hepatic metabolism, and biotransformation produces active metabolites. Clozapine and risperidone, two newer antipsychotics, are eliminated mainly through hepatic enzyme metabolism, with the exception of risperidone, a minor amount of which is also excreted renally.

For all first-generation antipsychotics (typical antipsychotics), postsynaptic blockade of brain dopamine D2 receptors appears to be the mechanism of action (14-16). In the central nervous system, first-generation antipsychotics bind with dopamine receptors nonspecifically. This explains their risk of extrapyramidal symptoms and prolactinemia. First-generation antipsychotics also have distinct effects on neuronal 5-HT2a, alpha-1, histaminic, and muscarinic receptors, which often correlate to their different side effect profiles.

Second-generation antipsychotics (atypical antipsychotics) vary from dopamine receptor antagonists (first-generation antipsychotics) as they have a high affinity for both serotonin 2A (5-HT2A) and dopamine (D2) receptors. Second-generation antipsychotics are also known as serotonin dopamine antagonists, newer antipsychotics, or atypical antipsychotics. Among atypical antipsychotics, some (i.e., clozapine, olanzapine, and quetiapine) are called multiple receptor antagonists while others (i.e., risperidone, sertindole, ziprasidone, and zotepine) are the more selective 5-HT2/D2 antagonists.

Side effects

The common side effects of antipsychotic medications include sedation, hypotension, anticholinergic effects (i.e., constipation, urinary retention, dry mouth, blurred vision and, at times, cognitive impairment), extrapyramidal symptoms (pseudo-parkinsonism, akathisia, acute dystonia, and tardive dyskinesia), hyperprolactinemia, sexual dysfunction, agranulocytosis, cardiac arrhythmias, seizures, and metabolic syndrome issues (such as weight gain and others).

Black-box warning

Antipsychotic drugs have no black box warning in the pediatric population. These medications are associated with an increased risk of death in elderly patients with dementia-related psychosis. Although the causes of death were varied, it appeared that most of the deaths were either cardiovascular (e.g., heart failure, sudden death) or infectious (e.g., pneumonia). Table 4 lists the commonly used antipsychotics, doses, and side effects.

Stimulants and non-stimulants

Stimulants are considered the first line of treatment for managing attention-deficit/hyperactivity disorder (ADHD) in the child and adolescent population (29,30). Still, it is essential to recognize that pharmacotherapy is only one part of a comprehensive treatment plan for ADHD. Other interventions include parent education programs, parent management training, social skills training, problem-solving skills training for children, group cognitive-behavioral therapies and, behavioral interventions in the classroom.

Table 4. Commonly used antipsychotics

Class	Agent	Avg. daily dose	Side effects
First-generation	Chlorpromazine	50-400 mg	Common side effects of first-generation antipsychotics include: sedation, orthostatic hypotension, anticholinergic symptoms, parkinsonism, dystonia, and akathisia
	Thioridazine	50-400 mg	
	Fluphenazine	2-10 mg	
	Perphenazine	5-40 mg	
	Trifluoperazine	2-20 mg	
	Haloperidol	2-10 mg	
	Loxapine	5-50 mg	
	Molindone	5-50 mg	
	Thiothixene	2-20 mg	
Second-generation			
	Clozapine*	25-300mg	Weight gain, hypercholesteremia, hyperprolactinemia, tardive dyskinesia
	Risperidone	1-4 mg	
	Olanzapine	5-20 mg	
	Quetiapine	200-600 mg	
	Ziprasidone	80-120 mg	
	Asenapine	5-20mg	
	Iloperidone	2-12mg	
	Paliperidone	3-12mg	
	Lurasidone	40-160mg	
Partial DA agonist	Aripiprazole	10-25 mg	Can exacerbate psychosis

* Side effects that are unique to clozapine: hypersalivation, tachycardia, increased risk of seizures, and agranulocytosis.

Before starting the pharmacologic treatment, it is essential to assess cardiovascular status by inquiring about any history of exercise syncope, chest pain, palpitations or family history of sudden cardiac death. Heart rate (HR) and blood pressure (BP) should be evaluated; also, an electrocardiogram (ECG) should be considered in individuals with any of the above risk factors. An assessment of the risk for potential drug misuse or diversion also should be a part of the comprehensive pre-treatment evaluation. The decision regarding which medication to use is based on any adverse effects experienced during previous trials, anticipated adherence issues, the potential for diversion, convenience (including whether a mid-day dose will be needed at school), and presence of comorbid conditions, including tics, seizures, and structural cardiac defects.

FDA approved indications

Stimulants are approved for the treatment of ADHD, narcolepsy, and exogenous obesity (body mass index at or above 95th percentile) in pediatric patients. Methamphetamine and benzphetamine are both approved for the treatment of exogenous obesity in 12-17-year-old patients. Dextroamphetamine IR (immediate-release), dextroamphetamine SR (sustained-release), and amphetamine mixed salts are approved for narcolepsy in 6-17 years old. Almost all stimulant medications are approved for the treatment of ADHD in children aged 6-17 years old, with two exceptions: amphetamine mixed salts and dextroamphetamine IR are approved for children 3 years and older. In comparison, dextroamphetamine IR and SR do not carry FDA approval for use in adolescents older than 16 years of age. The FDA has approved three non-stimulant medications for children and adolescents with ADHD: atomoxetine, extended-release guanfacine, and extended-release clonidine. Table 5 lists the commonly used medications, doses, and side effects for the treatment of ADHD.

Table 5. Commonly used medications, doses and side effects for the treatment of ADHD

		Formulation	Duration of action	Initial dose	Dose Increments	Maximum Dosage	Adverse Effects
STIMULANTS	Methylphenidate	Short-Acting	3 to 5 hrs	5 mg	5 mg/day every 3 to 7 days	≤25 kg – 35 mg 25 kg – 60 mg	Sleep problems Decreased appetite Weight loss Increased blood pressure Dizziness Headaches and stomachaches Rebound (irritability when the medication wears off) Moodiness and irritability Nervousness Tics Personality changes, like appearing dysphoric and not being as enthusiastic as usual
		Extended-Release	12 hrs	10-20 mg	10 to 20 mg/day every 7 days	60-100 mg	
	Dexmethylphenidate	Short-Acting	5 to 6 hrs	5 mg	2.5 to 5 mg/day every 3 to 7 days	20 mg	
		Extended-Release	12 hrs	5 mg	5 mg per dose every 3 to 7 days	40 mg	
	Amphetamine	Short-Acting	4 to 6 hrs	5 mg	2.5 mg/day every 7 days	40 mg	
		Extended-Release	12 hrs	2.5 or 5 mg	2.5 to 10 mg/day every 4 to 7 days	20 mg	
	Dextroamphetamine	Short-Acting	4 to 6 hrs	5 mg	5 mg/day every 3 to 7 days	≤50 kg – 40 mg >50 kg – 60 mg	
		Extended-Release	12 hrs	5 mg	5 mg/day every 3 to 7 days	≤50 kg: 40 mg >50 kg: 60 mg	
	Dextroamphetamine-amphetamine	Short-Acting	4 to 6 hrs	5 mg	5 mg/day every 3 to 7 days	≤50 kg – 40 mg >50 kg – 60 mg	
		Extended-Release	12 hrs	5 mg	5 mg per dose every 3 to 7 days	≤50 kg: 40 mg >50 kg: 60 mg	
		Extended-Release	12 hrs	5 mg	5 mg per dose every 3 to 7 days	≤50 kg: 40 mg >50 kg: 60 mg	
NON-STIMULANTS	Atomoxetine	Extended-Release	At least 10 to 12 hrs	0.5 mg/kg/day for a minimum of 3 days	Increase to 1.2 mg/kg per day after a minimum of 3 days (maximum 100 mg per day)	Lesser of 1.4 mg/kg or 100 mg	Weight loss, abdominal pain, decreased appetite, vomiting, nausea, dyspepsia, headache, dizziness, drowsiness, fatigue, irritability, Suicidal thinking, Tics, Liver Injury, increased HR, and BP.
	Viloxazine ER	Extended-Release	24 hrs	100-200 mg	Increments of 100 mg weekly	400 mg	
	Guanfacine ER	Extended-Release	At least 10 to 12 hrs	1 mg per day	Increments of 1 mg per day at no less than weekly intervals	≤12 years: 4 mg >12 years: 7 mg	

Stimulants and risk of priapism

In 2013, the US Food and Drug Administration (FDA) issued a warning regarding a possible link between the use of methylphenidate and priapism (painful erection lasting > 4 hours). There is still only limited information available, but the FDA has recommended updating drug labels to include mention of a "rare but serious risk of priapism." The FDA has identified 15 cases of priapism that occurred from 1997-2012; most cases (12) occurred in children younger than 18 years of age. These cases have presented under different conditions, including during use of short-acting methylphenidate, after discontinuation of methylphenidate, upon restarting the medication, and when there was a longer than usual interval between doses. The rarity of this side effect can be understood because in 2012 alone, 20 million prescriptions were written, and 4 million prescriptions were dispensed. However, physicians are advised to discuss this issue with parents and youth as well as recommend seeking immediate medical treatment if an erection lasts longer than 4 hours to prevent long-term problems.

Stimulants and risk of cardiovascular events

In 2005, awareness of the cardiovascular impact of stimulant medications was heightened when Health Canada suspended the distribution of Adderall XR after receiving reports of sudden cardiac death among children receiving the drug (29, 30). This ban was later lifted, and a warning was issued regarding the possibility of sudden cardiac death among children with known cardiac anomalies who are taking Adderall XR. The FDA also issued warnings about the use of stimulants in children with underlying cardiac disease; however, a 2006 FDA review acknowledged that no definite conclusions could be made about the association of stimulant use with sudden cardiac death. In 2011, the FDA announced that a large, recently completed study had not shown an association between the use of stimulants and adverse cardiovascular events such as stroke, myocardial infarction, and sudden cardiac death (29, 30).

The study under discussion was one of three studies sponsored by the FDA and the Agency for Healthcare and Quality (AHRQ), published in the November 1, 2011 issue of the New England Journal of Medicine (31). This study was a retrospective review of 1,200,438 children and young adults 2-24 years of age, followed for 373,667 person-years (sum of years that each person in the study was under observation) of ADHD medication use (31). Researchers reported no evidence of increased risk of cardiovascular events among individuals taking ADHD medications; however, the FDA continues to recommend periodic evaluation of HR as well as BP and advises avoiding the use of stimulants in individuals with serious cardiac problems.

Stimulants and risk of abuse and dependence

Stimulant medications are the most effective treatment for ADHD; however, their illicit use and diversion have become major public health concerns. According to the US Centers for Disease Control and Prevention (CDC), more than 20% of high school students have used prescription medications, including amphetamines and methylphenidate, without a doctor's knowledge (32). The prevalence of misuse increases to 35% among college-age individuals. The presence of conduct disorder or partially treated ADHD, immediate-release stimulant medications, and enrollment in a competitive college program are all risk factors for misuse.

The task of detecting and treating ongoing substance abuse in patients with ADHD is challenging. It is recommended that serial assessments of symptoms be performed, noting whether they present in a consistent pattern or are sporadic. Risk factors should be evaluated, and collateral information about the patient's behavior should be gathered from family members. Some of the telltale signs of a youth who may be abusing or diverting medications are a disheveled appearance, agitated behavior during sessions, unexplained and suspicious loss of medication bottles or prescriptions, repeated requests for increases in dose, requests to switch to immediate-release formulations, and unexplained accidents. Close observation and monitoring of symptoms in these situations are mandatory.

Atomoxetine and risk of hepatotoxicity, suicidal ideation, and priapism

Atomoxetine is a selective norepinephrine reuptake inhibitor that is FDA approved for the treatment of ADHD in the pediatric population (29, 30). The FDA has issued a "black box warning" regarding the increased rate of suicidal ideation among children taking this medication. If atomoxetine is chosen for the treatment of ADHD, then parents should be warned to watch for any adverse changes in behavior. Patients should be assessed at baseline and monitored at regular intervals for symptoms of worsening irritability, a gitation, or emerging suicidal ideation.

Atomoxetine also is associated with serum aminotransferase (AST) elevation (often >20 times normal) and has caused acute hepatic injury in a small number of cases. The onset of injury is usually within 3-12 weeks of medication initiation, and individuals present clinically with symptoms suggestive of acute viral hepatitis. Most cases are self-limited, but instances of acute liver failure have been noted in the literature. Atomoxetine should be discontinued if hepatic injury is suspected. Priapism is another known side effect of atomoxetine and appears to be more common among patients taking atomoxetine than those taking methylphenidate.

Conclusion

The last decade has seen numerous changes in the way pediatric psychopharmacology is conceptualized and practiced. With the advent of neuroimaging and genome mapping, the once farsighted goal of understanding the neurobiology of psychiatric disorders now appears to be within reach. There is also greater emphasis on evidence based psychiatric practice and on understanding the long-term effects of medications on the developing brain. However, there still is a clear need for further research to enhance our understanding of the complex treatment of these multifaceted disorders.

References

[1] Vitiello B. An international perspective on pediatric psychopharmacology. Int Rev Psychiatry 2008;20(2):121-6.

[2] Lin KM, Poland RE, Lesser IM. Ethnicity and psychopharmacology. Cult Med Psychiatry 1986; 10(2):151-65.

[3] McVoy M, Findling R. Child and adolescent psychopharmacology update. Psychiatr Clin North Am 2009;32(1):111-33.

[4] Koelch M, Schnoor K, Fegert JM. Ethical issues in psychopharmacology of children and adolescents. Curr Opin Psychiatry 2008;21(6):598-605.

[5] Vitiello B. Research in child and adolescent psychopharmacology: recent accomplishments and new challenges. Psychopharmacology (Berl) 2007;191(1):5-13.

[6] Martin A, Scahill L, Charney DS, James F, eds. Pediatric psychopharmacology: Principles and practice. New York: Oxford University Press, 2004:175–81.

[7] Celexa® (citalopram) prescribing information. URL: https://www.accessdata.fda.gov/drugsatfda_docs/label/2014/020822Orig1s046lbl.pdf

[8] Paxil® (paroxetine) prescribing information. URL: https://www.accessdata.fda.gov/drugsatfda_docs/label/2014/020031s071,020710s035lbl.pdf.

[9] Pexeva® (paroxetine mesylate) prescribing information. URL: https://www.accessdata.fda.gov/drugsatfda_docs/label/2014/021299s032lbl.pdf.

[10] Zoloft® (sertraline) prescribing information. URL: https://www.accessdata.fda.gov/drugsatfda_docs/label/2014/019839s084,020990s043lbl.pdf.

[11] Venlafaxine prescribing information. URL: https://www.accessdata.fda.gov/drugsatfda_docs/label/2014/076690s020lbl.pdf 14.

[12] US Department of Health and Human Services and US Food and Drug Administration. Revisions to product labeling. Drug Safety and availability: Information by drug class, 2007. URL: http://www.fda.gov/downloads/Drugs/DrugSafety/InformationbyDrugClass/UCM173233.pdf.

[13] Spiegel R, Aebi H-J. Psychopharmacology: An introduction. New York: Wiley Sons, 1983.

[14] Javaid JI. Clinical pharmacokinetics of antipsychotics. J Clin Pharmacol 1994;34(4):286-95.

[15] DeVane CL. Brief comparison of the pharmacokinetics and pharmacodynamics of the traditional and newer antipsychotic drugs. Am J Health Syst Pharm 1995;52(3 Suppl 1):S15-8.

[16] Marazziti D, Baroni S, Picchetti M, Piccinni A, Carlini M, Vatteroni E, et al. Pharmacokinetics and pharmacodinamics of psychotropic drugs: Effect of sex. CNS Spectrums 2013;18(3):118–27.

[17] Shulgin AT, Nichols DE. Characterization of three new psychotomimetics. In: Stillman RC, Willette RE, eds. The psychopharmacology of hallucinogens. New York: Pergamon, 1978:74–83.

[18] Muench J, Hamer AM. Adverse effects of antipsychotic medications. Am Fam Physician 2010; 81(5):617-22.

[19] Minjon L, Brozina I, Egberts TCG, Heerdink ER, van den Ban E. Monitoring of adverse drug reaction-related parameters in children and adolescents treated with antipsychotic drugs in psychiatric outpatient clinics. Front Psychiatry 2021;12:640377.

[20] Vitiello B. Research in child and adolescent psychopharmacology: Recent accomplishments and new challenges. Psychopharmacology (Berl) 2007;191(1):5-13.

[21] Vitiello B. An update on publicly funded multisite trials in pediatric psychopharmacology. Child Adolesc Psychiatr Clin North Am 2006;15(1):1-12.

[22] March JS., Szatmari P, Bukstein O, Chrisman A, Kondo D, Hamilton JD, et al. AACAP 2005 Research Forum: speeding the adoption of evidence-based practice in pediatric psychiatry. J Am Acad Child Adolesc Psychiatry 2007;46(9):1098-1110.

[23] Walkup J; Work Group on Quality Issues. Practice parameter on the use of psychotropic medication in children and adolescents. J Am Acad Child Adolesc Psychiatry 2009;48(9):961-73.

[24] Gleason M, Egger HL, Emslie GJ, Greenhill LL, Kowatch RA, Lieberman AF, et al. Psychopharmacological treatment for very young children: contexts and guidelines. J Am Acad Child Adolesc Psychiatry 2007;46(12):1532-72.

[25] Koelch M, Schnoor K, Fegert JM. Ethical issues in the psychopharmacology of children and adolescents. Curr Opin Psychiatry 2008;21(6):598-605.

[26] WohlfarthT, Kalverdijk L, Rademaker C, Schothorst P, Minderaa R, Gispen-de Wied C. Psychopharmacology for children: From off label use to registration. Eur Neuropsychopharmacol 2009;19(8):603-8.

[27] Harrison JN, Cluxton-Keller F, Gross D. Antipsychotic medication prescribing trends in children and adolescents. J Pediatr Health Care 2012;26(2):139-45.

[28] Thomas T, Stansifer L, Findling RL. Psychopharmacology of pediatric bipolar disorders in children and adolescents. Pediatr Clin North Am 2011;58(1):173-87.

[29] Greydanus DE, Nazeer A, Patel DR. Psychopharmacology of ADHD in pediatrics: current advances and issues. Neuropsychiatr Dis Treat 2009;5:171-81.

[30] March JS. The Preschool ADHD Treatment Study (PATS) as the culmination of twenty years of clinical trials in pediatric psychopharmacology. J Am Acad Child Adolesc Psychiatry 2011; 50(5):427-30.
[31] Cooper WO, Habel LA, Sox CM, Chan KA, Arbogast PG, Cheetham TC, et al. ADHD drugs and serious cardiovascular events in children and young adults. N Engl J Med 2011;365(20):1896-904.
[32] Kann L, McManus T, Harris WA, Shanklin SL, Flint KH, Hawkins J, et al. Youth risk behavior surveillance - United States, 2015. MMWR Surveill Summ 2016;65(6):1-174.

Section four: Acknowledgements

About the editors

Donald E Greydanus, MD, DrHC(Athens), FAAP, FIAP(Hon) is Professor and Founding Chair of the Department of Pediatric and Adolescent Medicine at the Western Michigan University Homer Stryker M.D. School of Medicine (WMED), Kalamazoo, Michigan, USA. He is also Clinical Professor of Pediatrics and Human Development at Michigan State University College of Human Medicine (East Lansing, Michigan, USA). Received the Mayo Clinic Distinguished Alumnus designation in 2017 from the Mayo Clinic Graduate School of Medicine, Rochester, Minnesota, USA.

Received the 1995 American Academy of Pediatrics' Adele D. Hofmann Award for "Distinquished Contributions in Adolescent Health", the 2000 Mayo Clinic Pediatrics Honored Alumnus Award for "National Contributions to the field of Pediatrics," and the 2003 William B Weil, Jr, MD Endowed Distinguished Pediatric Faculty Award from Michigan State University College of Medicine for "National and international recognition as well as exemplary scholarship in pediatrics." Received the 2004 Charles R Drew School of Medicine (Los Angeles, CA) Stellar Award for contributions to pediatric resident education and awarded an honorary membership in the Indian Academy of Pediatrics—an honor granted to only a few pediatricians outside of India. Was the 2007-2010 Visiting Professor of Pediatrics at Athens University, Athens, Greece and received the Michigan State University College of Human Medicine Outstanding Community Faculty Award in 2008. In 2010 he received the title of Doctor Honoris Causa from the University of Athens (Greece) as a "distinguished scientist who through outstanding work has bestowed praise and credit on the field of adolescent medicine (Ephebiatrics)." In 2010 he received the Outstanding Achievement in Adolescent Medicine Award from the Society for Adolescent Medicine "as a leading force in the field of adolescent medicine and health." In 2014 he was selected by the American Medical Association as AMA nominee for the ACGME Pediatrics Residency Review Committee (RRC) in Chicago, Illinois, USA. Past Chair of the National Conference and Exhibition Planning Group (Committee on Scientific Meetings) of the American Academy of Pediatrics and member of the Pediatric Academic Societies' (SPR/PAS) Planning Committee (1998 to Present). In 2011 elected to The Alpha Omega Alpha Honor Society (Faculty member) at Michigan State University College of Human Medicine, East Lansing, Michigan. Former member of the Appeals Committee for the Pediatrics' Residency Review Committee (RRC) of the Accreditation Council for Graduate Medical Education (Chicago, IL) in both adolescent medicine and general pediatrics. Numerous publications in pediatric and adolescent health as well as lectureships in many countries on adolescent health. Email: donald.greydanus@med.wmich.edu

Dilip R Patel, MD, FAAP, FSAM, FAACPDM, FACSM, is Professor and Chair, Department of Pediatric and Adolescent Medicine, Western Michigan University Homer Stryker M.D. School of Medicine, Kalamazoo, Michigan, United States. Dr Patel has subspecialty training and interests in neurodevelopmental disabilities, developmental-behavioral pediatrics, adolescent medicine and sports medicine. He has subspecialty training and interests in neurodevelopmental disabilities, developmental-behavioral pediatrics, adolescent medicine and sports medicine. Dr Patel also has interests and holds certifications in healthcare quality and healthcare management. He is a Vanguard Member of the American College of Physican Executives. Dr Patel has received many professional awards including the Adele Hoffmann Visiting Professor Award of the Society for Adolescent Medicine, and the William Weil Endowed Distinguished Pediatric Faculty Award of the Michigan State University College of Human Medicine. He is an elected fellow of the American Academy of Cerebral Palsy and Developmental Medicine as well as the American College of Sports Medicine. He has served on numerous national committees including the editorial board of American Academy of Pediatrics Developmental-Behavioral Pediatrics PREP Program. Dr Patel has published extensively and presented at numerous national and international professional and academic events. E-mail: dilip.patel@med.wmich.edu.

Ahsan Nazeer, MD, is the division chief of Child and Adolescent Mental Health Services at Sidra Medicine. He is leading an effort to improve access to psychiatric care for children and adolescents in Qatar, clinical and education services within the Division and working to broaden psychiatric awareness particularly in the area of prevention. Dr Nazeer joined Sidra Medicine in January of 2017. Before then, he was an Associate Professor of Child and Adolescent Psychiatry at Michigan State University and then at Western Michigan University, Homer Stryker MD School of Medicine, Kalamazoo, Michigan, United States.

Dr Nazeer went to medical school at Rawalpindi Medical College, Rawalpindi, Pakistan. He completed his psychiatry residency training at Kalamazoo Center for Medical Studies and fellowship in child and adolescent psychiatry from The University of Michigan, Ann Arbor. Dr Nazeer is certified by American Board of Psychiatry and Neurology (ABPN) in both adult and child and adolescent psychiatry.

Author of numerous articles and co-editor of two books, Dr Nazeer's research endeavors have focused on pediatric psychopharmacology and severe psychiatric disorders in youth. He is currently the co-principal investigator on a SIRF grant examining the Neurogenomics model of children with ADHD. Also, Dr. Nazeer is the PI and co-lead PI of numerous research studies ranging from investigating the validity of the rating scales to genetic underpinnings of ADHD and autism. Email: anazeer@sidra.org

Roger A Apple, PhD, is a licensed psychologist and Chief, Division of Pediatric Psychology, Director of the Autism Center and Associate Professor, Department of Pediatric and Adolescent Medicine, Western Michigan University, Homer Styker MD School of Medicine, Kalamazoo, Michigan, USA. He trained with Helen D Pratt, PhD. He has published numerous articles in pediatric psychology. Email: roger.apple@med.wmich.edu

Joav Merrick, MD, MMedSci, DMSc, born and educated in Denmark is professor of pediatrics, child health and human development, Division of Pediatrics, Hadassah Hebrew University Medical Center, Mt Scopus Campus, Jerusalem, Israel and Kentucky Children's Hospital, University of Kentucky, Lexington, Kentucky United States and professor of public health at the Center for Healthy Development, School of Public Health, Georgia State

University, Atlanta, United States, the medical director of the Health Services, Division for Intellectual and Developmental Disabilities, Ministry of Social Affairs and Social Services, Jerusalem, the founder and director of the National Institute of Child Health and Human Development in Israel.

Numerous publications in the field of pediatrics, child health and human development, rehabilitation, intellectual disability, disability, health, welfare, abuse, advocacy, quality of life and prevention. Received the Peter Sabroe Child Award for outstanding work on behalf of Danish Children in 1985 and the International LEGO-Prize ("The Children's Nobel Prize") for an extraordinary contribution towards improvement in child welfare and well-being in 1987. In 2017 appointed a Kentucky Colonel by the Commonwealth of Kentucky, the highest honor the governor can bestow to a person. Email: jmerrick@zahav.net.il

About the Department of Pediatric and Adolescent Medicine, Western Michigan University Homer Stryker MD School of Medicine (WMed), Kalamazoo, Michigan, United States of America

The medical school is a collaboration of Western Michigan University (WMU) and Kalamazoo's two teaching health systems—Ascension Borgess and Bronson Healthcare. The inaugural medical student class graduated in 2018 after completing an innovative, patient-centered, four-year curriculum that prepared them to be exceptional clinicians, leaders, educators, advocates, and researchers of tomorrow. WMed also offers three Master of Science degree programs in biomedical sciences, clinical informatics and medical engineering. More than 200 residents and fellows train in ten residencies and five fellowships accredited by the Accreditation Council for Graduate Medical Education. WMed residents and fellows serve patients throughout southwest Michigan in affiliate hospitals and in the WMed Health outpatient clinics. To support its mission to educate and inspire lifelong learners, WMed has Joint Accreditation for interprofessional continuing education, which incorporates accreditation by the Accreditation Council for Continuing Medical Education.

WMed Health is the clinical practice of the medical school with more than 330 providers (including residents and fellows) offering comprehensive primary care and specialty services in several locations throughout Kalamazoo and Portage. The 350,000 square foot educational building on the WE Upjohn MD Campus located in downtown Kalamazoo, that includes research laboratories and a state-of-the-art Simulation Center that is accredited by the Society for Simulation in Healthcare.

WMed is building upon Kalamazoo's century-long foundation of drug discovery and medical device development with a strategic investment in clinical, laboratory, community, and educational research. The Center for Immunobiology, Center for Clinical Research, WMed ForenTox, Research Histology Lab, Innovation Center, Division of Epidemiology and Biostatistics, and Human Research Protection Program contribute to WMed's advancement of knowledge through innovation and discovery.

The WMed Department of Pediatric and Adolescent Medicine, with over 100 faculty members, serves to deliver both undergraduate and graduate medical education, as well as a full range of comprehensive pediatric and adolescent medicine primary and subspecialty clinical care. The department faculty members have a long history of consistent engagement in research and scholarly activities and recognition at national and international levels. The faculty members have edited and authored numerous books and hundreds of peer-reviewed publications and served as invited presenters at national and international venues. The department has developed academic ties with a variety of international medical centers and organizations, including the Queen Elizabeth Hospital in Hong Kong, Indian Academy of

Pediatrics (New Delhi, India), the University of Athens Children's Hospital (First and Second Departments of Paediatrics) in Athens, Greece and the National Institute of Child Health and Human Development in Jerusalem, Israel.

Among the many published books, edited and authored by faculty members, include: Essential adolescent medicine (McGraw-Hill Medical Publishers), The pediatric diagnostic examination (McGraw-Hill), Pediatric and adolescent psychopharmacology (Cambridge University Press), Behavioral pediatrics, through 4th Edition (Nova Science, New York), Pediatric practice: Sports medicine (McGraw-Hill), Handbook of clinical pediatrics (Singapore: World Scientific), Neurodevelopmental disabilities: Clinical care for children and young adults (Dordrecht: Springer), Adolescent medicine: Pharmacotherapeutics in medical disorders (Berlin/Boston: De Gruyter), Adolescent medicine: Pharmacotherapeutics in general, mental, and sexual health (Berlin/Boston: De Gruyter), Pediatric psychodermatology (Berlin/Boston: De Gruyter), Substance abuse in adolescents and young adults: A manual for pediatric and primary care clinicians (Berlin/Boston: De Gruyter), Tropical pediatrics (New York: Nova), and Pediatric and adolescent sexuality and gynecology (New York: Nova Science).

The Department faculty members have served as invited guest editors for a number of peer-reviewed journal special issues. These include, the Pediatric Clinics of North America, Disease a Month, Pediatric Medicine, Annals of Translational Medicine, Translational Pediatrics, Adolescent Medicine State of the Art Reviews, Primary Care Clinics in Office Practice, Current Psychopharmacology, Indian Journal of Pediatrics, and International Journal of Environmental Research and Public Health.

Contact

Professor and Chair, Dilip R Patel, MD, MBA, MPH, Email: dilip.Patel@med.wmich.edu
and Professor and Founding Chair Donald E Greydanus, MD, Email:
Donald.greydanus@med.wmich.edu

Department of Pediatric and Adolescent Medicine, Western Michigan University Homer Stryker MD School of Medicine, 1000 Oakland Drive, D48G, Kalamazoo, Michigan 49008-1284, United States
Website: http://www.med.wmich.edu

About Sidra Medicine, Doha, Qatar

Sidra Medicine is a 400-bed women's and children's hospital and research center in Doha, Qatar. The hospital's outpatient facility debuted in 2016, and its inpatient hospital opened in January 2018. Sidra Medicine, is part of the Qatar Foundation for Education, Science, and Community Development (QF). Weill Cornell Medicine-Qatar, Georgetown University, Carnegie Mellon University and HEC Paris are among the leading international institutions in Education City, as are newly established national research institutes such as Qatar Biomedical Research Institute and Qatar Environment and Energy Research Institute.

The **Division of Child and Adolescent Mental Health Services (CAMHS)** in the Department of Psychiatry is one of the primary sources to provide child and adolescent mental health services in the State of Qatar. The division remains at the forefront of providing clinical service, professional education as well as research and the work of the division's faculty members covers a broad range of psychiatric illnesses with a focus on providing world-class care. The Division's multi-disciplinary approach to treatment, research, and education means that child and adolescent mental health services at Sidra Medicine has a strong foundation that spans the psychological underpinnings of diseases to the molecular basis of psychiatric disorders.

The mission of the Division is to advance clinical care, research and education by the exploration of psychopathology in children and adolescents and participating in state of the art research studies. The division is also actively involved in increasing community awareness of the pathophysiology of youth mental health concerns including mood, anxiety, ADHD and autism-related disorders by providing excellent care and community educational seminars.

With an expert team of child and adolescent psychiatrists and psychologists, all of whom are trained in excellent programs and universities abroad, the Division of Child and Adolescent Mental Health provides services to children and adolescents from 5 to 18 years of age. The services are provided through an out-patient clinic, inpatient consultation and liaison team and emergency department team. The target group includes young people with a diagnosable psychiatric disorder whose condition is detrimental to their growth or development and /or who have serious difficulties in their social group, school or family.

About the National Institute of Child Health and Human Development in Israel

The National Institute of Child Health and Human Development (NICHD) in Israel was established in 1998 as a virtual institute under the auspices of the Medical Director, Ministry of Social Affairs and Social Services in order to function as the research arm for the Office of the Medical Director. In 1998 the National Council for Child Health and Pediatrics, Ministry of Health and in 1999 the Director General and Deputy Director General of the Ministry of Health endorsed the establishment of the NICHD.

Mission

The mission of a National Institute for Child Health and Human Development in Israel is to provide an academic focal point for the scholarly interdisciplinary study of child life, health, public health, welfare, disability, rehabilitation, intellectual disability and related aspects of human development. This mission includes research, teaching, clinical work, information and public service activities in the field of child health and human development.

Service and academic activities

Over the years many activities became focused in the south of Israel due to collaboration with various professionals at the Faculty of Health Sciences (FOHS) at the Ben Gurion University of the Negev (BGU). Since 2000 an affiliation with the Zusman Child Development Center at the Pediatric Division of Soroka University Medical Center has resulted in collaboration around the establishment of the Down Syndrome Clinic at that center. In 2002 a full course on "Disability" was established at the Recanati School for Allied Professions in the Community, FOHS, BGU and in 2005 collaboration was started with the Primary Care Unit of the faculty and disability became part of the master of public health course on "Children and society". In the academic year 2005-2006 a one semester course on "Aging with disability" was started as part of the master of science program in gerontology in our collaboration with the Center for Multidisciplinary Research in Aging. In 2010 collaborations with the Division of Pediatrics, Hadassah Hebrew University Medical Center, Jerusalem, Israel around the National Down Syndrome Center and teaching students and residents about intellectual and developmental disabilities as part of their training at this campus.

Research activities

The affiliated staff have over the years published work from projects and research activities in this national and international collaboration. In the year 2000 the International Journal of Adolescent Medicine and Health and in 2005 the International Journal on Disability and Human Development of De Gruyter Publishing House (Berlin and New York) were affiliated with the National Institute of Child Health and Human Development. From 2008 also the International Journal of Child Health and Human Development (Nova Science, New York), the International Journal of Child and Adolescent Health (Nova Science) and the Journal of Pain Management (Nova Science) affiliated and from 2009 the International Public Health Journal (Nova Science) and Journal of Alternative Medicine Research (Nova Science). All peer-reviewed international journals.

National collaborations

Nationally the NICHD works in collaboration with the Faculty of Health Sciences, Ben Gurion University of the Negev; Department of Physical Therapy, Sackler School of Medicine, Tel Aviv University; Autism Center, Assaf HaRofeh Medical Center; National Rett and PKU Centers at Chaim Sheba Medical Center, Tel HaShomer; Department of Physiotherapy, Haifa University; Department of Education, Bar Ilan University, Ramat Gan, Faculty of Social Sciences and Health Sciences; College of Judea and Samaria in Ariel and in 2011 affiliation with Center for Pediatric Chronic Diseases and National Center for Down Syndrome, Department of Pediatrics, Hadassah Hebrew University Medical Center, Mount Scopus Campus, Jerusalem.

International collaborations

Internationally with the Department of Disability and Human Development, College of Applied Health Sciences, University of Illinois at Chicago; Strong Center for Developmental Disabilities, Golisano Children's Hospital at Strong, University of Rochester School of Medicine and Dentistry, New York; Centre on Intellectual Disabilities, University of Albany, New York; Centre for Chronic Disease Prevention and Control, Health Canada, Ottawa; Chandler Medical Center and Children's Hospital, Kentucky Children's Hospital, Section of Adolescent Medicine, University of Kentucky, Lexington; Chronic Disease Prevention and Control Research Center, Baylor College of Medicine, Houston, Texas; Division of Neuroscience, Department of Psychiatry, Columbia University, New York; Institute for the Study of Disadvantage and Disability, Atlanta; Center for Autism and Related Disorders, Department Psychiatry, Children's Hospital Boston, Boston; Department of Pediatric and Adolescent Medicine, Western Michigan University Homer Stryker MD School of Medicine, Kalamazoo, Michigan, United States; Department of Paediatrics, Child Health and Adolescent Medicine, Children's Hospital at Westmead, Westmead, Australia; International Centre for the Study of Occupational and Mental Health, Düsseldorf, Germany; Centre for Advanced Studies in Nursing, Department of General Practice and Primary Care, University of Aberdeen,

Aberdeen, United Kingdom; Quality of Life Research Center, Copenhagen, Denmark; Nordic School of Public Health, Gottenburg, Sweden, Scandinavian Institute of Quality of Working Life, Oslo, Norway; The Department of Applied Social Sciences (APSS) of The Hong Kong Polytechnic University Hong Kong.

Targets

Our focus is on research, international collaborations, clinical work, teaching and policy in health, disability and human development and to establish the NICHD as a permanent institute in Israel in order to conduct model research and policy.

Contact

Professor Joav Merrick, MD, MMedSci, DMSc
Director, National Institute of Child Health and Human Development, Jerusalem, Israel.
E-mail: jmerrick@zahav.net.il

Section five: Index

Index

D

E

F

G

H

I

J

K

L

M

N

O

P

Q

R

S

T

U

V

W

X

Z